Ruth Beecher

# Community Health Practitioners and Child Sexual Abuse in the Family, 1970s–2010s

palgrave
macmillan

Ruth Beecher
Birkbeck, University of London
London, UK

Wellcome Trust

ISSN 2730-9479 ISSN 2730-9487 (electronic)
Genders and Sexualities in History
ISBN 978-3-031-80051-1 ISBN 978-3-031-80052-8 (eBook)
https://doi.org/10.1007/978-3-031-80052-8



This Palgrave Macmillan imprint is published by the registered company Springer Nature Switzerland AG.
The registered company address is: Gewerbestrasse 11, 6330 Cham, Switzerland

*For Kim, my love*

# Series Editor Preface

In *Community Health Practitioners and Child Sexual Abuse in the Family, 1970s–2010s*, Ruth Beecher shows the different ways doctors, health visitors, and mental health practitioners responded to child sexual abuse in modern England and Wales. It is the first in-depth analysis of the impact of medical, nursing and psychiatric knowledge on the treatment of abused children, as well as seeking to explain why health practitioners were ambivalent about their role in identifying and intervening in the lives of children who were 'at risk.' Professionals in primary care settings found themselves enmeshed in wider debates about disciplinary boundaries, power, gender relations and familial functioning. Using archival sources, Beecher listens to what survivors of sexual abuse said about their attempts to get help and contrasts this with practitioners' memories which she captures in rich oral histories. The effect is a fascinating historical kaleidoscope of ideas and practices from medics, nurses, mental health practitioners and feminist/survivor activists.

The book is a sensitive and carefully argued history that explores the professional dilemmas and debates associated with child sexual abuse and how they were understood by community health professionals and by survivors. In common with many of the volumes in the 'Gender and Sexualities in History' series, *Community Health Practitioners and Child Sexual Abuse in the Family, 1970s–2010s* contributes to our knowledge of the past in relation to questions about medical authority, gender and child sexual abuse.

London, UK
Melbourne, VIC, Australia

Joanna Bourke
Sean Brady
Matthew Champion

Acknowledgements

I carried out this work as part of the Sexual Harms and Medical Encounters (SHaME) project at Birkbeck, surrounded by supportive colleagues in our research hub and in the wider School of Historical Studies. I am honoured to be part of Birkbeck's radical tradition. Thanks to the SHaME team: Rhea Sookdeosingh, Emma Yapp, Rhian Keyse, Allison McKibban and Cora Salkovskis, and particularly to Adeline Moussion Esteve, Stephanie Wright and George Severs for reading, re-reading, insights and great laughs. I am also grateful to the SHaME associates who gave advice at many events and work-in-progress sessions, especially Louise Hide, Caitlin Cunningham, Charlie Jeffries, Gethin Rees, Sameena Mulla and Mara Keire. For guidance from wise Birkbeck colleagues thanks to Matt Cook, Kate Retford, Sarah Marks, Jessica Reinisch and Hilary Sapire.

For excellence and unparalleled generosity in scholarship and mentorship, Joanna Bourke. You give so much of your time and energy to others; I valued every minute you gave to me and my work and I'm very, very grateful. Thanks also to my first academic mentor, the wonderful writer, teacher and broadcaster, Marybeth Hamilton.

For meticulous research and help with archiving, thanks to Alice Fox, Marcia Price and Anna Weedon.

Many individuals beyond Birkbeck helped me including Victoria Hoyle at the University of York whose ideas and advice were invaluable and here's to our future partnership projects on the histories of childhood. Thanks too to Emily Bridger for collaborating with me on the ethical and methodological challenges of research on sexual violence.

To my former colleagues in Islington Children's Services, my thanks for your great encouragement over the years, as well as your tenacious professionalism and good humour in the face of whatever hits you. And particular thanks to Laura Eden, an inspirational leader.

I was honoured to have the opportunity to record oral histories with the following practitioners about their experiences in relation to child protection. Thank you to (in order of recording) Gill Abramovich, Deborah Hodes, Peter Fuggle, Jane Bramwell, Anne Hackett,* Jane Hutcheson, Jennifer Xavier, Patricia Scowen, Stephen Frosh, Diana Quigley,* Chloe Duncan,* Danya Glaser, Michelle Cutland, Judith Trowell, Gerrilyn Smith, Arnon Bentovim, Sam Warner, Stephen Amiel, Kim Underhill,* Natasha Rahman.* To Suzy, thank you for sharing your experiences with medical and psychiatric services. Thanks also to those who gave up their time for background interviews, and/or made connections for me, and opened other doors and avenues for me to explore.

For access to archival materials, I am grateful to Liz Davies, Robert Dingwall, the Feminist Library, Liz Kelly at the Child and Woman Abuse Studies Unit at London Met, Corinne May Chahal and the NSPCC, the National Archive, the family of Rasjidah St John, Matthew Taylor at the Open University, Katy Mair at Wellcome, Sam Warner and Helen Wilson at the Association of Child Protection Professionals, the Women's Library at the LSE and Andrew Rackley at UCH.

I would not have been able to carry out the research on which this book is based without a postdoctoral research fellowship granted by the Wellcome Trust as part of the SHaME project [205378/Z/16/Z]. Thank you to Wellcome for supporting research that tackles the huge public health problem of sexual violence.

The friends and family who helped me get to the finish line have been incredibly patient and nurturing: my wife Kim Lawson, my incredible children Amy, Alice, Shannon and Joe Beecher and their dad Ian Olney, my beloved Mum and Dad and my brother Ads. Thanks to my dear friends Ailsa Russell, Evelyn Kerrigan Lebloch, Abi Gbago, Phil Tooher, Eve Olney and Morty McCarthy.

*Ethics* This study was performed in line with the principles of the Declaration of Helsinki. Approval was granted by the Ethics Committee of Birkbeck, University of London and followed the College's research integrity code of practice and ethical framework. Informed consent was freely given by participants in relation to participation and publication.

## Praise for *Community Health Practitioners and Child Sexual Abuse in the Family, 1970s–2010s*

"This challenging, probing book poses a difficult question – why do those in contact with sexually abused children fail to understand what they are seeing, despite training and policy guidelines that task them with vigilance? The history of community health professionals, working on the front line of tacking child abuse, provides some answers. Beecher sensitively explores children's disclosures of abuse and the lack of culture change within community health that has made responding so inadequate."

—Lucy Delap, Professor in Modern British and Gender History, *University of Cambridge, UK*

"In this exceptional book, Ruth Beecher pieces together the 'messy, complicated and contested' story of how community health practitioners built up knowledge of child sexual abuse in the family and how they tried to help children – but also how children were often failed by individuals and by systems. It's a story that is painful to read at times and will often induce anger, but in her unflinching determination to place children's rights and needs at the centre of this history, Beecher performs an urgent and necessary task. In refusing to turn away from this story of harm, Beecher breaks a myth of children's silence, shows how often adults refuse to listen, and performs her own quiet activism in urging readers not to turn away either. It's a work of brilliant and empathetic scholarship that is sensitive and brave in equal measure, that will shape the field for years to come."

—Tracey Loughran, Professor of History, *University of Essex, UK*

"In a subject shrouded in societal unease, this remarkably comprehensive book sheds light on the historical contexts of child sexual abuse. Understanding these perspectives is crucial for influencing current practices and making impactful changes in children's lives. Relevant, accessible, and significant, this book delivers an unmistakable message: we can, and must, do better. As a survivor of child sexual abuse within the family, this book offers hope for a better way forward."

—Sophie Olson, survivor activist and author, founder of *The Flying Child CIC, UK*

"An important and compassionate book that rigorously chronicles attempts to recognize, and intervene, in cases of child sexual abuse since the 1980s – and the politics and professional interests that have shaped them."

—Robert Dingwall, author of The Protection of Children: State Intervention and Family Life, UK

# Contents

# About the Author

**Ruth Beecher** is an historian and applied researcher. Her interests include the history of British and American health and social care, with an emphasis on the history of children and families and the professions that work with them, as well as the history and politics of gender, sexuality and sexual violence.

Prior to retraining as an historian, Beecher was a leader within local government where she programme managed local policy initiatives as well as translating national policy into successful practice on the ground, both in children's services and working across into other sectors particularly housing, health and employment.

CHAPTER 1

# Introduction

In 2015–2016, over fifty sexually abused children and young people aged six to nineteen were interviewed by researchers. Their evidence would form part of an inquiry initiated by the Children's Commissioner for England into child sexual abuse in the family environment.[1] The usual methods of inquiry (a systematic review of the literature, an analysis of government data, site visits, oral evidence) would not have captured the opinions of those who had been sexually abused. There was a silence, a dearth of children's voices in the body of research on child sexual abuse that mirrored 'the cultures of silence in which abuse and impunity flourish.'[2] The final report concluded that the fact that professionals and other adults continued to miss the signs of child sexual abuse placed an

[1] The definition of child sexual abuse in the family environment used here is that of the Children's Commissioner UK: sexual abuse perpetrated or facilitated in or out of the home, against a child under the age of 18, by a family member, or someone linked to the family, whether or not they are a family member. Perpetrators may be close to the victim (e.g. father, uncle), or less familiar (e.g. family friend, babysitter). Children's Commissioner, 'Protecting Children from Harm: A Critical Assessment of Child Sexual Abuse in the Family Network in England and Priorities for Action' (2015), 2.

[2] Camille Warrington et al., 'Making Noise: Children's Voices for Positive Change after Sexual Abuse' (Beds: University of Bedfordshire in partnership with the NSPCC, 2017), 167, 172.



R. Beecher, *Community Health Practitioners and Child Sexual Abuse in the Family, 1970s–2010s*, Genders and Sexualities in History, https://doi.org/10.1007/978-3-031-80052-8_1

unfair responsibility on children and young people to find help. Young people spoke up about what could be different. An eighteen-year-old said:

> There is more of a chance that somebody would admit to it if you asked them outright I think rather than [waiting for] them coming forward to you … there would've have been more of a chance I would have if somebody had just been like, 'is this happening?'
>
> *Young woman aged 18 years, 2015.*[3]

Twenty years earlier, an adult survivor of child sexual abuse wrote to a previous national inquiry, about being regularly raped by her male cousin:

> As it turns out, the signs were there although slightly hidden. I was forever at the doctors with urine infections and other problems 'down there.' I don't blame anybody for not noticing what was happening. I was so terrified of him carrying out his threats [to kill her if she told] that I had probably subconsciously gone out of my way to behave as normally as possible. I had always had excellent reports from school and wasn't a 'problem' child.
>
> *Woman, age unknown, 1995*[4]

These young women spoke about two possible means by which someone could have helped them and stopped the abuse: encouraging them to speak or noticing the possible signs. In the lexicon of social welfare and medicine, or what some historians have called 'something approaching a freestanding child abuse profession' that has developed since the early 1970s,[5] 'noticing' and 'encouraging children to speak' have been formalised into the language of 'identification' and 'disclosure.' Health professionals based in the community, whether doctors, nurses or therapists, are well placed to see and hear what is happening to children. As one of the survivors above said, she was 'forever at the doctor.' And yet those professional groups rationalise the fact that they do not identify the possible signs of sexual abuse in the family context by citing a range of barriers.

In relation to disclosure, some say they believe that children are unlikely to disclose to them no matter how they behave as professionals. Children

[3] Ibid., 66.

[4] Letter from a female survivor to the National Commission of Inquiry into the Prevention of Child Abuse (NCIPCA), 6 Mar 1995.

[5] Philip Jenkins, *Moral Panic: Changing Concepts of the Child Molester in Modern America* (New Haven and London: Yale University Press, 1998), 128.

and young adult survivors say the opposite, that adults can and should listen and pay attention to the signs. A twelve-year-old told researchers in 2015 that

> when all this is happening and someone doesn't really take any notice and you should always make people feel like they're noticed. It makes me angry that they didn't notice this before.
>
> *Girl, aged 12 years, 2015.*[6]

In 1995, a young adult survivor wondered why nobody displayed any curiosity about the illness that caused her to miss a year of school:

> I had a year's illness, aged fourteen, which was diagnosed as ME, because no one knew what it was but this was a cry for help. The symptoms were chronic tiredness and general aches and pains….. The cause was explained by Doctors as psychological, but nobody questioned further. WHY??? … Every signal, ideally, should be noticed.
>
> *Young woman, aged about 20 years, 1995.*[7]

The universal health services are an essential means of promoting children's health and wellbeing and protecting them from abuse (whether physical, emotional, sexual abuse or neglect). This has been an accepted proposition within the health services in the United Kingdom for decades. From the 1970s, the community-based health professions accepted the protection of children from what was then called 'battering' as one of their core responsibilities. By the 1980s, child sexual abuse was acknowledged and included in this. I will say more about this in Chap. 2. It has been the subject of reams of policy and procedure, as well as a topic for training materials and guidance.

In part, community health professionals have ended up with child protection as a core responsibility because they believe that people would want to confide in them. Our ideas about the sanctity of the relationship between patients and their nurse, doctor or therapist have changed over time and they do not apply equally or in the same way to all members of our societies. Poor and marginalised families may see a healthcare

[6] Warrington et al, 'Making Noise: Children's Voices for Positive Change after Sexual Abuse,' 65.

[7] Letter from female survivor (age approximately twenty) to NCIPCA, 1995.

professional less often or only in an emergency situation.[8] Undocumented families without a legal right to be in the country may avoid all services for fear of arrest and deportation.[9] Barriers of race, disability and gender undoubtedly affect whether and from whom patients seek help.

Nevertheless, long traditions of a trusting contract between patients and their health practitioners suggest that people will confide in them. Family members can be seen in a private space (which is not the case for teachers or youth workers) and the accepted territory of their conversations includes intimate bodily functions and worries about physical or mental health. Seeking advice not only about one's own health but about that of another family member is not uncommon. Family doctors, paediatricians, health visitors and school nurses have different types and levels of training, but each profession learns about anatomy and physiology. Because they understand the way the body looks and functions, they are well situated to spot the physical signs that might indicate sexual abuse. Similarly, they and to a greater extent community-based psychologists and psychiatrists are trained to observe behaviour and the emotions, which ideally positions them to be alert to the presence of concerning symptoms.

And yet the child who is sexually abused by a family member is not well served by the health practitioners that they are most likely to see in their day-to-day lives: their family doctor, health visitor, school nurse or mental health practitioner. We have statements such as those above from child and adult survivors that testify to this. Although we have to exercise caution with quantitative data, it tells a similar story. There have been fluctuations in public awareness of child sexual abuse in the family since the 1970s but overall, children's disclosure rates have not improved.[10] Through data on referral sources to child protection services, we can be certain that not

[8] There are fewer GPs in poor areas, people find it difficult to get an appointment and are less likely than those financially better off to have a good experience of visiting their GP. 'Poor areas left behind on standards of GP care, research reveals,' https://www.nuffieldtrust.org.uk/news-item/poor-areas-left-behind-on-standards-of-gp-care-research-reveals, 24 Dec 2018.

[9] Melanie Griffiths and Colin Yeo, 'The UK's Hostile Environment: Deputising Immigration Control,' *Critical Social Policy* 41, no 4 (2021): 521–544.

[10] Kathleen Coulborn Faller, 'The Child Sexual Abuse Disclosure Controversy: New Perspectives on an Abiding Problem,' *Child Abuse & Neglect* 99 (2020).

only do health professionals not receive disclosures, they very rarely identify concerns of sexual abuse either.[11]

This is a cause for considerable concern. Sexual abuse has a lasting and severe impact on mental and physical health, relationships and behaviour throughout a person's childhood, adolescence and adulthood. Beyond the effects on an individual's health, delay in recognising that a child is being abused creates a subsequent financial burden on the state and particularly health services.[12] The extent of the damage depends on many factors including the frequency of the sexual assault, the duration of the abuse, the identity of the abuser and the level of secrecy and coercion. The types of health problems associated with sexual abuse include depression and anxiety, risk of suicide, self-harm, eating disorders, substance misuse and post-traumatic stress symptoms such as intrusive thoughts, avoidance of remembering or thinking about the event(s), alterations in cognition or mood, or in arousal and activity exemplified by irritability, angry outbursts or self-destructive behaviour.[13] There can also be direct physical effects including sexually transmitted diseases, pelvic and gynaecological problems at all stages of a girl and woman's life. In fact, there are long-term physical health consequences for both girls and boys.[14] These problems are not inevitable and should not be weaponised by pathologising adult survivors. To help avoid these problems as children grow up, speaking to children and noticing their distress should be prioritised by professionals, but it seems that it is not.

This book takes seriously children's expressed wish that we tackle 'the cultures of silence in which abuse and impunity flourish.' Within it, I examine more closely the context and history of the involvement of doctors, nurses and therapists in community settings in protecting children from sexual abuse. They are the primary contact for children and families'

[11] Debra Allnock and Pam Miller, 'No One Noticed, No One Heard: A Study of Disclosures of Childhood Abuse,' (London: NSPCC, 2013, 23–24).

[12] Olumide Adisa, Megan Hermolle, and Fiona Ellis, 'Denial, Disbelief and Delays: Examining the Costs on the NHS of Delayed Child Sexual Abuse Disclosures in England and Wales,' (Suffolk: Survivors in Transition and University of Suffolk, 2023).

[13] This is a sample of the symptoms and signs, for a straightforward list from the psychiatric perspective, see 'What is PTSD?' https://www.psychiatry.org/patients-families/ptsd/what-is-ptsd#section_0, accessed 29 Jan 2024.

[14] Sarah Nelson, 'Surviving Well,' (Scotland: Wellbeing Scotland, 2020); Leah Irish et al., 'Long-term Physical Health Consequences of Childhood Sexual Abuse: A Meta-analytic Review,' *Journal of Pediatric Psychology* 35, no 5 (2010): 450–461. https://doi.org/10.1093/jpepsy/jsp118.

health issues on a day-to-day and non-emergency basis and are in a position to intervene early in a family where a child has been sexually abused and therefore to reduce the amount of harm done to the child. By deliberately centring community health practitioners' own experiences and understanding, this book explores why, despite encouragement and training to be vigilant in relation to the physical and behavioural signs of sexual abuse, their rates of identification of child sexual abuse within the family environment did not rise over time.

## Professional Silences

There has been no in-depth exploration of this particular quandary. Reasons for these silences include the common myth that children do not or cannot tell; the fact that the potential of the role of community health professionals in child protection is overlooked; the way the public, media and politicians erroneously associate all aspects of child abuse with social workers and to a lesser extent with the police. I will examine these reasons further before explaining why it is an essential area for further investigation.

Some commentators argue that the reason that health professionals do not hear disclosures is obvious. Children rarely tell anyone about sexual abuse. The small proportion of children who do disclose before their eighteenth birthday usually confide in a relative or person they know socially and trust. This may include their mother (unless she is involved in the abuse) or a friend, for example. They may speak to a teacher or counsellor at school. Very few tell a doctor, nurse or therapist based in their community. Most apparently do not entrust the information to anybody at all until they are an adult,[15] although a recent UK research study has challenged this.[16] A 2015 research review of prevalence studies confirmed that few children who have been sexually abused receive help from official agencies such as social services. These international studies estimate a rate of 127 per thousand for sexual abuse in self-reported studies (when adults

[15] Noel Smith, Cristian Dogaru, and Fiona Ellis, *Hear Me. Believe Me. Respect Me. A Survey of Adult Survivors of Child Sexual Abuse and Their Experiences of Support Services* (Suffolk: Survivors in Transition and University Campus Suffolk, 2015), 13–17; Ben Mathews, 'The Context of Child Sexual Abuse, and Points of Departure,' in *New International Frontiers in Child Sexual Abuse: Theory, Problems and Progress* (Switzerland: Springer Nature, 2019), 21–25.

[16] Allnock and Miller, 'No One Noticed, No One Heard,' 16.

were asked 'were you ever sexually abused during childhood?') but only four per thousand for reported sexual abuse (informants such as medical professionals, child protection workers or teachers reporting on the abuse experiences of children with whom they were in touch). In other words, adults asked whether they were abused as children report that they were at a much higher proportion than is observed by professionals during their childhood. However, the same review demonstrated that most child abuse *of any type* [emphasis mine] is unknown to statutory agencies and remains outside official statistics.[17] The many survivors who gave evidence to the UK National Commission of Inquiry into the Prevention of Child Abuse in 1995 also testified to that effect.[18]

Thus, whilst we acknowledge that sexual abuse brings additional layers of secrecy and shame, we can recognise too that it is not unique in comparison to other forms of abuse in being largely hidden from services. We should also admit that the statistics and adult survivor reports that children did not disclose any form of abuse may mask many efforts to tell. Eighty per cent of sixty young adult survivors of all forms of abuse in the UK said they had tried to tell someone.[19] Furthermore, as Ramonia Alaggia and colleagues have highlighted, the research has to date produced more knowledge on inhibitors and barriers than on understanding the conditions that can better promote and facilitate earlier disclosures.[20] We have much more to learn about the conditions in which children can and do tell and there is more to discover about how health settings can make that easier for children, young people and non-abusing carers.

I argue that the potential of the role of community health professionals—in identifying child sexual abuse within the family early and responding to it in ways that assist children and young people in getting help—is overlooked. This affects not only the practitioner responses to children

[17] Marije Stoltenborgh et al, 'The Prevalence of Child Maltreatment across the Globe: Review of a Series of Meta-Analyses,' *Child Abuse Review* 24, no 1 (2015).

[18] Corinne Wattam and Clare Woodward, 'And Do I Abuse My Children? No!,' in *Childhood Matters: Report of the National Commission of Inquiry into the Prevention of Child Abuse. Vol 2: Background Papers* (London: The Stationery Office, 1996), 104–105; 'Childhood Matters: Report of the National Commission of Inquiry into the Prevention of Child Abuse. Volume 1,' (Great Britain: Department of Health, 1996).

[19] Allnock and Miller, 'No One Noticed, No One Heard,' 16.

[20] Ramona Alaggia, Delphine Collin-Vézina, and Rusan Lateef, 'Facilitators and Barriers to Child Sexual Abuse (CSA) Disclosures: A Research Update (2000–2016),' *Trauma, Violence & Abuse* 20, no 2 (2019).

but is also responsible for a gap in the research. Since the early 1990s, the role of health practitioners in child sexual abuse is portrayed as either forensic or therapeutic. Forensically in that nurses, medics and therapists' roles are interpreted as incorporating the examination of a child where a suspicion of sexual abuse has already come to light, and the production of an evidential record of that is to inform the social workers planning for care or criminal proceedings.[21] Therapeutically in that medics are seen as mainly there to treat symptoms arising from the abuse. Although it is accepted in policy terms that community-based nurses, doctors and therapists are well-placed to identify sexual abuse in the course of their daily duties, this is eclipsed in the research agenda by more captivating topics for exploration such as 'false memory syndrome.'[22]

Within the health professions too, community practitioners generally have a lesser status and less research is carried out on their activities. They stand at the nexus of different groups in terms of their role and function. They are not specialists in investigation, diagnosis, assessment or treatment. Rather, they are generalists operating at the early stages of patient care or working alongside specialists to support the treatment plan following a diagnosis. They are part of the health landscape but are set apart from other health professionals by virtue of their location dispersed in the community. Their orientation is different as it leans towards public health and prevention rather than 'curing' the sick. In the case of the health visitor, that public health role has a long history dating back to nineteenth century efforts to reduce child mortality and prevent infectious diseases. With other professional groups, for example, general practitioners in the UK during the 1970s, taking on a more preventative and public health role was a new initiative that met with some resistance. Either way, it marks

[21] Nigel Parton and Corinne Wattam, eds., *Child Sexual Abuse: Responding to the Experiences of Children*, Wiley Series in Child Protection and Policy (Chichester: Wiley, 1999), 6.

[22] D. M. Bernstein and E. F. Loftus, 'How to Tell If a Particular Memory Is True or False,' *Perspectives on Psychological Science* 4, no 4 (2009); M. Garry et al, 'Imagination Inflation: Imagining a Childhood Event Inflates Confidence That It Occurred,' *Psychonomic Bulletin and Review* 3 (1996); E. F. Loftus and M. J. Guyer, 'Who Abused Jane Doe? The Hazards of the Single Case History. Part 1,' *Skeptical Inquirer* 26, no 3 (2002); E. F. Loftus and J. E. Pickrell, 'The Formation of False Memories,' *Psychiatric Annals* 25, no 12 (1995); L. Patihis et al, 'Are the "Memory Wars" Over? A Scientist-Practitioner Gap in Beliefs About Repressed Memory,' *Psychological Science* 25, no 2 (2014); I. van Damme et al, 'Emotion and False Memory: How Goal-Irrelevance Can Be Relevant for What People Remember,' *Memory* 25, no 2 (2017).

them out as different within health institutions and pulls them away from medicine and towards what was referred to in the 1970s (and sometimes for decades after that) as 'social medicine' and is now usually called 'social care.'

Another reason that community health is overlooked is that, since the latest wave of professionalisation of child protection in the 1970s, it has come to be seen as a multidisciplinary endeavour led by social workers and the police. Although health is purportedly the third side of this equilateral triangle of institutions, its status in child protection has somewhat diminished since the late 1980s (I will return to the reasons for this in Chap. 5). Studies focus more on social work and police practice or on the multi-agency workforce (including healthcare) as it operates across different professional groups and organisations. These studies tend to be similar to that of government inquiries, paying attention to the ways such practitioners work as part of the multi-agency network in terms of clarity of function, adherence to procedures and communication across institutional boundaries.[23]

In fact, the public, practitioners and scholars alike often associate the identification of potential child sexual abuse and early responses to it erroneously with social workers rather than doctors, nurses or therapists based in primary care. This is a basic misunderstanding of the role of social workers in the UK who rarely come into direct contact with a child who might make a disclosure or exhibit the signs of sexual abuse unless they are already 'case-working' the child and family. They operate at a more specialist level, dealing with families already identified as having children whose welfare or development is compromised in some way and are at higher risk of harm. A member of the public or another professional will alert them to the suspicion of abuse. In other words, most social workers cannot contribute to 'noticing' the sexual abuse or 'encouraging a child to speak' unless that family is already known to them because of other welfare concerns.

These are some of the reasons why scholars have not taken the potential of community-based practitioners to identify child sexual abuse seriously.

[23] Christine Hallett and Olive Stevenson, *Child Abuse: Aspects of Interprofessional Co-operation* (London and Boston: Allen & Unwin, 1980); Olive Stevenson, ed. *Child Abuse: Public Policy and Professional Practice* (Herts: Harvester Wheatsheaf, 1989); Carolyn Davies and Harriet Ward, *Safeguarding Children across Services: Messages from Research*, Safeguarding Children across Services Series (London: Jessica Kingsley, 2012).

There is a final reason why there has not been an investment into research in this area. Many commentators maintain that there is such an accumulation of obvious social, cultural, political, professional and personal disincentives that prevent health professionals from noticing the signs of sexual abuse that further investigation is unnecessary. Their professional status may be fragile (gender plays a part here with a high and growing proportion of women in the community health professions); they may be disorientated by frequent restructures or the privatisation of services; worn down by the stress of managing high-risk cases and the spectre of public inquiries when things go wrong; or fatigued by policy and initiative overload. Their behaviour may be affected by conflicting feelings about state intervention versus family privacy. These ebb and flow over time but have certainly been present to a certain degree since the 1960s in the UK and the US. Fear of complaints against them or negative press coverage may increase their reluctance to intervene. A belief that children may suffer greater harm if removed from their family into care may affect them, especially in the context of funding constraints. They may hold certain prejudices against children such as stereotypes of them as unreliable witnesses or wayward, promiscuous adolescents. These labels are typically exacerbated by racial or other prejudices. By virtue of their community base, they are in close proximity on a daily basis to families, including perpetrators. They may lack the courage to challenge potential abusers who intimidate them because they are violent or powerful individuals who wield great influence in the community. There are also intra- and inter-professional hierarchies and rivalries at play; examples include professional jostling between social workers and health visitors in the 1970s and between child psychotherapists and clinical psychologists in the 1980s. These have changed over time, it is important to contextualise them but they are always present to some degree.

Practitioners at the frontline are also inhibited from protecting children by the impact of the unprecedented backlash against them following crises and scandals where they are criticised for doing too little to protect children (for example, in all child death inquiries and in child sexual exploitation inquiries, particularly Rochdale), or being overzealous and trampling on parents' rights (particularly in the Cleveland and Orkney Inquiries in the UK (1987 and 1991)).[24] I will examine Cleveland in greater detail in

[24] Department of Health and Social Security, *Child Abuse: A Study of Inquiry Reports 1973–1981* (London: HMSO, 1982); Department of Health, *Child Abuse: A Study of*

Chap. 5. Suffice to say here that the excoriation of the paediatricians involved reduced the confidence of medics to identify the physical signs of sexual abuse whilst the controversy in relation to interviewing children left a legacy of challenges in relation to disclosures.

These are not minor problems. Prior to 2005, there was no certainty that parents who had been wrongly accused of child abuse would not sue doctors or social workers for negligence in carrying out their investigations. The subsequent Lords ruling that professionals owed a duty of care to the child alone and not to the parents may not have assuaged all fears of litigation.[25] Furthermore, practitioners require a high level of professional confidence to ask difficult questions. As a consultant community paediatrician commented in 2019:

> People are really, really terrified about asking children if they are being sexually abused. The nurse isn't going to say to that child who comes in with tummy ache, 'and has anybody done anything you don't like,' because that's what I teach people to ask but I don't even know if they dare ask that. Because the police would say 'you put ideas into their head, didn't you?'
> *Deborah Hodes, paediatrician, 2019.*[26]

There appears to be a firm consensus across institutions at national and local government levels that community health practitioners have an important job to do in relation to identifying child sexual abuse. This is asserted by professional bodies such as the Royal Colleges, commissioners and managers of health services, leaders of health provider organisations, management at all levels and practitioners themselves. Why does policy and practice guidance tell them that is their role? Why do we dissemble about our expectations of disclosure and identifications if in reality we do not believe that a community-based nurse, doctor or therapist will identify the physical, emotional and behavioural symptoms of child sexual abuse and take action? Are we to renege on these ethical responsibilities to

*Inquiry Reports 1980–1989* (London: HMSO, 1991); Alexis Jay, 'Independent Inquiry into Child Sexual Exploitation in Rotherham 1997–2013,' (Rotherham Metropolitan Borough Counci, 2014); Elizabeth Butler-Sloss, 'Report of the Inquiry into Child Abuse in Cleveland 1987: Presented to the Secretary of State for Social Services by the Right Honourable Lord Justice Butler-Sloss,' (London: HMSO, 1988); James J. Clyde, *The Report of the Inquiry into the Removal of Children from Orkney in February 1991* (Edinburgh: HMSO, 1992).

[25] JD (FC) (Appellant) v. East Berkshire Community Health NHS Trust and others (Respondents) and two other actions (FC), UKHL23 (2005).

[26] Oral history interview with Deborah Hodes by author, 31 May 2019.

children? And what about children who are least able to tell: children too young to speak, children with physical or intellectual disabilities, those trying to communicate across racial, religious, ethnic or cultural barriers, those whose families are marked out as different owing to poverty, substance misuse, domestic violence or mental health problems or those who are subject to prejudice because of their sexuality or transgender identity? A system that operates to prevent us from seeing and hearing children's distress is oppressive. If we are not working to dismantle it and think differently, are we colluding to preserve it?

## Professional Thoughts, Emotions and Actions

Each one of these professional groups has an individual history that affects their engagement with debates about protecting children and in turn affects their practice. They also have a shared history. What are the underlying factors that have affected them since the late 1960s and in what ways have those factors changed their thoughts, emotions, utterances and actions over that period? How influential was the US in transmitting ideas to UK health professionals and did those ideas transfer in near identical forms or were they altered? To what extent did a medical model or feminism influence health practitioners? The barriers identified by health professionals and the notion that children cannot articulate their distress are presented ahistorically in the literature. Have these ideas been constant since the 1970s or did they change due to external factors along the way? And what about examples of health professionals who have listened or acted? How have they arrived at a difference stance and practice? How have their situations—whether organisational, geographical, racial or otherwise—affected their disposition towards sexual abuse and in what ways can we understand this?

A historical perspective can help us dissect the strange coexistence of surface acquiescence to, and apparent compliance with, laws, statutory guidance, policy and procedures with a generalised reluctance to recognise sexual abuse. As Sarah Nelson has pointed out, written documents, guidance and regulation will 'in themselves neither protect nor identify children at risk. It is like giving people the furniture and fittings before the floors and walls of the house are built.'[27] With the exception of those with

[27] Sarah Nelson, 'Preparing for the Special Challenge of Sexual Abuse,' in *Safeguarding Children in Primary Care*, ed. Julie Taylor and Markus Huber (London: Jessica Kingsley Publishers, 2009).

a 'designated' child protection role or a special interest in child abuse, practitioners state that being alert to the possibility of child sexual abuse is an accepted part of the job, whilst admitting that they have never, or only once or twice, encountered a case of child sexual abuse in their own careers. A health visitor explained that:

Quigley*: In terms of sexual abuse, I think that's an interesting one because although we know that children as young as whatever can be subject to sexual abuse, I think it would be more likely that we would have been perhaps supporting a mother or indeed a father who might have experienced that type of abuse rather than seeing it in the preschool child. Which isn't saying it doesn't exist there because it does but, you know …

Beecher: I was also surprised by the statistics around age … Because in terms of children who are registered [on a child protection plan with primary reason as sexual abuse], there is quite a high proportion of children under five —

Quigley: There are, yeah.

Beecher: And I wondered how much health visitors had been told about that really?

Quigley: Yeah, I think they are now, yes.[28]

This particular person had held a specialist child protection role and yet she still found it difficult to accept that health visitors could spot the signs of sexual abuse in babies and young children and act. And yet, it was policy for her and her colleagues across Britain to do so.

Is it impossible for health professionals to take on this responsibility? Our societies pay lip service to children's agency and autonomy and claim that it is imperative to 'listen to children.' Meanwhile, children are silenced. They have fewer relationships outside the family now than they had in the 1970s due to increased fear of strangers.[29] As a society, we have once again retreated from an acceptance that sexual danger for children exists within

[28] Oral history interview with Diana Quigley* by author, 23 Jan 2020. Pseudonyms are used where requested by interviewees and are marked * on first use.

[29] The language of paedophilia and alarm about sexual abuse became common after the mid 1970s leading to 'a closing down of a physical landscape beyond the home.' Mathew Thomson, *Lost Freedom: The Landscape of the Child and the British Post-War Settlement* (Oxford: Oxford University Press, 2013), 154.

the family and trusted close relations. Inquiries into child sexual exploitation and institutional abuse are happening all over the world. They are necessary but also circle us back to older ideas about 'stranger danger' outside of the home and away from the most frequent serious and long-term abusers: father-figures, brothers, cousins. The child who is groomed or threatened into sexual activity today will be less able to speak out if their father, brother or cousin is the perpetrator. Who will they confide in?

Within the formal and rigid structures of child protection, there are additional barriers. Families and communities who may suspect abuse are encouraged to believe that only professionals should get involved, while professionals who are generalists and located in the community think that only specialists can ask about sexual abuse. As a clinical psychologist commented in 2019:

> there's a profound complication for children which is that we ask them to receive help from strangers. Now the whole social— the whole social adaptability, the whole kind of way that it works outside of the professional system is you seek help from people you know. You don't— nobody seeks help from strangers, that's the weirdest idea and … we … overcome it because we go to lawyers or we go to GPs. We have titles that protect us and make us feel safe. But for children, it's the weirdest thing. The more distressed you are, the more strangers you go and see. And that seems to me, that inhibits this kind of capacity. When they're just about to tell you, you're in the context of often— often with strangers, even kind— it can be very kind strangers but they're still strangers.
>
> *Peter Fuggle, clinical psychologist, 2019.*[30]

The ultimate impact is on children who, if they are brave enough to signal for help or to speak up to someone they trust, are passed on to a different professional, usually someone totally unknown to them. Processes are designed from adult perspectives and usually to protect adult interests; often these adults are the professionals in contact with the child, often these processes inadvertently protect the perpetrator of the abuse.

[30] Oral history interview with Peter Fuggle by author, 6 Jun 2019.

## Selective Statistics

The quantitative data about the incidence, prevalence and impact of child sexual abuse is complicated and contested. Different interest groups at different points in time since the 1970s have set out to use the data to scaffold their arguments about sexual abuse. Medics saw child abuse as a syndrome and wanted epidemiological studies to evaluate its incidence and distribution and devise a plan to control it. Social scientists wanted to understand the extent and nature of the social problem faced while feminists, moral conservatives and survivors wanted data to support their lobbying efforts.

Prior to the late 1970s, there were few efforts to obtain an accurate picture of the extent of child maltreatment generally or sexual abuse specifically. Alfred Kinsey's random study of 5000 women in the early 1950s asked them about their sexual experiences. Some scholars focused on his finding that a quarter of the women had experienced an inappropriate sexual advance from an adult before the age of thirteen.[31] Others cited a different finding that 6.5 per cent of the women interviewed said they had been sexually abused by their father or stepfather.[32] The former encompasses a wider range of predatory behaviours, the latter is narrowly defined—I cite them both here as an example of the way in which 'high/low' figures have been deployed which create confusion and sometimes scepticism about the actual extent of child sexual abuse. Historians have demonstrated that this tendency to selectively cite low or high data is common when linked to sites of political contention.[33] Sexual abuse data was difficult to capture and interpret, came with caveats and required cautious interpretation. Because the topic was emotionally charged, such care was rarely applied; some used the data negligently or selectively and doubters treated the data as highly contentious.

After Kinsey, US sociologist David Finkelhor's late 1970s survey of college students was one of the first attempts to establish prevalence. He found that nineteen per cent of the women and just under nine per cent

[31] Alfred C. Kinsey et al, *Sexual Behavior in the Human Female* (Philadelphia: Saunders, 1953); Mary MacLeod and Esther Saraga, 'Challenging the Orthodoxy: Towards a Feminist Theory and Practice,' *Feminist Review*, 28, no 1 (1988): 76.

[32] Lynn Sacco, *Unspeakable: Father-Daughter Incest in American History* (Baltimore. Md: Johns Hopkins University Press, 2009), 214.

[33] For a fraught numbers debates on a very different topic, see Charles C. Mann, '1491,' *The Atlantic Monthly*, March 2002.

of the men interviewed had a sexual experience of some kind with an adult during their childhood.[34] In 1997, Kevin M. Gorey and Donald R. Leslie carried out a quantitative meta-analysis of prior US research reviews. They estimated that between twelve and seventeen per cent of girls and five to eight per cent of boys had been sexually abused in childhood.[35] A few years later, Bolen and Scannapieco carried out a similar meta-analysis arriving at different estimates of thirty to forty per cent of girls and more than thirteen per cent of boys.[36] The US population was 281 million in 2000 so even a few percentage points represented many children and altered the scale of the problem significantly. The methodological difficulties and the contentious nature of high vs low estimates are demonstrated in the highly technical debate between these two groups of scholars in the pages of *Social Science Review*.[37] I will address what was at stake within these disputes about the validity of the data below, but first a brief description of the UK situation.

In 2022, there is still no national and consistent monitoring of the incidence (cases reported within a year) or prevalence (within a child's lifetime) of sexual abuse generally or of specific types of sexual abuse in the UK. The most cited data on prevalence is a study commissioned by the National Society for the Protection of Cruelty to Children (NSPCC) published in 2011. Over 4000 young people aged eleven to seventeen and young adults aged eighteen to 24 were selected randomly and interviewed. A total of 2160 parents or guardians also spoke on behalf of their children aged under eleven to a market research company. Eleven per cent of eighteen to twenty-four-year-olds said they had experienced contact sexual abuse in childhood.[38] In terms of gender, eighteen per cent of the

[34] David Finkelhor, *Sexually Victimized Children* (New York: Free Press, 1979), 53.

[35] Kevin M Gorey and Donald R Leslie, 'The Prevalence of Child Sexual Abuse: Integrative Review Adjustment for Potential Response and Measurement Biases,' *Child Abuse & Neglect* 21, no 4 (1997).

[36] Rebecca M. Bolen and Maria Scannapieco, 'Prevalence of Child Sexual Abuse: A Corrective Metanalysis,' *Social Service Review* 73, no 3 (1999): 299.

[37] Kevin M. Gorey and Donald R. Leslie, 'Debate with Authors. Working toward a Valid Prevalence Estimate of Child Sexual Abuse: A Reply to Bolen and Scannapieco,' *Social Service Review* 75, no 1 (2001).

[38] The percentages were lower for under elevens (0.5 per cent) and for eleven to seventeen-year-olds (five per cent). Contact sexual abuse includes including assault by penetration (for example, rape or oral sex) or non-penetrative acts such as masturbation, kissing, rubbing and touching outside of clothing. Non-contact activities include involving children in looking at, or in the production of, sexual images, watching sexual activities, encouraging children to

eighteen to twenty-year-olds were young women and five per cent were young men. A very large proportion of the abuse (just under 66 per cent) was reportedly perpetrated by other children aged under eighteen. A very tiny proportion (less than two per cent) reported contact sexual abuse by a parent or guardian.[39]

The NSPCC methodology was subsequently criticised because parents could control most aspects of the interviews. Their consent was required for participation, they answered on behalf of children under eleven and they were present when the eleven to seventeen-year-olds were interviewed. They may have perpetrated the abuse themselves, protected another perpetrator or have simply been unaware of it.[40] Although other research indicates that juvenile assault is common, the presence of parents may have skewed the data about its extent as it may be less frightening for children to suggest that than to accuse an adult.

The NSPCC study focused only on contact sexual abuse but if we return to the US meta-analysis by Bolen and Scannapieco (1999) described above, we find that the studies they reviewed included the estimated lifetime prevalence of both contact and non-contact sexual abuse.[41] We cannot compare these findings as they are not measuring like for like. As far back as 1980, US social worker Patricia Mrazek cautioned that the data was subject to criticism because 'definitions are vague and distinctly different types of sexual experiences are combined into a single category.'[42] The combining of categories made comparison of change over time challenging—were more children abused or were different behaviours included? It also led commentators to question whether non-contact incidents such as exposing the genitals should be considered as harmful.

Historian Philip Jenkins claimed the statistics deployed by US feminists in the 1980s suggested 'an incredible frequency not just of molestation

behave in sexually inappropriate ways or grooming a child in preparation for abuse (including via the internet). Lorraine Radford and National Society for the Prevention of Cruelty to Children, 'Child Abuse and Neglect in the UK Today' (2011).

39 'Child Abuse and Neglect in the UK Today.'

40 Nelson, *Tackling Child Sexual Abuse: Radical Approaches to Prevention, Protection and Support*, 28; For a recent summary of methodological issues, Liz Kelly and Kairika Karsna, 'Measuring the Scale and Changing Nature of Child Sexual Abuse and Child Sexual Exploitation - Scoping Report' (London: Centre of Expertise on Child Sexual Abuse, London Metropolitan University, 2021).

41 Bolen and Scannapieco, 'Prevalence of Child Sexual Abuse: A Corrective Metanalysis.'

42 Patricia Beezley Mrazek, 'Sexual Abuse of Children,' *Journal of Child Psychology and Psychiatry* 21, no 1 (1980).

but of the most extreme forms of rape and incest, a process of inflation accomplished by the familiar mid-century device of expansive definition and of assimilating all minor forms of deviancy with the most threatening acts of sexual predation.'[43] Feminists lobbied for definitions of sexual violence that went beyond forced sexual intercourse. But in Jenkins' opinion, by making 'abuse a matter of subjective definition, [they] eroded distinctions between violent or incestuous assaults and acts like exhibitionism.'[44] The examples put forward in the landmark feminist self-help book *The Courage to Heal* included being 'forced to listen to sex talk' or 'fondled, kissed or held in a way that made you uncomfortable.'[45] Jenkins appears to suggest that these actions should not 'count' as child sexual abuse because '[b]ased on these criteria, it would be amazing if incest and abuse were not reported on a vast scale.'[46]

Of course, his assumption is that the harm of sexual violence against children can be conceptualised as a hierarchy, with exhibitionism as the least harmful act and violent rape as the most damaging violation. Liz Kelly has formulated a different way of theorising the impact of sexual violence. She describes a continuum that ranges from behaviours that the criminal justice system might classify as 'minor' through to those that would be legally classified as sexual assault or rape. The common characteristics of 'abuse, coercion and force' are present at all points of the continuum, deployed in the vast majority of cases by men and experienced by (mostly) women and girls. Kelly's formulation explains the varying responses of women and children that 'cannot be read off simplistically from the form of sexual violence' they experience. In other words, certain supposedly minor acts may cause lasting harm and, depending on the victim's experiences, the extent of the harm may change over time.[47]

The studies reviewed by Gorey, Leslie, Bolen and Scannapieco were based on adult retrospective surveys. In the years 2003, 2008 and 2011, Finkelhor carried out national telephone surveys with a total of 2293

[43] Jenkins, *Moral Panic: Changing Concepts of the Child Molester in Modern America*, 119.

[44] Here Jenkins follows Hacking: 'Vice is conquering our society, not because we are more vicious but because we are declaring a vastly wider range of acts to be wicked.' Ian Hacking, 'The Making and Moulding of Child Sexual Abuse,' *Critical Inquiry* 17, no 2 (1991), 280.

[45] Ellen Bass and Laura Davis, *The Courage to Heal: A Guide for Women Survivors of Child Sexual Abuse* (New York: Perennial Library, 1988).

[46] Jenkins, *Moral Panic: Changing Concepts of the Child Molester in Modern America*, 130.

[47] Liz Kelly, 'Continuum of Sexual Violence,' in *Women, Violence and Social Control*, ed. J. Hanmer and M. Maynard (London: Macmillan Press Ltd, 1987), 46–60.

fifteen to seventeen-year-olds in the US. These estimated the likelihood of contact sexual abuse and sexual assault by age seventeen at 27 per cent for girls and five per cent for boys. The youth survey aimed to capture accurate data closer in time to the abusive incident(s) and hence understand the contemporary picture (rather than referring to non-recent abuse as was the case with the retrospective self-reported adult studies). Finklehor's surveys consistently indicated higher rates of lifetime abuse than other methods and found significantly higher rates than the UK NSPCC study. He argued that his methodology captured a more complete picture because levels of abuse rise sharply in the late teens especially for young women who are much more vulnerable as they approach eighteen. The surveys asked separate questions about 'a grown up you know' and 'a grown up you did not know,' about 'other kids' and about attempts to force sexual acts. While less than two per cent of the NSPCC's UK cohort reported contact sexual abuse by a parent or guardian, Finkelhor's data was six per cent for girls and one per cent for boys. However, again the data cannot be directly compared as the Finkelhor studies' category of family contact abuse included parents and carers, uncles, cousins and grandparents. At 66 per cent, the NSPCC study was starkly different in terms of juvenile abuse, Finkelhor recorded eighteen per cent for girls and three per cent for boys.[48]

Contentiously, Finkelhor and Lisa Jones have argued that there has been a large decline in sexual abuse in the US since the early 1990s. They cited quantitative data from child protective services (as measured by the National Child Abuse and Neglect Data System), self-reporting surveys and the National Incidence Study (NIS) of cases known to professionals. They judged their results to be 'about as well established as crime trends can be in contemporary social science.' Discounting the possibility that the figures could be lower due to decreases in funding for investigations or the exclusion of certain categories of victim or offender, they claimed that the NIS findings were reliable as they used identical criteria and standards at different points in time.[49] Although there is no consistent measure in the UK, indicators or proxy measures suggest the same trajectory for

[48] David Finkelhor et al, 'The Lifetime Prevalence of Child Sexual Abuse and Sexual Assault Assessed in Late Adolescence,' *Journal of Adolescent Health* 55, no 3 (2014): 329–333.

[49] David Finkelhor and Lisa Jones, 'Have Sexual Abuse and Physical Abuse Declined since the 1990s?,' (New Hampshire: Crimes against children research centre, 2012).

sexual abuse incidence, in that the cases reported to social services have dropped. However, in the same time period, reports to the police for sexual crimes against children have risen.[50] In one of the few recent books to advocate for a renewed effort to tackle child sexual abuse in the UK, feminist researcher Sarah Nelson was adamant that the decline in the numbers recorded did not represent a lower prevalence but a reduction in the level of protection afforded to children. On the international stage, for example, there is a proliferation of online (often sadistic) images of children being sexually abused. At the national level, there have been shifts in priorities and resources from child protection to family support.[51] Local authority budgets have been cut and although children's services spending is up, this relates to crisis spending on late intervention.[52]

Over the last fifty years, the data about child sexual abuse has been heavily contested. Why do these statistics matter and how do they relate to the work of community health professionals and to this study? The fact that it was not simple to measure the extent of sexual abuse as a 'social problem' and subsequently to monitor whether progress had been made in mitigating or reducing it made it a 'harder sell' than physical abuse to medics, who prided themselves on following a scientific route. Measuring progress in tackling sexual abuse as a public health problem could not be achieved in the way that medical officers or health visitors had in the past addressed infant mortality or tuberculosis. As Nigel Parton points out, there are complications in taking a public health approach. Identifying risk accurately is challenging. Epidemiological population studies identify relevant risk factors which are subsequently misapplied through being directed at community, familial or individual levels rather than population level. These inaccurately identify a high level of false positives (children said to be at high risk) and a 'small but significant number of false negatives (children who are at high risk but who are adjudged as safe).' The increased surveillance necessitated by a public

[50] Kelly and Karsna, 'Measuring the Scale and Changing Nature of Child Sexual Abuse and Child Sexual Exploitation - Scoping Report,' 19, 31–33.

[51] Liz Davies, 'Reforms have been imposed at the expense of protecting children,' *The Guardian*, 2 Dec 2008.

[52] Franklin, Jon, Jack Larkham, and Mariam Mansoor. 'The Well-Worn Path: Children's Services Spending 2010–11 to 2021–22.' London: Pro Bono Economics, 2023. https://media.actionforchildren.org.uk/documents/Childrens_Services_Spending_Report.pdf. Accessed 30 Sep 2024.

health approach reduces confidentiality and encroaches on civil liberties. Thus, it can deter families from seeking help or engaging with services.[53]

To some, the statistics indicated that the problem existed on a huge scale in US and UK society. To others, the methodological challenges in data collection and the conflation of different types of abuse into one overarching category of child sexual abuse seemed disingenuous at the least and deliberately misleading at the worst. The lack of 'trustworthy' data made it very difficult for a health visitor or community doctor to get a sense of how often they were likely to encounter a child who was being sexually abused within the family. It meant that practitioners lacked clear information about the characteristics of children that might have supported their practice. For example, health visitors rarely had access to data on age patterns in relation to sexual abuse specifically. This could lead to a misapprehension that babies and pre-school aged children were unlikely to be sexually abused and hence to a lower level of vigilance on their part. Disabled children were missing altogether from the statistics despite being more vulnerable to abuse.[54] Research found under-reporting of sexual abuse in some minority ethnic communities in proportion to population.[55]

Debates about the prevalence of child sexual abuse in the family have been displaced by the extent of child sexual abuse in institutions that has been exposed by survivors over the last decade. What we can say is that scholars have reached a consensus on certain matters. Firstly, child sexual abuse in the family occurs more frequently and to a greater degree that reports to child protective services would suggest. This means that many children's feeling that 'abuse and impunity flourish within cultures of silence' is supported by the data as is my argument that we need to take a hard look at those services that come into contact with children on a day-to-day basis—we cannot cast blame on social services for failing to help children outside of their orbit. Secondly, due to 'a strong cultural taboo' surrounding female-perpetrated child sexual abuse in the family, there may

[53] Nigel Parton, 'Changing and Competing Conceptions of Risk and Their Implications for Public Health Approaches to Child Protection,' in *Re-Visioning Public Health Approaches for Protecting Children*, ed. B. Lonne et al, Child Maltreatment (Switzerland: Springer Nature, 2019), 74–75.

[54] David Miller and Jon Brown, '"We Have the Right to Be Safe:" Protecting Disabled Children from Abuse' (London: NSPCC, 2014).

[55] Nelson, *Tackling Child Sexual Abuse: Radical Approaches to Prevention, Protection and Support*, 35–36.

be underreporting.[56] However, the vast majority of the abuse is perpetrated by men. It is mainly directed at girls, but also includes a significant proportion of boys. Therefore, the feminist analysis of rape and child sexual abuse as an abuse of male power and authority is still relevant. Thirdly, while unclear about the exact proportions, the data demonstrates that much of this abuse is perpetrated by young males aged under eighteen within the family context, especially by brothers.[57] Lastly, we can say that the lack of trust in the data has been a constant factor in the debates. However, arguments about incidence and prevalence form only part of the picture. Child sexual abuse has generated profound silences and ferocious controversies over the last half century and to begin to understand these, we have to revisit how the most recent discourses began.

## Origin Stories

The public's awareness of adults engaging children in sexual activity coalesces, breaks apart and is submerged repeatedly over time. Different aspects of the phenomena (physical abuse, emotional maltreatment, sexual abuse in various manifestations) surface in different periods. Some scholars have explained this ebb and flow in denial or recognition as caused by wider social issues, others cite the media or the influence of feminism in different historical periods. Some have taken an objectivist, empiricist or positivist stance, looking for verifiable 'facts' about abuse as a concrete phenomenon that we can come to 'know,' arguing about how it can be measured in terms of its extent and its impact and how we can draw robust conclusions about its wider meanings. Others have taken a social constructionist position, attempting to understand how and why claims about child sexual abuse are constructed and justified at different historical junctures. Another binary opposition in the literature is between empiricists

[56] A Gekoski, J C Davidson, and M A H Horvath, 'The Prevalence, Nature, and Impact of Intrafamilial Child Sexual Abuse: Findings from a Rapid Evidence Assessment,' *Journal of Criminological Research, Policy and Practice* 2, no 4 (2016). See Joanna Bourke on sexually violent women and motherhood: '[The concept of motherhood] was used both as proof that she could not have committed the sexual crimes (because she was … 'very nice, a mother hen') and proof that, if she had ordered the rapes and murders, she was particularly odious.' Joanna Bourke, *Disgrace: Global Reflections on Sexual Violence* (London: Reaktion Books, 2022).

[57] Gekoski, Davidson, and Horvath, 'The Prevalence, Nature, and Impact of Intrafamilial Child Sexual Abuse: Findings from a Rapid Evidence Assessment.'

and those more interested in a psychoanalytic understanding of child sexual abuse and its significance in society.

In seeking to understand why child sexual abuse came to such prominence on both sides of the Atlantic in the 1970s, a common 'origin story' in the literature cites its genesis in Denver, Colorado and its chief publicist as paediatrician Dr Henry C. Kempe. In 1961, Kempe provocatively attributed the name 'battered babies syndrome' to cases where babies had been physically injured by their parents.[58] In the late 1970s, he urged paediatricians to use their professional curiosity to unearth another hidden problem, namely, sexual abuse. Kempe noted that

> [t]he runaway who is simply asked 'Why did you run away?' will say, 'I had a fight with my folks.' The next question is 'What was your fight about?' The answer, 'I was out late.' Most professionals stop right there, but that's where we should all start ... One needs to lead up to the relationships with the child's mother and father, and then one finally has to ask some direct questions, in as kind a way as possible, in order to give the child permission to relate his/her loneliness, shame, and fears.[59]

An alternative 'awakening' is situated in a speech delivered by social worker and feminist Florence Rush to a conference on rape sponsored by the New York Radical Feminists in 1971.[60] Rush had been sexually assaulted as a child and she gave personal testimony along with a critical analysis of the various theories that had been expounded on sexual abuse up to that time. Her credibility was bolstered by her extensive direct experience in working with survivors of abuse. In different ways, Kempe and Rush were among the vanguard of those enabling a 'new' awareness of child sexual abuse in the US. However, as Richard Krugman (himself a protegé of Kempe) points out, the women's movement and rape crisis approach preceded the Kempe paper and were based on a different ethos. Feminists sought to ensure that the perpetrator was prosecuted and that his victims (daughters and mothers) were supported to build a safe and loving home without him. Kempe's goal was to ensure the child was in a

[58] C. Henry Kempe et al, 'The Battered-Child Syndrome,' *JAMA* 181, no 1 (1962).

[59] C. H. Kempe, 'Sexual Abuse, Another Hidden Pediatric Problem: The 1977 C. Anderson Aldrich Lecture,' *Pediatrics* 62, no 3 (1978).

[60] See for example, Joseph E. Davis, *Accounts of Innocence: Sexual Abuse, Trauma, and the Self* (Chicago, London: University of Chicago Press, 2004), 26–27; Jenkins, *Moral Panic: Changing Concepts of the Child Molester in Modern America*, 127.

place of safety before providing a therapeutic intervention that could rehabilitate the family.[61] Both approaches would influence feminists, paediatricians and psychiatrists in the UK to push for greater child protection intervention over the ensuing decade.

We can see the link between feminist activism on adult rape and child sexual abuse in Susan Brownmiller's foundational text *Against Our Will: Men, Women and Rape*. In fact, Brownmiller relied on Rush for much of the material she presented about incest. Referencing a range of studies to describe the characteristics of 'father rapists,' she analysed what was known about the prevalence and effects of incest. Brownmiller was not a victim-survivor of child sexual abuse but she humanised the child victim and the non-abusing mother through her use of primary sources, most memorably an extensive excerpt from African American author and activist Maya Angelou's autobiography *I Know Why the Caged Bird Sings*. In it, Angelou described not only how her mother's boyfriend repeatedly sexually assaulted her but also its aftermath—the court case, his murder and the feelings of guilt which led her to become an elective mute.[62]

When Rush's *The Best Kept Secret* was published in 1980, it was prefaced by a personal recounting of a sexual assault by her family dentist and her family's refusal to accept that it had happened. She contrasted her family's resistance to the 'respectable' dentist's culpability with her father's overreaction when she told him a shop clerk was paying her friendly attention. It was clear that the perpetrator's respectability and social standing had a large part to play in whether children were to be believed. Rush's book comprised an episodic history of sexual abuse (the Christians, the Greeks and the Victorians) alongside a sociological dissection of the structural and social contortions required to keep child molestation concealed (in political systems, legislation and popular culture).[63] By the late 1970s, women publicly testifying to childhood molestation had become a trope. One could almost forget that until Rush told the story of her own abuse

[61] Richard D. Krugman, 'Chapter 20 Introduction and Commentary: Child Sexual Abuse,' in *C. Henry Kempe: A 50 Year Legacy to the Field of Child Abuse and Neglect*, ed. Richard D. Krugman and Jill E. Korbin (Netherlands: Springer, 2013).

[62] Susan Brownmiller, *Against Our Will: Men, Women, and Rape* (New York: Bantam, 1975), 271–280.

[63] Florence Rush, 'The Sexual Abuse of Children: A Feminist Point of View,' in *Rape: The First Sourcebook for Women*, ed. Noreen Connell and Cassandra Wilson (New York: New American Library, 1974); 'The Freudian Cover-Up,' *Chrysalis* (1977); *The Best Kept Secret: Sexual Abuse of Children* (New York: McGraw-Hill, 1980).

at the 1971 conference, 'no socially recognized story of victimization existed that would warrant such a public telling or provide the terms in which to do so.' Clinical accounts of individual experiences had been recorded by psychiatrists and the victim experience had been surveyed, but first-person narrations did not exist. The notion of telling a personal story in public had been revolutionary at the beginning of the decade.[64]

It was not surprising that women were speaking out publicly about childhood abuse. The disbelief that they encountered from their families in childhood was routinely echoed in the consulting rooms of the psychoanalysts they visited in adulthood. Therapists were trained to classify disclosures as fantasies. One of Rush's lengthiest chapters exposed what she dubbed the 'Freudian cover-up.' Sigmund Freud had treated women exhibiting what the Victorians called 'hysteria,' a category encompassing a range of physical symptoms with no discernible organic cause. Freud listened to his patients' traumatic memories of childhood sexual assault and concluded they were causal factors in their adult neuroses. In 1896 he outlined his thoughts in a paper called 'On the Aetiology of Hysteria' to the Society for Psychiatry and Neurology in Vienna. Freud's feelings about his father led him, according to Rush, to ultimately reject the idea of the father as 'seducer.' He decided that these stories of fathers were 'defensive fictions' and arrived instead at the Oedipus complex. She noted that Freud's seduction theory which 'incriminated incestuous fathers' emerged from the experiences of the women who spoke to him. The Oedipal theory which 'insisted that seduction was a fantasy, an invention, not a fact' came not from his clinical practice with a range of patients but from his own memories, dreams and experiences, marked as they were by his individual personality, gender and class. Thus, he denied the 'reality of female sexual abuse' which he instead 'projected into a universal infantile-parental hostility.' Rush accused him of 'gaslighting' not only the individual female patients who were made to doubt the reliability of their own memories, but 'gaslighting an age into ignoring a devastating childhood reality and a very serious social problem.'[65]

In 1984, Jeffrey Masson alleged that for complicated personal reasons, Freud suppressed his earlier understanding that 'a sexual seduction was a real sexual act forced on a young child who in no way desired it or encouraged it.' This precipitated a bitter controversy amongst psychoanalysts and

[64] Davis, *Accounts of Innocence: Sexual Abuse, Trauma, and the Self*, 27–28.

[65] Rush, *The Best Kept Secret: Sexual Abuse of Children.*

historians that went beyond academic journals to the mainstream press. Criticisms of Masson ranged from the intellectual (he did not understand the history of psychoanalysis) to the factual (his claims that Freud was ostracised by his peers for years after his 1896 talk were false). Masson saw himself as standing alongside American feminists like Rush, Louise Armstrong and Diana Russell to expose the extent of child sexual abuse and the further harm inflicted on individuals by their therapists. He concluded that analysts trained in the Freudian tradition were predisposed to believe that their patients' memories of abuse were fantasies. Therefore 'no matter how benevolent' they were in other ways, their practice did 'violence to the [patient's] inner life' and was in 'covert collusion with what made her ill in the first place.'[66] Janice Haaken agreed that Freud's retreat was influenced by social convention but noted that he also came to see 'unconscious fantasy' as important in 'reworking' childhood memories. He thought that hysterical illness was a 'disguised enactment of unbearable conflict,' and that the onset of adult sexuality brought with it an awareness of moral judgments and created retroactive trauma. Steven Angelides challenged the Rush/Masson interpretation which, he argued, 'simplifies and misrepresents the psychoanalytical notion of trauma by attempting to impute a traumatic essence to a single sexual act' (that is, a sexual assault).[67]

Feminists are credited with exposing child sexual abuse and its concomitant harm in the 1970s and for advocating for stronger action against perpetrators and more appropriate assistance for their victims. Paediatricians and psychiatrists were also influential but set out with the distinct goal of rehabilitating the family. It is significant that even though rape crisis centres raised the profile of child sexual abuse because mothers spoke to them about their daughters, the public testimony from survivors was not that of children but of adult women remembering childhood violation. This association of policies to eradicate child sexual abuse with feminism rather than with medics and with adult women survivors rather than children would play a part in the conflict about the phenomenon that would emerge in the late 1980s.

[66] Jeffrey M. Masson, *The Assault on Truth: Freud's Suppression of the Seduction Theory* (London: Faber, 1984); 'Freud and the Seduction Theory: A Challenge to the Foundations of Psychoanalysis,' *The Atlantic*, February 1984.

[67] Janice Haaken, *Pillar of Salt: Gender, Memory, and the Perils of Looking Back* (London: Free Association, 1998), 64; Steven Angelides, *The Fear of Child Sexuality: Young People, Sex, and Agency* (Chicago: The University of Chicago Press, 2019), 62.

## Waves of Awareness

Historians have established that child sexual abuse was not 'discovered' in the 1970s with the arrival of second-wave feminism.[68] George Behlmer, Harry Ferguson, Carol-Ann Hooper, Louise Jackson, Stephen Robertson, Linda Gordon and Lucy Delap have each in different ways exposed earlier waves of awareness. In fact, as sociologist Carol Smart reminds us, the 'idea that adult-child sexual contact existed in an objective fashion but that it was systematically ignored or covered up' is not conducive to a better understanding of its history. She suggests that it is more productive to see it as 'a discursive conflict going on in which some actors attempted to give prominence to the view that adult-child sexual contact was extremely harmful to the child (morally, physically and psychologically), destructive of childhood, and highly damaging to society as a whole.'[69]

Changing ideas about 'the child' were also important. In his history of working-class New Yorkers engaged with the criminal courts in relation to sexual violence against children, Stephen Robertson describes the clashing views on children's nature espoused in the late nineteenth century. On one hand, they were seen as 'creatures of primitive vitality and imagination, who needed to be able to pursue their instincts free of adult interference,' while on the other, they were 'impressionable creatures' with developing bodies who required parental control. Robertson argues that a combination of these opposing images was applied to prepubescent children and adolescent boys up until the 1930s. Attitudes to working-class teenage girls were more complex. Reformers attempted to define them as

[68] George Behlmer, *Child Abuse and Moral Reform in England, 1870–1908* (Stanford, Ca: Stanford University Press, 1982); Harry Ferguson, 'Protecting Children in Time: A Historical Sociological Study of the Abused Child and Child Protection in Cleveland from 1880 to the 'Cleveland Affair' of 1987,' (University of Cambridge, 1992); Carol-Ann Hooper, 'Child Sexual Abuse and the Regulation of Women: Variations on a Theme,' in *Gender Violence: Interdisciplinary Perspectives*, ed. Laura L. O'Toole, Jessica R. Schiffman, and Marge L. Kiter Edwards (New York: New York University Press, 2007); Louise A. Jackson, *Child Sexual Abuse in Victorian England* (London: Routledge, 2000); Stephen Robertson, *Crimes against Children: Sexual Violence and Legal Culture in New York City, 1880–1960* (Chapel Hill, NC: University of North Carolina Press, 2005); Lucy Delap, '"Disgusting Details Which Are Best Forgotten:" Disclosures of Child Sexual Abuse in Twentieth-Century Britain,' *Journal of British Studies* 57, no 1 (2018); Linda Gordon, *Heroes of Their Own Lives: The Politics and History of Family Violence Boston, 1880–1960* (London: Virago, 1989).

[69] Carol Smart, 'A History of Ambivalence and Conflict in the Discursive Construction of the "Child Victim" of Sexual Abuse,' *Social & Legal Studies* 8, no 3 (1999): 393.

'simply children' but they could not interpret their behaviour as 'innocent' and jurors, prosecutors and their own families did not treat them in the same way as younger children.[70]

Gordon's extensive research in the casefiles of Boston child protection agencies covers the period from the late nineteenth century up to the 1960s. She discovers a shift in the interpretation of abuse by the 1920s when it was redefined as an act that occurred outside the home and was perpetrated by a stranger.[71] Erna Olafson, David Corwin and Roland Summit note that the child molester was now portrayed as 'radically different from other men, pathological, and properly the province of the treating professionals.'[72] This was accompanied by a reclassification of the victim. No longer an 'innocent betrayed,' she was now considered 'a sex delinquent.' Fears of feminism, Bolshevism and unfettered sexuality were at a peak after the first World War and reformers attempted to bolster the authority of the father. The 'carnal abuse' of fathers faded from public discourse, to be replaced by the 'moral neglect' of mothers. Their unsupervised daughters lost their innocence and were subsequently labelled as juvenile sex delinquents.[73]

Robertson claims that by the 1920s, New York reformers searched for a theoretical framework that could help them to devise a new strategy in relation to teenage girls. They reached for psychologist G. Stanley Hall's book *Adolescence* (1904). Hall's delineation of adolescence as a new period of development in which girls were physiologically developed and yet psychologically immature could be used as the rationale to protect their morality through girls' clubs, bolster parental authority and protect the age of consent. For sexuality was 'a deep unconscious instrument that the child would not understand, and that needed to be sublimated in order for an individual to successfully attain adulthood.'[74]

[70] Robertson, *Crimes against Children: Sexual Violence and Legal Culture in New York City, 1880–1960*, 7–8.

[71] Linda Gordon, 'The Politics of Child Sexual Abuse: Notes from American History,' *Feminist Review*, 28, no 1 (1988): 57–60.

[72] Erna Olafson, David L. Corwin, and Roland C. Summit, 'Modern History of Child Sexual Abuse Awareness: Cycles of Discovery and Suppression,' *Child Abuse & Neglect* 17, no 1 (1993): 13.

[73] Gordon, 'The Politics of Child Sexual Abuse: Notes from American History,' 57–60.

[74] Robertson, *Crimes against Children: Sexual Violence and Legal Culture in New York City, 1880–1960*, 119, 133–134.

Harry Hendrick argues that historically the rhetoric of concern about abused children 'as subjects' is dubious and that in fact children are treated 'merely as objects in the struggles and ambitions of professions, and as figures in expressions of ideological and cultural value systems.'[75] Historian of childhood Stephen Mintz concurs and sees concern about child sexual abuse increasing across society when women enter the workforce and specific groups lobby to 'bring a pressing problem to public light.' Thus, in the US, the fast-paced urbanisation and rising immigration in the period just after the Civil War led to anxiety and activism on the issue of child sexual abuse from the 1880s.[76] As the era of Progressive reform commenced in earnest in the 1890s, a wide range of activists pushed for government intervention to alleviate the ills ushered in by industrial capitalism. Their concerns were broad and included child labour, temperance, divorce, sexual immorality, prostitution, the family and juvenile delinquency. Historians dispute their motivations. According to Daniel T. Rodgers, Progressives revolted against ideas of the 'autonomous man,' with his 'individualistic excesses,' preferring a rhetoric of social cohesion. This drove them to take an avid interest in 'the discovery of new forms of social sinning and corresponding new measures of social control, and a vivid, nervous concern with social cohesion.'[77] Similarly, the foundation of the National Society for the Prevention of Cruelty to Children (NSPCC) in London in 1884 instituted a central nationalised network of inspectors visiting families at home. According to historian Harry Ferguson, it became in effect a systematic surveillance mechanism to regulate families' morality and behaviour.[78]

Although Linda Gordon characterises the attitudes of upper-class female 'child-savers' of the late nineteenth century in the US as a 'mixture of prudish, feminist, anti-immigrant and anti-pauper,' they did recognise incest as common 'quintessentially male crimes against girls.' The increasingly professionalised social workers of the 1920s and 1930s tended to

[75] Harry D. Hendrick, *Child Welfare: England: 1872–1989* (London: Routledge, 1994), 242.

[76] Steven Mintz, 'Placing Childhood Sexual Abuse in Historical Perspective,' https://tif.ssrc.org/2012/07/13/placing-childhood-sexual-abuse-in-historical-perspective/. Accessed 24 Sep 2024.

[77] Daniel T. Rodgers, 'In Search of Progressivism,' *Reviews in American History* 10, no 4 (1982): 124–125.

[78] Harry Ferguson, *Protecting Children in Time: Child Abuse, Child Protection and the Consequences of Modernity* (Hampshire: Palgrave Macmillan, 2004), 36.

blame mothers and daughters to a much greater extent.[79] Regina Kunzel demonstrates that female social workers jostled for professional power through adopting a scientific language which pathologised young unmarried pregnant women. Where the charity workers had depicted them as 'fallen women' who could potentially be saved, the social workers saw them as potentially irretrievably 'feeble minded' or 'sexually delinquent.'[80]

At the end of the nineteenth century, feminists, churchmen and sex reformers on both sides of the Atlantic grouped together to campaign against incest on the basis that it cut across all social classes. Most historians argue that prejudicial ideas about the working class, immigrants and people of colour made it much easier to acknowledge what Gordon dubs 'problems unmentionable by standards of Victorian propriety.' In her Boston research, incest could be acknowledged by the 'child-savers' because it was a problem safely sequestered in the overcrowded homes of the Catholic immigrant poor. Most Victorian writing about incest associated it with poverty, the foreign-born and the sexually promiscuous.[81] Lynn Sacco explores the high prevalence of vaginal gonorrhoea infection in young girls in the late nineteenth century US which physicians found 'unspeakable.' She particularly attributes their denial to class and racial biases—they could not accept the implications when they found infection not only in the vaginas of poor, immigrant and African-American girls but also in those of middle-class white girls. Their prevalence could not be acknowledged as it would destroy the myth that incest was a working-class phenomenon.[82] Roger Davidson examines the 'pernicious delusion' described by medical 'experts' testifying in child abuse prosecutions in the Scottish courts in the early twentieth century that sex with a virgin could cure a sexually transmitted disease. This belief was not generally expressed directly by the Scottish working-class men on trial but instead served as a

[79] Gordon, *Heroes of Their Own Lives: The Politics and History of Family Violence Boston, 1880–1960*, 215–222.

[80] Regina G. Kunzel, *Fallen Women, Problem Girls: Unmarried Mothers and the Professionalization of Social Work, 1890–1945*, Yale Historical Publications (New Haven: Yale University Press, 1993), 52–54.

[81] Gordon, 'The Politics of Child Sexual Abuse: Notes from American History,' 56; Olafson, Corwin, and Summit, 'Modern History of Child Sexual Abuse Awareness: Cycles of Discovery and Suppression,' 8–9.

[82] Sacco, *Unspeakable: Father-Daughter Incest in American History.*

sort of insulation to the medics, protecting them from admitting the extent of incest within their society.[83]

Psychiatry, sexology and other secular professions formed alongside a wave of controversy about women, families and sexuality in Europe and America in the late nineteenth century. On the one hand, there were 'feminist fictional utopias,' on the other there were depictions of a brutish and sexually aggressive masculinity. The controversy discussed above in relation to Freud's retraction of his seduction theory can be better understood in the context of a psychiatric discourse that trivialised what female patients said to their analysts. It was not only the professionalising field of female social workers who discredited the feminists, reformers and religious men, but also the expanding psychiatric professions who depicted them as 'man-hating, frigid, and possibly lesbian "prudes" who threatened to "desex" society.'[84] Rather than redefining sexuality in a way that responded to feminist demands for respectful sexual behaviours, modernism brought a new aggressive notion of masculine entitlement.[85]

Under the banner of sexual freedom and 'modern' attitudes, psychoanalysts wondered whether children might in fact seek out sex with adults. Lauretta Bender and Abram Blau wrote in 1937 that 'frequently we considered the possibility that the child might have been the actual seducer rather than the one innocently seduced.' Remarking that children's sexual experiences with adults appeared to incur minimal negative effects, they nevertheless criticised mothers for negligence in failing to protect their children.[86] There is a strain of thought here that Rush would describe in her invocation of 'the demon nymphette' and James R. Kincaid explores

[83] Roger Davidson, '"This Pernicious Delusion:" Law, Medicine, and Child Sexual Abuse in Early Twentieth-Century Scotland,' *Journal of the History of Sexuality* 10, no 1 (2001); Jackson found similar tendencies in eighteenth century England. The class of the victim and defendant was important in a criminal trial. Jackson showed that despite stereotypes the poor were not 'desensitised to morality,' but that within the criminal justice system, the likelihood of a conviction depended on the social class, reputation and status of both the defendant and the victim. Jackson, *Child Sexual Abuse in Victorian England*, 6–8.

[84] Olafson, Corwin, and Summit, 'Modern History of Child Sexual Abuse Awareness: Cycles of Discovery and Suppression,' 12–13.

[85] Sheila Jeffreys, *The Spinster and Her Enemies: Feminism and Sexuality, 1880–1930* (London: Pandora Press, 1985), 14.

[86] Lauretta Bender and Abram Blau, 'The Reaction of Children to Sexual Relations with Adults,' *American Journal of Orthopsychiatry* 7, no 4 (1937): 514, 511.

in detail in his study of the 'erotic' or 'carnal' child.[87] As Corry Azzopardi, Ramona Alaggia and Barbara Fallon show, the shift of culpability from abusing father to non-abusing mother continued with early 'family systems' thinking which broadened 'the circle of blame' to all members of the family unit. Therapists believed that when the mother failed to meet her husband's sexual needs and renounced her wifely duties, her daughter stepped into the role.[88] Mothers were understood as consciously or unconsciously colluding with the incestuous relationship. Attachment theory originating from Bowlby and Ainsworth also included an element of mother- and child-blaming explanations for the causes and effects of child sexual abuse. The different types of attachment difficulties were each considered to create additional risks. An insecure attachment increased the risk that a child would be victimised and might result in the abuse continuing over time, and influence its impact. This was because the non-abusive avoidant attachment mother might be less emotionally available to her child and the child, feeling unloved, might be less able to protect themselves. Mothers with a resistant attachment might be less attuned to their child's needs and their children might be more vulnerable to the abuser's grooming. Mothers with disorganised attachments might be too enmeshed in their own historical trauma or chaotic lifestyle to see that the abuse was occurring and equally their children might see the abuser as representing security in a life of chaos.[89]

Azzopardi and her colleagues acknowledge feminist analyses that show how gendered power imbalances perpetuates male entitlement and male violence in all forms against women and children. They see that the idea of the 'all-knowing, all-sacrificing, and all-powerful mother, who instinctually ought to know when sexual abuse is occurring and ought to be able to stop it, permeates institutional practices, policies, and attitudes.' This is despite empirical research that demonstrates that most mothers are protective of their children and increasing evidence of the 'unrelenting grooming strategies' abusers use to build trust and gain access to children. Critiques of a 'grand feminist narrative' of male privilege underestimate

[87] James R. Kincaid, *Erotic Innocence: The Culture of Child Molesting* (Durham: Duke University Press, 1998).

[88] Corry Azzopardi, Ramona Alaggia, and Barbara Fallon, 'From Freud to Feminism: Gendered Constructions of Blame across Theories of Child Sexual Abuse,' *Journal of Child Sexual Abuse* 27, no 3 (2018): 257–260.

[89] 'From Freud to Feminism: Gendered Constructions of Blame across Theories of Child Sexual Abuse,' 257–260.

individual pathology and agency, fail to explain why only a small number of men sexually offend and refuse to engage with (albeit the very small proportion of) female sexual abusers. They optimistically offer up ecological theory as a more useful lens for viewing sexual abuse as it integrates the individual, family, community and wider society in its analysis. The emphasis is no longer heavily weighted towards mothers' responsibilities but spread across the ecosystem and best understood as a way of weighing risks against protective factors.[90]

Writing in the late 1990s, Jenkins made the forceful claim that in the US feminist influence was so strong in lobbying for child protection from the mid-1970s that it led to 'a perception that all American children were sexually at risk.' Jenkins avowed that he was reluctant to discount as 'groundless panic' the testimony of millions of Americans who said they were victims of sexual assault. Yet his language suggests that he believed it was an unsubstantiated 'panic' stemming from feminist hyperbole. He described the writings of Florence Rush, Diana Russell, Ann Burgess, Judith Herman and other feminists as arriving in a 'cascade' from 1977 and reaching 'flood proportions' by 1984. As noted above, Jenkins was critical of the statistics they wielded, depicting them as 'ambitious,' 'embellished,' 'remarkable' and after 1974, 'swelled' by mandatory reporting.[91] His phraseology supported his overarching thesis of 'moral panic' and undermined the legitimacy of feminist activism. Even as he accepted that child sexual abuse was prevalent, his language implied otherwise. 'Panic' implies an irrational reaction to a sudden crisis. Jenkins used words such as 'flood' and 'epidemic' to imply a 'suddenness' in the emergence of the problem which compromises its credibility. Other critics agreed that some of the statistics he challenged were inflated but he failed to set those in their proper context of some degree of scholarly consensus about the scale of child sexual abuse as set out above.

Jenkins saw the feminist movement as immensely successful in infiltrating popular culture where depictions of incest, child murders and abductions became commonplace and self-help literature proliferated. This opinion was supported by Adrian Bingham's research on the media in the UK. He demonstrated that journalists from the 1970s portrayed sexual abuse in a new way—as a specific harm—and this change was influenced

[90] Ibid., 60–264.

[91] Jenkins, *Moral Panic: Changing Concepts of the Child Molester in Modern America*, 118–120.

by the ideas and language of social work and feminism.[92] According to Jenkins, the feminist movement was 'authentically revolutionary' in transforming attitudes. It replaced the myth that sexual abuse was perpetrated by pathological 'sex psychopaths' and exposed instead 'quite ordinary men' who molested (their own) children whilst societal attitudes to male sexuality shielded them from censure.[93] As Brownmiller had put it in 1975, the men who raped their daughters were not a 'subspecies of brute monster,' but rather there was 'nothing at all special' about them. Paul Gebhard's researchers at the Institute for Sex Research founded by Kinsey claimed they were actually 'conservative, moralistic, restrained and religiously devout.'[94] Ultimately, Jenkins claimed that feminists succeeded in embedding their views about child abuse 'as a component of social orthodoxy.' He argued that their success came in part from alliances with social welfare organisations and moral conservatives. Thus, the figure of the 'helpless child' was ultimately projected to the wider society to campaign not only against child sexual abuse, but against any sexual activity that threatened the narrow orthodoxy of traditional marriage (such as homosexuality, pornography and sex education).[95]

In a similar vein, Angelides saw the 1980s as 'a sex panic of epic proportions.' He criticised 'radical feminists' for stifling debate about children's sexual agency and ultimately desexualising childhood.[96] He objected to concepts of child sexuality which characterised it as immature play or experimentation on the path to a mature adult sexual expression. Furthermore, because 'many children firmly believe in their own power and control in sexual encounters with adults,' feminist practitioners who tried to convince a child that the sexual abuse is not their fault may,

[92] Bingham see continuities in reporting styles from prior decades that perpetuated suspicions of female sexuality and shifted responsibility onto victims to protect themselves from assault. There was an ongoing concentration on individual 'sex beasts' which minimised discussion of the wider structural power imbalances. Adrian Bingham, '"It Would Be Better for the Newspapers to Call a Spade a Spade": The British Press and Child Sexual Abuse, C. 1918–90,' *History Workshop Journal* 88 (2019): 102–106.

[93] Jenkins, *Moral Panic: Changing Concepts of the Child Molester in Modern America*, 120–121.

[94] Brownmiller, *Against Our Will: Men, Women, and Rape*, 280–281.

[95] Jenkins, *Moral Panic: Changing Concepts of the Child Molester in Modern America*, 120–121.

[96] Note that Angelides includes a broad range of child protection practitioners including sociologists, psychologists and social workers under the banner of radical feminism. Angelides, *The Fear of Child Sexuality: Young People, Sex, and Agency.*

according to Angelides, harm the child by causing shame and guilt about an act they may feel they have participated in by choice. Arguing that adults or children who are 'purportedly in submission' can actually exercise power to 'varying degrees' unless they are in a state of complete bondage, Angelides deplored what he saw as a blanket denial of the sexuality of a child who at the cusp of adulthood did not jump from 'a position of powerlessness to one of (adult) power, or from a position of sexual ignorance to a position of sexual knowledge.'[97]

Historicising and theorising responses to child sexual abuse have not been the sole preserve of historians. In fact, due to the difficult ethical restrictions relating to research about children (to which I will return), much of what has been written about the phenomena in the twentieth century has been generated by medical doctors and psychiatrists, sociologists, social workers, cultural theorists and media scholars. Although there has been common ground across disciplines, it has been a contested and heavily politicised field of scholarship. Whenever the high prevalence of childhood sexual abuse and its impact on children's wellbeing are debated, a strong reaction ensues.

## The Backlash

Stories about false allegations of child sexual abuse emerged in the US as early as the mid-1980s. In *The Battle and the Backlash*, journalist David Hechler reprinted a full page advertisement by 'the friends of the McMartin pre-school defendants.' Enormous headlines compared the prosecution of eight people accused of child abuse in Manhattan Beach, California, in 1985 to the 'innocent lives lost or ruined because of the false accusations of the infamous Salem witch hunts' of the seventeenth century. Warning readers not to be complacent and think that this sort of thing could not happen in America, the advertisers stated: 'It could happen to you. All it takes is for someone to point a finger.'[98] The backlash was played out in the courts where defence lawyers questioned the reliability of children's testimony in criminal cases, care and divorce proceedings. Journalists asked whether children were coached by over-zealous professionals or

[97] *The Fear of Child Sexuality: Young People, Sex, and Agency*, 52–56.

[98] David Hechler, *The Battle and the Backlash: The Child Sexual Abuse War* (Lexington, Mass.: Lexington Books, 1988).

mothers in custody disputes attempting to deprive fathers of the right to see their children.[99]

Adult women survivors claimed to remember long-buried details of childhood sexual assault during therapy. Their accounts formed part of canonical feminist texts such as Judith Herman's *Father Daughter Incest* (1981) and self-help guides such as Ellen Bass and Laura Davis's *The Courage to Heal* (1988), which emphasised the seriousness of sexual abuse as a social issue.[100] But by the mid-1990s, adult survivors' credibility was under attack. Articles appeared in newspapers and magazines about 'false memories.' Some were sponsored by the False Memory Syndrome Foundation, an organisation founded in 1992 by parents who claimed to be falsely accused by their adult children. Psychologists joined with journalists to write full-length studies cautioning against the 'science' of repressed memories.[101] Two major studies appeared in 1994: one led by Elizabeth Loftus, the other by Richard Ofshe. Both had testified for the defence of alleged abusers in the courts. Neither denied that sexual abuse occurred and could be suppressed, but they emphasised the 'labile' and 'dynamic' nature of human memories. A 'historic truth' existed but it was accompanied by a 'narrative truth' of the memory as it was retold. *The New York Times* hailed their critiques as a 'frightening indictment' of the practices of at least some members of the 'burgeoning therapy industry' which had a 'heads-I-win and tails-you-lose approach to moral rectitude' and strong 'capacities for self-delusion.'[102]

While agreeing that some of these 'retrieved' memories of abuse are untrue, historian Janet Walker believes that 'the breadth and vehemence of their denial' do not arise solely from an antifeminist backlash. They also indicate an 'unproductive rejection of any possible relationship between fantasy and historical truth.' Although she understands why the deconstructionist approaches of Hayden White, Michel Foucault and others may be questioned in the face of widespread denial, she cautions against

[99] Louise Armstrong, *Rocking the Cradle of Sexual Politics: What Happened When Women Said Incest* (London: Women's Press, 1996), 115–200.

[100] Judith Lewis Herman and Lisa Hirschman, *Father-Daughter Incest* (Cambridge, Mass: Harvard University Press, 1981); Bass and Davis, *The Courage to Heal*.

[101] Elizabeth F. Loftus and Katherine Ketcham, *The Myth of Repressed Memory: False Memories and Allegations of Sexual Abuse* (New York: St. Martin's Press, 1994); R. Ofshe and E. Watters, *Making Monsters: False Memories, Psychotherapy, and Sexual Hysteria* (New York: Charles Scribner, 1994).

[102] Steven Rose, 'Two types of truth.' *The New York Times*, 26 Feb 1995, Section 7, 20.

turning wholesale to empirical historical studies to prove 'beyond a doubt that incest was and is an abuse of epidemic proportions.' Instead she argues that 'external trauma' can modify remembered details that cultural conventions invalidate in determinations of truth. She cites as an example a Holocaust survivor who was an eyewitness to the Auschwitz uprising. The woman recalled four chimneys blowing up when in fact only one had exploded. The misremembered details caused some historians to doubt her veracity, but Walker argues that her testimony articulated an historical truth. The memory though exaggerated preserved the 'true import' of the event.[103] Haaken agrees that 'recovered' memories may not be a literal recounting of the truth but can represent the emotional reality of women's experiences.[104]

## Reflections on the Literature

This overview of the literature began with two 1970s origin stories. Kempe defined sexual abuse as a medical problem involving a sick caregiver. The aim was to make the child safe, heal the perpetrator and rehabilitate the family. The feminist origins story looked very different; Rush and other key feminists told of their personal experiences of child sexual abuse. They sought to ensure perpetrators were prosecuted and women helped each other. When they sought therapeutic support, it was empathetic and humanistic in contrast to what they perceived as an incredulous and detached style of psychoanalysis that had developed after Freud. Personal testimonies of childhood rape and sexual assault came as a reaction not just to a blanket silence about sexual violence, but as a response to the fact that women's voices had been suppressed in society more generally. Conscious of the old stereotypes of women's emotionality and irrationality, feminists cited research and statistics to support their activism. Looked at retrospectively, those statistics were exaggerated in some cases but there was not a clear body of research about prevalence in the 1970s and 1980s.

Most of the recent historiography focuses on child sexual abuse as a discursive conflict and a circular narrative of 'discovery.' The 1970s was not the first decade in which the phenomena were exposed. Changing ideas about the nature of the child can be traced alongside shifting

[103] Janet Walker, 'The Traumatic Paradox: Documentary Films, Historical Fictions, and Catacylismic Past Events,' *Signs* 22, no 4 (1997): 805–808.

[104] Haaken, *Pillar of Salt: Gender, Memory, and the Perils of Looking Back.*

attitudes to incest and other forms of sexual abuse. Was the child innocent and creative? Should they be free to explore the world and their sexuality? Or impressionable, vulnerable and requiring close surveillance? Were they innocents or delinquents? Or were they merely objects onto whom professionals and the wider culture could project whatever image suited their own needs? Class, race and poverty played a part in what professionals and the public 'saw' when their gaze fell upon a child and their family. Medics and other 'child-savers' of the late nineteenth and early twentieth century could acknowledge the physical signs of child abuse only when they were sited in poor, immigrant or Black families. Middle-class deviance was denied. As social work and psychiatry professionalised in the first part of the twentieth century, they silenced not only the voices of girls and women patients but also the voices of those earlier feminists, churchmen and reformers who had argued that incest could be found at all societal levels.

Sexual modernism brought an aggressive male sexuality and less societal concern about incest.[105] Where it was identified, mothers' apparent failure to protect their daughters was deplored. This trend rose in the course of the twentieth century and can be seen in early family systems theory and to a certain degree in attachment theory as well. As I will explore in Chap. 4, these modes of thinking are remarkably persistent in professional formulations of family 'problems' and in the challenges practitioners face in their day-to-day work in health and childcare settings.

To varying degrees, Jenkins, Angelides and others are critical of feminist activism since the 1970s which they see as creating the figure of the 'helpless' child and involuntarily creating a space for moral conservatives to lobby against any 'unorthodox' sexuality. Angelides takes this further and blames feminists for stifling discourse on child sexuality. Indeed, scepticism about various aspects of child sexual abuse has tended to focus on adult women and feminists: whether they are survivors who allegedly recover false memories, therapists who use unprofessional methods and apparently make vast profits, wives in custody disputes, doctors who are too ready to see physical symptoms as signs of assault or child protection professionals whose methods for interviewing children encourage false disclosures. Psychologists such as Loftus have exposed the risks in

[105] In sexual modernism, sexuality is characterised as a 'powerful, continuous, compulsive and irrestible force in human life, which is dangerous as well as wholesome, and with which everybody has to come to terms.' Harry Oosterhuis, 'Sexual Modernity in the Works of Richard Von Krafft-Ebing and Albert Moll,' *Medical History* 56, no 2 (2012).

uncritically accepting adult memories of childhood trauma. Others like Haaken have tried to complicate simplistic notions of a truth/fiction dichotomy by exploring more sensitively the role of fantasy in this conflictual discourse.

These writings form the backdrop to the practice of community nurses, doctors and therapists in the UK and the themes outlined above will resurface in the narratives that unfold from the archives and from their own memories of the past decades of their practice. Before I outline the structure of my exploration of their changing thoughts, emotions and actions, I set out a brief explanation of the terminology and methodologies I employ.

## Terminology

Delap outlines how, prior to the 1980s, various individuals and groups in the UK were concerned about sexual acts involving children and sometimes referred to them as abusive. However, they used a range of terms including 'molesting, tampering, flashing, fondling, and ill-usage.' It was not until the late 1980s that the concept of 'child sexual abuse' became a stable category.[106] As Bingham explains, it is a concept that is 'discursively constructed in relation to changing understandings of gender, sexuality and age, and with references to different legal regimes.'[107] In the US, it came to be understood in a particular way a little earlier when by the end of the 1970s it became associated with 'connotations of betrayal of trust, hidden trauma, and denial.'[108] The term certainly implied greater harm than sexual assault per se as it connoted an adult in a position of trust corrupting their position of power and the duty of care to the child, as well as abusing their physical body.

'Child sexual abuse' is considered to encompass a broad range of sexual acts perpetrated by adults upon children including contact and non-contact forms as defined above. This study focuses on child sexual abuse in the family setting. In the late 1960s when this study begins, this was generally referred to as 'incest' and this term lingered into the 1980s. It

[106] Delap, '"Disgusting Details Which Are Best Forgotten:" Disclosures of Child Sexual Abuse in Twentieth-Century Britain,' 81.

[107] Bingham, '"It Would Be Better for the Newspapers to Call a Spade a Spade": The British Press and Child Sexual Abuse, C. 1918–90,' 90.

[108] Jenkins, *Moral Panic: Changing Concepts of the Child Molester in Modern America*, xi.

usually referred to those who were biologically and directly related to the child, although it was increasingly extended to sexual assault by other close family members such as stepfathers as societal norms about marriage and divorce began to shift in the 1970s.

I have chosen to refer to sexual abuse in the family environment following the UK Children's Commissioner definition:

> sexual abuse perpetrated or facilitated in or out of the home, against a child under the age of 18, by a family member, or someone otherwise linked to the family context or environment, whether or not they are a family member. Within this definition, perpetrators may be close to the victim (e.g. father, uncle, stepfather), or less familiar (e.g. family friend, babysitter).[109]

I will use this term or refer to child sexual abuse 'in the family or the child's close network.' I choose not to use the term 'interfamilial' child sexual abuse which masks the gender politics as this is a crime perpetrated almost entirely by men and boys and suggests to a certain degree the historical tendency of officials and medics to assign blame to mothers and daughters for the sexual violence inflicted upon them.

Children are described as 'children who have been sexually abused' or sometimes for brevity, 'sexually abused children,' although I dislike the latter for its implication that the sexual abuse completely consumes all of the other parts of children's complex identities. I use the term adult 'survivor' in most cases, with an appreciation that not everyone survives and that some people identify as victims for reasons that include garnering attention for activism relating to sexual violence and gaining access to resources.[110]

## Methodology and Ethics

Louise Jackson defines the historian's methodology as

[109] Children's Commissioner. 'Protecting Children from Harm: A Critical Assessment of Child Sexual Abuse in the Family Network in England and Priorities for Action.' 2015, 2.

[110] Roxani Krystalli and Philipp Schulz, 'Taking Love and Care Seriously: An Emergent Research Agenda for Remaking Worlds in the Wake of Violence,' *International Studies Review* 24, no 1 (2022).

> interpreting statements and uncovering diverse and complex sets of meanings in relation to wider political, cultural and linguistic structures, but also with an awareness of individual initiative, agency and resistance.[111]

Jackson's considerable skills as an historian enabled her to use the records of courts, child welfare agencies and the wider rhetoric about children in the Victorian period to reveal 'the ways of telling, explaining, or denying what would otherwise be left unsaid in the public realm' in relation to child sexual abuse.[112] There are significant challenges in attempting to explore the more recent histories of child sexual abuse in the family.

In published historical writing, methodology and ethics often sit off stage and are not on show to the book's readers. However, histories of sensitive topics that involve living or recently deceased subjects carry a number of risks, including damaging an individual's reputation, causing them distress, loss of privacy or even putting them at risk of violence or abuse. Hence, I will briefly sketch out some of the ethical and methodological issues here.

This book draws on my background in service development and leadership within children's services, as well as my training as a social researcher and historian. My experience in early years and children's social care services often involved me in processes designed to aid the early identification of vulnerable children and in safeguarding and child protection, as well as engaging me in interagency collaboration across health care, housing, youth justice and education. I have drawn on this to explore the motivations, emotions and practices of community health practitioners in relation to children who have been sexually abused in the family.

Investigating the recent histories of child abuse is challenging. Access to sources is restricted because data holders (governments, services, archives) fear they will breach individuals' rights to privacy, and/or fall foul of regulations relating to data protection. Information relating to living individuals is normally closed for 100 years from their date of birth or until proof of death. However, the historical perspective is valuable, and it can counter the tendency of the social sciences literature to generalise and to assume continuity over time.[113] Historical methods can complicate

[111] Jackson, *Child Sexual Abuse in Victorian England*, 9.

[112] Lydia Murdoch, review of Child Sexual Abuse in Victorian England by Louise A. Jackson, *Victorian Studies* 44, no 3 (2002): 542.

[113] Peter J. Buckley, 'Historical Research Approaches to the Analysis of Internationalisation,' *Management International Review* 56, no 6 (2016); Some social work scholars (like Harry

simplistic narratives of chronological progress and interrogate the roles of different actors; they can pay careful attention to subtle and major shifts over time, and to the variability in context that affects processes, policies, decisions and emotions. Insights can be gained into the roles of individuals or professional groups, as well as particular causal events or factors.

Two main sources and methods were used to produce this book. The first was archival historical research using trade and professional journals; books published by medics, feminists, scholars, survivors and activists; documentation from public inquiries; videos and recordings from conferences or interviews; policies and practice guidance from professional bodies, local and national government and published research or interviews representing the views of survivors of child sexual assault and community health professionals. Each of these sources was produced with a particular purpose in mind, delivered in a particular style and tone and must be considered within its wider context. Class, race, gender and politics affected both their production and their reception by their intended audiences. They may have been constructed with a greater degree of vigilance that was usual practice, because of the sensitive and often controversial nature of child sexual abuse. I have approached them with caution as socially constructed artefacts within the book. Nevertheless, as Paul Thompson has pointed out, 'there is a remarkable amount of unexploited personal and ordinary information' in these sorts of sources,[114] which can contribute to the historical record of health practitioners' involvement in child sexual abuse.

The second aspect of the methodology comprises short interviews and longer oral history interviews I conducted with community health professionals between 2018 and 2023, mainly in England. I interviewed over fifty individuals informally and recorded oral histories with twenty practitioners aged between 40 and 80. This enabled the collection of rich

Ferguson and Nigel Parton) and sociologists (e.g. Carol Smart and David Finkelhor) have historicised child abuse and child protection. Ferguson, *Protecting Children in Time: Child Abuse, Child Protection and the Consequences of Modernity*; Nigel Parton, *Governing the Family: Child Care, Child Protection and the State* (Hampshire: Palgrave, 1991); *Safeguarding Childhood: Early Intervention and Surveillance in a Late Modern Society* (Hampshire, New York: Palgrave Macmillan, 2006); *The Politics of Child Protection: Contemporary Developments and Future Directions* (Basingstoke: Palgrave Macmillan, 2014).

[114] Paul Thompson, 'The Voice of the Past: Oral History,' in *The Oral History Reader*, ed. Robert Perks and Alastair Thomson (London and New York: Routledge, 2003), 23.

information about the changing context and direct experiences of health professionals who had trained and worked with children and families over the last fifty years. The short interviews took place on the telephone or face-to-face; the oral histories were recorded at a venue of the narrator's choosing which was usually their home or office. Although the gender dynamics of the professions I researched changed over the period (a great deal for doctors and psychiatrists and only marginally for health visitors and clinical psychologists), in the main, these professions and their practitioners have been under-researched. Therefore, I aimed to give narrators the opportunity to talk about their careers in working with children as fully as they wished, rather than ask a series of questions about child sexual abuse; some spoke about family background and formative personal experiences as well as the ethical, technical and affective aspects of their training and practice in the child protection field. Furthermore, as oral histories their identities will be public in the archive and in this book unless they have specified that they wish to use a pseudonym. The intention is to enable pride in the interview and a celebration of the narrator's life and work as well as to increase the social and historical value of the information they imparted.[115] This naming practice was unfamiliar to many of the narrators who were more familiar with the anonymisation of social sciences research, but the rationale for naming individuals in the historical record and ways of mitigating any risks associated with that were fully discussed with participants.

The interviews varied in terms of length, subject matter and atmosphere. Some were recorded during the Covid pandemic which brought its own challenges.[116] I had protocols in place in case participants became distressed or a safeguarding issue arose but most of the narrators had encountered violence, abuse and trauma in their daily working lives for many years and had developed their own support systems. I used the oral histories with an awareness of how they might be inflected by the dynamics between us in the interview and by their experiences and the contextual changes that had unfolded since the period under discussion.[117]

[115] Paul Thompson and Joanna Bornat, *The Voice of the Past: Oral History*, Fourth edition ed. (Oxford: Oxford University Press, 2017), 337.

[116] Tracey Loughran, Kate Mahoney, and Daisy Payling, 'Reflections on Remote Interviewing in a Pandemic: Negotiating Participant and Researcher Emotions,' *Oral History* 50, no 1 (2022).

[117] Lynn Abrams, *Oral History Theory* (Abingdon: Routledge, 2010), 58; Anna Sheftel and Stacey Zembrzycki, 'Only Human: A Reflection on the Ethical and Methodological Challenges of Working with "Difficult" Stories,' *The Oral History Review* 37, no 2 (2010).

I sought to gather survivor testimonies about their experiences with health professionals from archival sources through a collaboration with Anna Weedon (an experienced practitioner in sexual assault services and children's advocacy). We approached survivor organisations across Britain, seeking published and unpublished material in which survivors commented on help-seeking as we wished to find what they had to say about their encounters with community-based doctors, nurses or those who provided psychological support. Unfortunately, the information available was sparse, it appears that although smaller organisations regularly consult with their service users, the material is often destroyed due to lack of office space, concerns about confidentiality or a failure to see the importance of the material. Therefore, survivor perspectives came from an assembled archive, including memoirs and reports, often mediated by other researchers for a different purpose. The most significant primary source to which I had access was a collection of letters sent by survivors to the National Commission of Inquiry on the Prevention of Child Abuse in the mid-1990s. I analysed those and drew out references to experiences that would have brought the survivors into contact with health practitioners while they were children. I did not keep records of those survivors' names or geographic locations in my own field notes and they obviously do not appear in the book.

Lastly, in writing this book, I have tried to avoid replicating the violence that has been inflicted on children and young people by those who sexually abused them. I have tried not to display the abused child as spectacle, but equally I wished to avoid reproducing the silences that are enforced upon children. I also did not want to enable the perpetrators of the abuse and the injuries and harm they caused to disappear. In parts of the book, therefore, the reader will encounter some distressing descriptions of child abuse.

## Structure of the Book

The book begins with the perspectives of survivors of childhood sexual abuse. In Chap. 2, I examine what survivors have said about the strategies they (and in the best-case scenario, a protective adult in their lives) took to protect themselves and whether they tried to seek help from a health professional. How did they perceive the attitudes, feelings and practices of doctors, nurses, psychologists or psychiatrists towards them? I consider the body and mind of the child and young person—survivors' views about the emotional and behavioural symptoms, the physical signs of abuse and the extent to which health practitioners should be able to recognise them. Despite historical and contemporary evidence that children and young people *do* attempt to speak out or indicate through their behaviour that they are victims of repeated sexual assault within the family, health practitioners often deny that and there is little evidence that they identify suspected sexual abuse. Can we see changes over time in how children felt practitioners responded to them or has failure to 'see' abuse been the status quo since vigilance against child sexual abuse was established as a practitioner's responsibility in UK policy in the 1980s?

Chapter 3, 'Bring it out from the shadows,' considers the messages that medical and nursing practitioners on the ground encountered about the emergence (or as historians have more accurately described it, the re-emergence) of child maltreatment as a social issue from the late 1960s, emphasising the reasons for their ambivalence about working in 'child protection.' This is in the context of the considerable upheavals that they experienced in those decades, as national policy dramatically reshaped organisational structures in health and local government services. Sweeping social changes affected how practitioners (and the wider public) thought, not only about children and families but also about sex and violence. I look at the ways in which child sexual abuse was represented in academic journals and the more informal trade 'magazines' of the various community health professionals and critique the rather caricatured depiction of practitioner awareness relating to child sexual abuse rising to a 'frenzy' until the Cleveland scandal and then subsiding swiftly because of professional fears of the negative consequences for themselves.

Chapter 4 'Colonising the Field' explores the very different understandings of child *sexual* abuse that came to the fore in the 1980s; in feminist and/or survivor circles on the one hand, and in medical and psychiatric circles on the other. These created schisms in thinking about how it should be identified and treated. I trace the transatlantic trajectory of knowledge and activism from key players in America to the UK. Why did these rigid factions form in this period and what were the consequences in the community settings where general practitioners and health visitors were asked to respond to children who had been sexually abused by a family member?

Chapters 5 and 6 look closely at the motivations, training and workplace experiences of health visitors, family doctors, paediatricians and child mental health practitioners who worked in family homes and community clinics. I investigate what encouraged them to choose to work with children and families in community health settings and the supports that were in place for them to do so, whether it was formal, in-service or specialist training and supervision, or other resources that supported their professional functions. What did practitioners experience in the workplace in relation to sexual abuse and how did their professional culture help or hinder them in fulfilling expectations about protecting children? Chapter 5 considers particularly the influence of the Leeds Sexual Abuse team and the way the reliability of the physical signs came to dominate conversations about child sexual abuse in the late 1980s and particularly in relation to the Inquiry into child abuse in Cleveland. The main focus of Chap. 6 is on mental health services for children and young people and primarily clinical child psychology, where some practitioners have been heavily involved in responding to child sexual abuse whilst the profession overall has been largely oblivious to it.

Finally, in the conclusion, I revisit the book's key themes and the implications for survivors, as well as for the different community-based health professions tasked with protecting children. I argue that the history of community health practitioners' involvement in protecting children between the 1970s and the 2010s was messy, complicated and contested, and cannot be contained within a neat narrative of linear progress. Their effectiveness was affected by context and contingency and changed over time but was ultimately hampered by a lack of strategic leadership, poor structural and institutional investment in those engaged in frontline practice and the legacy of a misogynistic culture that operated at multiple levels. Finally, I call for a renewed feminist stance in which all adults take responsibility as active protectors of children.

CHAPTER 2

# Silenced Voices, Invisible Bodies: Survivor / Practitioner Encounters

## Introduction

On 18 November 1994, a letter arrived at the east London office of a British charity, the National Society for the Prevention of Cruelty to Children (NSPCC). Readers of newspapers or magazines, as well as viewers of breakfast television shows, had been asked to share their experiences of abuse with a new National Commission of Inquiry into the Prevention of Child Abuse (NCIPCA). They were told 'HERE'S your chance to help other abused children. The NSPCC wants to hear from victims of abuse.' This particular letter was from Jo Mary Stafford who asked the Inquiry to read her autobiography *Light in the Dust* and consider it within the body of evidence that they would examine.[1] She wanted them to know about her childhood, made miserable by poverty and the various forms of tyrannical cruelty her father wielded over the family. The Inquiry received almost a thousand letters and over seven hundred of them were from people who told of their own experiences of childhood abuse of all forms. Nearly all of those who wrote in had been sexually abused by family members or people they knew well.

Most of the chapters in this book deliberately centre health practitioners' experiences, exploring why, despite encouragement and training to

[1] Letter to the National Commission of Inquiry into the Prevention of Child Abuse (NCIPCA) from Jo Mary Stafford, 18 Nov 1994.



R. Beecher, *Community Health Practitioners and Child Sexual Abuse in the Family, 1970s–2010s*, Genders and Sexualities in History, https://doi.org/10.1007/978-3-031-80052-8_2

be vigilant in relation to the physical and behavioural signs of sexual abuse, their rates of identification did not rise over time. To understand why there was little improvement, we need to make some effort to see things through practitioners' eyes. How did they perceive and react to the messages targeted at them and what support did they receive to fulfil their responsibilities? First, in this chapter I set out to gain a sense of what children themselves lived through and felt and what adult survivors remember. How can their views help us to interpret the causes of this stagnation in terms of the early identification of child sexual abuse in the family?

Ideally, what follows would be a chorus of children, young people and adults' voices. Their views would form the central point of this history and serve as a touchstone alongside archival and professional reflections. Born in different places and at different times, the survivors would be fully present in this history; describing their childhoods, the strategies they adopted to protect themselves, and who, if anyone, they asked for help, whether directly or obliquely. For example, did they seek to confide in a health practitioner—a doctor, nurse or mental health worker they encountered at school, a health centre or another local venue? Although the frequency and consistency vary over time, most children come into contact with health practitioners in the course of their daily lives: their GP, health visitor, school nurse or counsellor, perhaps a community paediatrician. As they move towards greater independence, young people come into contact with other types of community health practitioners too: for example, sexual health workers, psychologists, health promotion staff, drugs education workers. How have children and young people who have been sexually abused perceived the attitudes, feelings and practices of these health practitioners towards them? The intention of such an approach would not be to expose professional failures, but rather to understand more about the circumstances in which swift intervention might have been possible and children might have felt listened to and respected.

But such testimonies, whether positive, negative or mixed, are hard to find. There is currently no central archive in England or Wales that preserves the first-person testimonies of those who have experienced sexual abuse. It may sometimes feel that survivors' stories proliferate in magazines, newspapers, memoirs and through public inquiries, recounting familiar tales of abuse, secrecy and suffering. But these, in fact, are often brief accounts or decontextualised excerpts that omit or obfuscate specific details that could help us to situate experiences temporally or geographically. The Independent Inquiry into Child Sexual Abuse (IICSA 2015–22) website contains many survivor accounts, each one accompanied by a note that states 'all names and identifying details have been changed.' The segments are depersonalised and disconnected from other information; they may tell us something about the abuse and about the survivor's age, ability or disability, race, religion, class, sexuality or gender, but because they are untethered from their historical context, we are often prevented from answering specific questions about when the abuse happened, what else was happening in society at that time, how one survivor's experience differed from someone else's and possible reasons why that was the case.[2] Slivers of survivors' stories can be found scattered and submerged within other historical documents. Fuller accounts of abuse are often sealed, categorised as too sensitive and distressing to be made available for public scrutiny.

Historians therefore have to 'assemble' survivor archives by combining accounts found in autobiographies, memoirs, interviews given to magazines or other media, oral histories or testimonies given to researchers or policymakers.[3] In some circumstances, individuals explicitly state or imply that they want the story of what happened to them to be known, for example, when they answer an appeal such as that from the National Commission of Inquiry (NCIPCA) in the mid-1990s (more of this below) or IICSA. For others, the abuse was not the part of their life that they would have wished others to remember. Historian Lucy Delap rightly warns scholars against 'fragmenting [survivors'] lives and imposing labels.' Despite her reservations, Delap collected scraps and snippets of lives because this was the only route she could take to challenge notions that rape and abuse were inescapable and relentless.[4] As Joanna Bourke put it, sexual abuse and rape are 'culturally constructed' and vary 'across time and place.'[5] Interrogating what survivors say about the context in which abuse was perpetrated and what enabled them to stop it or what circumstances allowed it to continue unchallenged can help us to tackle descriptions of it as pervasive and unchanging.

[2] https://www.iicsa.org.uk/victims-and-survivors/experiences-shared.html, static website, last updated Jan 2023.

[3] Jennifer Crane, *Child Protection in England, 1960–2000: Expertise, Experience, and Emotion* (Cham, Switzerland: Palgrave Macmillan, 2018), 201–209, 161.

[4] Lucy Delap, 'Disgusting Details Which Are Best Forgotten:' Disclosures of Child Sexual Abuse in Twentieth-Century Britain,' *Journal of British Studies* 57, no 1 (2018): 79–107.

[5] Joanna Bourke, *Disgrace: Global Reflections on Sexual Violence* (London: Reaktion Books, 2022), 8.

A large portion of this chapter looks at correspondence sent to the NCIPCA in 1994 and 1995 by adult survivors of abuse. Most of those who wrote in were abused prior to 1980, in a period when child sexual abuse rarely appeared in the popular media or in materials aimed at health, social care and other professionals. Some subsequent studies that included survivor feedback are also considered, although those only provide published reports (i.e. secondary data). It has not been possible to extract many contemporaneous children's voices or indeed to compare children's experiences before and after the 1980s based on the adult survivor feedback available. One study gives the views of young adults who had experienced sexual abuse in the more recent years. Others include survivors of sexual abuse across a very broad time period. But the materials are still invaluable, they give a good sense of what mattered to survivors and which of their experiences with health practitioners were consistent across time. Some of the methodological and ethical challenges relating to historical research that seeks data from survivors of sexual abuse are described in Chap. 1. Here, I will briefly state my belief that all of the individuals whose views are represented in this chapter wanted, by telling their own stories, to contribute to protecting other children and I include them with that shared intention.

## Part 1: The Memoir

The memoir that Jo Mary Stafford encouraged the Inquiry to read included a vivid description of how she came to be sexually abused. Seven-year-old Jo Mary and her older sisters were sent out to play in the garden on Sunday afternoons so that the house would be quiet while their father took a nap after a drinking session in the local pub. On one such occasion, their entertainment was cut short when Jo Mary cut her knee and ran sobbing to find her mother. She heard her father call out to her but as she ran towards the stairs to go up to him, her mother grabbed her and 'hauled [her] back into the living room, slamming the door behind her.' She proceeded to give her a 'dreadful warning' telling her to 'never, never goo to yer dad's bed, or let 'im touch ya … stay safe. Stay away from 'im … 'e might 'urt ya like me dad did me.'

Jo Mary's mother told her that when she herself was a child, her own father 'had started to … interfere' with her. He 'pushed 'is peter inside me tummy,' she said, and 'told me not to tell nobody or 'e'd kill me.' The rape was repeated when her 'mom wuz out a lot cleaning' and she was left alone with her father until, aged ten, she was admitted to hospital with scarlet fever and 'some doctor noticed a swelling at the top of me leg.' He asked her mother about it and the assaults stopped.[6]

In an effort to protect Jo Mary, her mother told her, '[y]our dad knows what me dad done to me, and 'e says 'e'll do it to you gairls if I don't do everything 'e says.'[7] Jo Mary's sister also tried to protect her, telling her that 'when me dad calls ya to cum to 'is bed or anything, yer'll 'ave to act like ya ain't 'eard like me and Josy do.' But when, a short time later, her father called her to the bedroom in a 'purring and gentle' tone, Jo Mary obeyed him. She had 'forgotten mom's warning,' or she supposed that subconsciously she 'didn't want to believe it anyway.' She described explicitly in her memoir how her father's cuddles shifted to sexual assault. Afterwards, she 'struggled free,' 'raced to the doorway' and shouted back 'you'm a dirty man, aint ya dad?' In a different authorial voice that indicated her adult self reflecting back on the childhood abuse, she recalled sitting in the garden and beginning to 'piece together a sort of jigsaw in my mind.' She realised that this incident 'had not been the first time dad had tried to interfere with me. Funny how I had pushed it out of my mind until now.'[8]

Certain aspects of this family's story were common to many of the letters the Inquiry received from people who had experienced abuse. These included an innocent child, an overbearing and cruel father figure and a childhood affected by various forms of abuse including emotional deprivation, physical cruelty and neglect. Jo Mary's understanding of what had happened to her and the narrative she told was also obviously influenced by contemporary psychiatric theories. The first edition of the memoir was published in 1990 and Jo Mary had clearly absorbed ideas about 'the cycle of abuse' that had been disseminated by medics and psychiatrists in the previous decade.[9] She wrote that she was 'tainted twice over through two

[6] Jo Mary Stafford, *Light in the Dust* (Hants: Caric Press Ltd, 1990), 46–47.

[7] *Light in the Dust*, 47.

[8] *Light in the Dust*, 48–49.

[9] See, for example, J. Garbarino and D. Sherman, 'High-Risk Neighborhoods and High-Risk Families: The Human Ecology of Child Maltreatment,' *Child Development* 51 (1980); B. F. Steele, 'Violence within the Family,' in *Child Abuse and Neglect: The Family and the Community*, ed. Ray Eugene Helfer and C. Henry Kempe (Cambridge, Mass.: Ballinger Publishing Co., 1976); A. Sharma and R. Sunderland, 'Increasing Medical Burden of Child Abuse,' *Archives of Disease in Childhood* 63, no 2 (1988).

generations. Later I would learn about the third generation. I wondered if it was hereditary.'[10]

The manner in which Jo Mary's father manipulated her mother, with the blatant threat that he would sexually abuse their daughters if the mother did not follow his orders, was not frequently found in other submissions to the Inquiry. It may be that the survivors had not been aware of such threats as children. Jo Mary's mother's frankness with her daughter was also unusual. Most letter writers did not describe their mothers warning them in a direct way about the risk of sexual abuse. Jo Mary's mother gave her a 'dreadful warning,' her sisters issued similar admonishments and the explicit language used by all three made it clear precisely what sexual assault was, and that Jo Mary must avoid it. Unfortunately, verbalising the risk was not enough to protect the youngest daughter; she was so emotionally deprived that she responded to any sign of affection from her father.

Jo Mary's memoir recreated the small and often miserable world of her childhood. She was born in 1939. At the outbreak of war, her father signed up immediately and she reflected that 'for certain children the years of wartime would encompass the only peace they would ever know.' On his return, he was filled with bitterness about his failures in life and put his own needs ahead of those of his family on every occasion. They often lacked the basic necessities of life such as food and clothing and every family member seems to have been vulnerable to his physical and sexual attacks. But her book was also full of the games and the dramas that made up the fabric of her childhood. All of it—joyful and dismal—conveyed the insularity of her social world and the limited options she had in terms of people she could talk to about the pervasive cruelty she experienced at home.

Contemporary research tells us that *if* a girl feels able to disclose abuse, the person she will most commonly confide in is her mother. But Jo Mary's mother already knew the risks and took protective, albeit ineffective, action. Regardless of how explicit the warning was, it was not likely to have much chance of adequately protecting a young child of seven from an adult male. But given that her husband had control of every aspect of their home life, we might surmise that the consequences of seeking outside help (if such a thought ever occurred to her) could well have been life threatening for her and her children. As far as we, the readers, are told, she never sought any such support.

[10] Stafford, *Light in the Dust*, 47–48.

Nor was there any sense of a professional 'outsider' paying attention to whether anything was amiss in the family. Jo Mary wrote of the local midwife who gossiped to neighbours at their garden gates about the gory details of each birth on their estate. There was no mention of a health visitor. Poor families had limited access to healthcare before the establishment of the National Health Service (NHS). Insurance schemes provided some coverage for working men, but as the Minister of Health noted in the House of Commons, they provided 'no personal doctor for the wives and dependants of insured persons.'[11] Alexander Walkden, the MP for Bristol South, called attention to the millions of women and children with no coverage.[12] After the establishment of the NHS in 1948, things improved and by 1952 nearly a third of GP patients were children.[13] But in Jo Mary's infancy and childhood, she would probably have been taken to the local hospital in an emergency and otherwise had very little contact with doctors. Perhaps someone at school could have asked questions. The memoir did not address that possibility, although it criticised the school's failure to provide her and her siblings with a reasonable education. Contemporary research suggests that children, particularly girls, sometimes chose to confide in teachers but none of the teachers at Stafford's school seemed to have taken an interest in the circumstances of these children's lives.

Jo Mary's mother's story was quite different. A childhood illness (which likely took place in the 1910s or early 1920s) brought her into contact with a vigilant doctor who noticed an injury, a potential sign of abuse and asked Jo Mary's grandmother about it. We do not know whether the doctor spoke directly to Jo Mary's grandfather or whether they informed 'authorities' in the police or a voluntary sector social welfare agency that a ten-year-old girl had been sexually assaulted. Perhaps just knowing that the doctor had asked the question was enough to make Jo Mary's grandfather fear that his actions would be discovered. Either way, the doctor's question was life changing for Jo Mary's mother. Her father stopped raping her.[14]

[11] HC Deb 16 Mar 1944, vol 398, col 430.

[12] HC Deb 16 Mar 1944, vol 398, col 472.

[13] Victor Neale, *The British Paediatric Association 1952–1968* (London: Pitman Medical, 1970), 4.

[14] August has described working-class women's tactics in resisting abuse and intimidation by male heads of household in this period. Andrew August, 'A Culture of Consolation? Rethinking Politics in Working-Class London, 1870–1914,' *Historical Research* 74, no 184 (2001): 193–219.

Stafford's is just one survivor account. But perhaps the memoir format allows a fuller and more nuanced story to be told than can be gleaned from other sources. To some extent, her book was a challenge to those who assume that, as the twentieth century progressed, attitudes to abuse became increasingly enlightened. Her descriptions of the frank way her mother and sisters spoke to her about her father's predatory behaviour contradict claims that such matters were not spoken about in families prior to the 1970s. Her story undermines certain stereotypes, including that of the 'colluding mother' propagated by medics and psychiatrists and critiqued by feminists in the 1980s.[15] To some extent, it also calls into question psychiatry's portrayal of the deeply damaged victim because Jo Mary's story was ultimately one of resilience; she overcame the abusive environment of her home. And perhaps most interestingly in relation to early intervention and health practitioners was the fact that in the first third of the twentieth century, a doctor's intervention had a powerful effect in protecting a child from further sexual abuse (Jo Mary's mother); two decades later, when Jo Mary herself was sexually assaulted by her father, no-one from outside the Stafford household was alert to any signs at all.[16]

## Part 2: The Inquiry

Most of the survivors who contacted NCIPCA used a ballpoint pen and paper torn out of a notebook to write their letters. Some were written clearly, others were scrawled and almost indecipherable. The authors were all adults, most well into adulthood, and yet some had never previously described their experiences to anyone. There were brief and somewhat vague accounts that suggested that their writers could not find the right words to describe what had been done to them or felt too much shame to

[15] Ruth S. Kempe and C. Henry Kempe, *Child Abuse*, ed. Jerome Bruner, Michael Cole, and Barbara Lloyd, The Developing Child (London: Fontana/ Open Books, 1978), 66; Mary MacLeod and Esther Saraga, 'Challenging the Orthodoxy: Towards a Feminist Theory and Practice,' *Feminist Review*, 28, no 1 (1988).

[16] By contrast, when Lynette Gould (born in 1979) told her mother 'what dad had done to me,' her mother questioned her father with Lynette in the room. Her mother believed him when he said, 'little girls make up stories like this,' and the brutal sexual assaults carried on. Looking back Gould wrote, 'All she had to do was take me to the doctor for a check up. That would have told them something was wrong, but she never did.' Lynette Gould and Stephen Richards, *Heart of Darkness: How I Triumphed over a Childhood of Abuse* (London: John Blake Publishing Ltd, 2007).

express it. Other letters were long, comprising page after page of painful memories while one or two contained graphic descriptions of obscene acts of cruelty. Approximately 721 of the letters that were sent to the Inquiry described personal experiences of abuse; 80 per cent of their writers had been sexually abused. It was rarely just sexual. Rather it was similar to what Stafford had endured, part of a childhood experience of multiple and combined forms of abuse. But the sexual abuse was a central focus of their letters; it tended to 'be serious involving penetration' and it had usually been done to them over a long period, thus destroying a great portion of their childhood.[17]

Throughout the twentieth century, public inquiries were used as a mechanism to investigate issues of public concern in the UK, and NCIPCA fitted into this category and followed on from several inquiries related to child abuse. It was distinctive in two ways, however. Firstly, most child abuse inquiries up to that date had arisen as a response to a specific child's death or serious incident(s),[18] but the NCIPCA Inquiry did not emerge from a particular crisis or scandal. Rather it was the result of extensive lobbying by the NSPCC who were eager to promote a national conversation about child abuse. The charity also funded the Inquiry. Secondly, this was the first Inquiry to reach out beyond 'expert' views and ask victims and survivors to describe their experiences ('HERE'S your chance to help other abused children') in order to inform the findings and recommendations for the future.

There had been a noticeable shift in attitudes towards children in the 1980s, which was reflected in European policy. In the UK, the Children Act 1989 was intended to shift the balance of power away from parents and towards children themselves if they were at risk of 'significant harm.' Children's wishes and feelings were, at least theoretically, given more weight in child protection practice. In the same year, the United Nations General Assembly adopted the Convention on the Rights of the Child and called on member states to sign up. The UK government ratified the Convention on 16 December 1991. Article 12 stated that 'every child has the right to express their views, feelings and wishes in all matters affecting

[17] Corinne Wattam and Clare Woodward, 'And Do I Abuse My Children? No!,' in *Childhood Matters: Report of the National Commission of Inquiry into the Prevention of Child Abuse. Vol 2: Background Papers* (London: The Stationery Office, 1996), 56.

[18] See Department of Health and Social Security, *Child Abuse: A Study of Inquiry Reports 1973–1981* (London: HMSO, 1982); Department of Health, *Child Abuse: A Study of Inquiry Reports 1980–1989* (London: HMSO, 1991).

them, and to have their views considered and taken seriously.' To some extent, the legislation and guidance codified a shift towards children's participation that had taken place in the previous two decades. Interest in consulting with children and in understanding their experiences and emotions had been growing since the 1970s and child protection work by the NSPCC and smaller charities encouraged children themselves to speak out. However, for the most part, 'adults remained mediators of child expertise,' advocating for them.[19] Even so, by the 1990s, there was a stated commitment in many service settings to support children, listen to them and encourage their 'participation' on multiple levels, especially in relation to their own wellbeing and care and in matters concerning practice and policy improvements.

Adult survivors' views also began to emerge. In particular, magazine and newspaper 'agony aunts' began to publish and respond to survivors' experiences from the 1980s,[20] and the NCIPCA's appeals for contributors to the Inquiry were placed alongside their columns. The notices ran in a wide range of publications: in newspapers, both broadsheet and tabloid, in magazines and on television shows. The Inquiry's advisory members included Deidre Sanders, who, at the time of the Inquiry was the problem page editor of *The Sun* newspaper, and claimed to send out responses to up to a thousand readers per week.[21] She had written a number of books for the general reader including the very widely read *The Woman Report on Love and Sex* and *The Woman Report on Men*.[22]

These books demonstrated a new willingness to air emotional and sexual problems. Their descriptions of 'incest' were frank. By this time, survivors' stories appeared regularly in the British media, but it was still very unusual to hear men's descriptions of being sexually abused by their fathers, mothers, grandfathers, older sisters, uncles and other relatives. When men did speak out, they reported that as children they had not understood what was happening or had been too frightened to tell anyone. Some, like Rory, described his own resistance. His grandfather

[19] Crane, *Child Protection in England*, 16.

[20] *Child Protection in England*, 164–166.

[21] 'Childhood Matters: Report of the National Commission of Inquiry into the Prevention of Child Abuse. Vol I,' (London: The Stationery Office, 1996), 156.

[22] Deidre Sanders, *The Woman Book of Love and Sex* (London: Sphere Books Limited, 1985); *The Woman Report on Men* (London: Sphere Books Limited, 1987).

molested him but, at a certain stage, Rory refused to do what was asked and 'after that I wouldn't let him near me.' As Sanders warned, many people presumed boys could 'take care of themselves, but their hopes of future happiness can be damaged by such experiences, just as much as women.'

Descriptions of various abusive incidents perpetrated on boys and young men in *The Woman Report on Men* culminated in Sander's statement that 'the risk is that the abused children become abusing adults' in 'a grim pattern repeated down the generations.' The section continued with Gordon who, having been abused at age twelve by his brother-in-law, went on to abuse his own step-daughter when she was the same age. Finally, we were introduced to Alex who abused his children for six years from age nine. He placed the blame on his daughter (for failing to 'object'), God (for not stopping him sooner in answer to his prayers) and the 'sexual urges [that] used to take control of me.' Sanders felt his justifications were 'typical of this type of abuser.'

Sanders' prevention strategy was fairly innocuous. It included teaching 'all our children to say no to any form of touching that makes them feel uncomfortable' and making sure they had 'the opportunity to discuss sex outside of the home.[23]' However, she was integral to the Inquiry's aim of getting survivors' views. She had an enormous public presence and influence. *The Woman Report on Love and Sex* and *The Woman Report on Men*[24] were based on surveys completed by thousands of women and men, all of whom were recruited through *Woman* magazine, which at the time claimed a readership of six million.[25]

Once the letters sent to the NCIPCA had been collated, sociologists Corrine Wattam and Clare Woodward coded and analysed them and produced a report of their findings for the Inquiry. They provided a composite picture of survivors' experiences interspersed with extracts from individual survivors' letters.[26] The majority of the letter-writers were between twenty and fifty-five years old and details in their letters indicated that most had been abused between the early 1940s and the early 1980s. Nine out of ten were women. The circumstances and context of the abuse

[23] *The Woman Report on Men*, 165–168.

[24] *The Woman Book of Love and Sex*; *The Woman Report on Men.*

[25] *The Woman Report on Men*, 2.

[26] For a thorough synopsis of Wattam and Woodward's findings, see Crane, *Child Protection in England*, 170–172.

that survivors had experienced were summarised, including who (if anyone) they had tried to tell, the support they had sought out and the impact on their later lives. The combined data demonstrated the extent to which young children were victimised: 67 per cent of writers reported that the onset of abuse had been when they were below the age of eleven. Most reported that the abuse had gone on unchecked for years. And, in the majority of cases, the abuse was very serious, involving penetrative sex. In nearly all cases (91 per cent), the perpetrator was known to the victim and they were often a member of the victim's own family (64 per cent of the cases). The perpetrator was usually a man (74 per cent of cases) but in a small proportion of cases, it was a man and a woman. Thus, the letters highlighted that children were most at risk in the supposed safety of the domestic space, and safety campaigns that emphasised stranger danger were off the mark.[27]

The survivors' letters demonstrated that they rarely thought to seek help from a locally based nurse, doctor or mental health practitioner during their childhood or adolescence. Only five per cent of those who wrote to the Inquiry had spoken to a counsellor, medical professional, nurse or similar. In fact, fewer than a third of victims had told anyone about the abuse while they were still children. Of those who felt able to confide in someone, just over a third chose their mothers. Many of the adult survivors' letters emphasised that there were indications that they were being neglected and abused, but no one posed questions to them about any possible cause. As Wattam and Woodward noted, 'the reverse was more the case, that people would write about how they must have been giving off signs, but no-one bothered to ask what the matter was.'[28] The practitioners who are the subjects of this book were either oblivious to the 'signs' or ignored them.

In most of the nearly six hundred letters that referred to sexual abuse, the distressing and sometimes life-threatening experiences forced upon the children (who were nearly all girls) are set down on the page using few words, with little description or context. In a few, the details of cruelty and violence are lengthy, graphic, and I will not reproduce them here.[29] Thirty

[27] Wattam and Woodward, 'And Do I Abuse My Children? No!,' 59.

[28] 'And Do I Abuse My Children? No!,' 69.

[29] See discussion of the ethics of representing interpersonal violence and abuse in Chap. 1 (Introduction).

of these letters specifically referred to health issues that would have required medical attention and would have provided an opportunity for a curious or concerned health practitioner to ask questions about the child's circumstances. The content of these thirty letters is examined below.

One of the letters was from an adult woman who described when her mother brought her to a hospital because her anus was bleeding. She had been sexually assaulted by a male relative who coached her to tell hospital staff that she 'had fallen on spiked railings while climbing.' She complied. She hoped that even though she was forced to lie about the circumstances of her injury, doctors would ask questions and discern the truth. No one asked anything on that occasion, but when her mother brought her back to the hospital for a follow-up outpatient appointment, the doctor took her aside. The two adults went into an office, leaving the girl outside. In her letter to the Inquiry, the adult survivor wrote, 'I now know that doctor asked my mum was there any chance I was being abused and she dismissed that from their minds.' The hospital staff did not speak to her alone or ask her about what had happened to her. 'By them not asking me,' she commented, 'that gave my stepfather a meal ticket to carry on for the next five years.'[30]

Often questions were not asked even when the physical signs were incontrovertible. The most common physical sign of sexual abuse that the adult survivors wrote about was pregnancy. Eight out of the thirty letters about health issues referred to pregnancy, miscarriages or abortions experienced by girls when they were between the ages of eleven and eighteen years old. One woman recalled how, in the late 1940s, she was taken to the hospital where she sat on a bucket with 'all this blood coming away from me.' There was no sense that anyone explained what was happening to her or offered her any comfort. Instead, she 'heard the doctors tell my auntie I had been completely ruined.'[31] She had experienced a miscarriage at eleven years old.[32] She had been let down by adults as her letter to the

[30] Letter to NCIPCA, LL0023.

[31] For a discussion of the emotional and economic impact of being a 'ruined' girl in the Victorian period, see Joan Jacobs Brumberg, '"Ruined" Girls: Changing Community Responses to Illegitimacy in Upstate New York, 1890–1920,' *Journal of Social History* 18, no 2 (1984): 250; Susan Mumm, '"Not Worse Than Other Girls:" the Convent-Based Rehabilitation of Fallen Women in Victorian Britain,' *Journal of Social History* 29, no 3 (1996).

[32] Letter to NCIPCA, LL0009.

Inquiry explained, for when her mother died, her father 'did not want us.' She and her sister were sent away to live in separate households with people they did not know where she was terrorised by one of those adults who would

> drag me in the bedroom and put a pillow in my face. I will never forget it. I was threatened if I told anyone, he could kill me and put me under a tree as no one would know that my father did not want me. I could not turn to anyone. I was terrified.

Despite the threats, she eventually told this man's wife and was sent back to her aunt's house. It was then that she had the miscarriage. She wrote nothing of how confusing and terrifying the ordeal must have been for her at age eleven, but in her letter she informed the Inquiry that her adult life was full of unhappiness and loss.

Another girl became pregnant aged twelve following five or six years of abuse. She was taken to a mother and baby home where her son was forcibly removed from her. Although we cannot precisely date her experience, mother and baby homes and forced adoptions were most frequently used between the 1950s and the 1970s.[33] She spent two years in and out of homes, while her abuser was sentenced to just six months in prison. She stated that she had been given no help, 'no-one talked to me, no-one told me I was a victim and that what happened wasn't my fault.'[34]

The letters sent to the NSPCC were often brief and the descriptions matter of fact, but they described deeply distressing events in these young girls' lives: pregnancies brought about by rapes perpetrated by their fathers, stepfathers or brothers; premature and sickly babies; babies who died; and babies taken away for adoption. There were other punishments and penalties that came after the abuse was exposed, one of which was expulsion from the family home.

Some girls, like the twelve-year-old described above, were despatched to mother and baby homes, but survivors were also expelled to other places. One girl who was sexually abused by her brother (probably in the

[33] Gillian Clark, 'The Role of Mother and Baby Homes in the Adoption of Children Born Outside Marriage in Twentieth-Century England and Wales,' *Family & Community History* 11, no 1 (2008); Leanne McCormick et al, *Mother and Baby Homes and Magdalene Laundries in Northern Ireland, 1922–1990* (London: Department of Health, 2021).

[34] Letter to NCIPCA, LL0010.

1970s) merely stated that she was sent away from the family home when she became pregnant at thirteen and that she tried to commit suicide twice, once at eleven and once at fifteen.[35] It seems that the banishment and how it made her feel were the important details for her, rather than where she was sent to live. Another survivor divulged that her stepfather had raped her over a four-year period, which culminated in her becoming pregnant at fifteen. She recalled her abuser trying to persuade her to have an illegal abortion. When she eventually told her mother, she was expelled from the family home to stay with relatives. In her letter, she chose not to recount what had happened to her baby or indeed whether she had given birth, stating only that she had 'no counselling and in fact felt as though I was the guilty party, being told at one point that "no decent man would want me now."'[36]

In some cases, the survivors reported that no one had noticed that they were being abused, but a professional had later picked up signs in relation to their younger siblings. For example, a woman wrote to say that the sexual assaults inflicted on her by her father went on for many years and was not detected until she was twenty-three years old. The abuse was not recognised until her younger sister attempted suicide and was referred to a psychiatrist who called in social services to investigate. She recalled that when the social worker visited, her father was drunk and had a young boy aged about eleven with him. Even though her father admitted to being responsible for sexually abusing his daughters, the only action taken was to refer him to see the psychiatrist as well. His daughter told NCIPCA that he went on abusing children (girls and boys, within and outside the family network) for years.[37] Another survivor was 'only offered help when [her] father was arrested, charged with … vaginal damage to his two stepdaughters.' Her own distress had gone unnoticed.[38]

There were silences and omissions in the letters in relation to certain physical signs. For example, we know from other sources that sexually transmitted diseases (STDs) would have been a symptom of abuse and yet there was no explicit mention of it in the letters.[39] The woman in Chap. 1

[35] Letter to NCIPCA, LL0017.
[36] Letter to NCIPCA, LL0025.
[37] Letter to NCIPCA, LL0002.
[38] Letter to NCIPCA, LL0005.
[39] 'Physical Signs of Sexual Abuse in Children: A Report of the Royal College of Physicians,' (The Royal College of Physicians, 1991).

(Introduction) who wrote about having been 'forever at the doctors with urine infections' and 'other problems down there' as a girl was likely alluding to an STD.[40] Researcher Sarah Nelson cited a similar example:

> My doctor knew I was being abused – I told him when I was ten. It was awkward for him because he was friendly with my family. I had a urinary infection from it – he gave me antibiotics but didn't do anything else. It was the start of a history of these infections, with sometimes unbearable pain.[41]

These sorts of details were deeply personal and infused with feelings of shame.[42] Although there was more openness about sexual matters and family violence in various forms featured more frequently in the media in the 1990s, it was often presented in a rather abstract way, disconnected from embodied experiences of rape and abuse. These survivors wrote to the Inquiry about the abuse they had experienced, but there was a lot of detail related to its visceral reality that they did not feel able to share even in anonymous letters to strangers.

The letters demonstrate that pregnancy was a conspicuous marker of sexual activity for these survivors who had been sexually abused prior to the 1980s. These accounts show that pregnancy could be the event that led to the abuse stopping, although rarely without further negative consequences for the victim. Being pregnant did not make the adults around these girls take a supportive stance. Even in the face of this in disputable proof of abuse, the adults in these girls' lives punished them rather than treat them as potential victims forced to participate in sexual activities through coercion, threat or violence. The professionals they encountered rarely asked questions about what had happened to them.

Although there is not a similar collection of letters available in relation to girls who experienced sexual abuse after 1980, the surveys and other forms of consultation discussed in part three of this chapter with survivors of (mostly) post-1980 abuse barely mention pregnancy. It may be that, when discussions about sex, sexuality, contraception and abortion became more open (a process that had begun in the 1960s but developed

[40] Letter to NCIPCA, LL0001.

[41] Sarah Nelson, 'Surviving Well,' (Scotland: Wellbeing Scotland, 2020), 26.

[42] Anne Hanley, '"I Caught It and Yours Truly Was Very Sorry for Himself:" Mapping the Emotional Worlds of British VD Patients,' in *Patient Voices in Britain, 1840–1948.*, ed. A. Hanley and J. Meyer, Social Histories of Medicine (Manchester, England: Manchester University Press, 2021).

unevenly),[43] abusers took precautions to avoid impregnating their victims. But the reduction in child and teen pregnancies may have had the unforeseen consequence of hiding one of the overt signs of child sexual abuse.

Letter writers reported that their emotional distress was ignored or wrongly attributed by doctors and psychiatrists. Worrying changes in their behaviour were overlooked or disregarded. One woman remembered that from the age of eight, she had regular bouts of sickness, she overdosed twice and experienced dramatic weight loss. She was referred to a psychiatrist at fourteen. She explained that 'after about one year of being on antidepressants and tranquillizers,' she felt able to tell them that she had been abused by a neighbour. She received counselling over a period of three years.[44] It had taken her a while to get help but when compared with others who wrote to the Inquiry, her experience might be rated positively. Her distress signals were noticed by the adults around her, she was able to place her trust in a psychiatrist, she eventually disclosed to that clinician and received appropriate treatment.

For others, the response to potential signs did not lead to support, but rather to labelling and sometimes to criminalisation. One young woman was taken to a police cell when the abuse was exposed 'as if I was the one who had committed the crime.'[45] Another girl wrote that she had been taken to the doctor who reported 'the matter' to the police. She recalled that she was then

> taken to the Police station, then off to '[redacted] Prison' for the weekend, then a Mrs [redacted] came and took me to a home for correction ... I was in there for three years, I was very upset, as my half-brother [who had abused her] was let off...[46]

Some girls were told that their removal from the family home was necessary to protect them from the abuser but the supposed places of safety could feel like sites of punishment. A girl who told her school counsellor

[43] Hera Cook, *The Long Sexual Revolution: English Women, Sex, and Contraception, 1800–1975* (Oxford: Oxford University Press, 2004); Caroline Rusterholz, *Women's Medicine, Sex, Family Planning and British Female Doctors in Transnational Perspective (1920–70)* (Manchester: Manchester University Press, 2020).

[44] Letter to NCIPCA, LL0007c.

[45] Letter to NCIPCA, LL0004.

[46] Letter to NCIPCA, LL0026.

that she was being molested found that 'next thing I know I'm put in a children's home for two years and nobody came to see me.'[47]

In other circumstances, survivors described how adults in the family and those in authority failed to keep them safe from sexual violence. As a consequence, their behaviour worsened contributing to their eventual criminalisation. A survivor who was abused by her step grandfather from the age of five to fifteen (in the 1980s) wrote that 'my school teachers and my parents knew.' They banned the step grandfather from the house for six months, during which time the girl did well at school but, she wrote, 'as soon as he was allowed back into the house it all started up again.' Her behaviour spiralled, she was taken into care and subsequently incarcerated in a reformatory for young offenders. She described spending

> a period of time in [redacted] Prison doing Borstal and still everyone thought that I was just a crazy child trying to get attention all the time by whatever means I could. In and out of hospital with depression being given labels every time when all I needed was for someone to look that little bit closer, harder.[48]

In this case, the girl wanted other people to notice her distress because the adults who knew about the abuse (her parents and the school authorities) failed to protect her. Instead, she was imprisoned and labelled as an attention seeker with mental health problems.

She was not the only survivor who reported that her experience was known but ignored. Another survivor stated that she

> had no help to date. When my dad did what he did, it came to a social worker and a doctor's attention…. nothing was done. I gradually came to believe it was my fault… I've been to doctors on and off over the years with the symptoms. I don't and haven't ever trusted another doctor since I was 12–13 and wasn't believed…[49]

This survivor had a very negative first experience as the social worker and doctor did not believe or support her, which had a longer-term effect on her ability to engage with healthcare. Wattam and Parton pointed out

[47] Letter to NCIPCA, LL0013.

[48] Letter to NCIPCA, LL0003a.

[49] Wattam and Woodward, 'And Do I Abuse My Children? No!,' 80.

that the fear of not being believed was exacerbated if the abuser was female or if the victim was a boy.[50] But, as this case shows, the effects were already severe.

Some survivors described serial encounters with health practitioners that established, rather than dismantled, barriers to help. A woman who had been abused by her grandfather as 'a small child around seven years of age' told the Inquiry that her parents were suspicious that something was wrong and asked her 'had he done anything.' She said 'no.' A 'breakdown at fourteen' led to her hospitalisation. She did not give any information about that admission, but her letter implied that she was not asked anything about the causes of her mental distress or that, if she was asked, she did not feel able to speak about it. In her late teens when she sought help for depression, her (female) GP dismissed her, telling her you 'should stop drinking coffee!' She persisted in her efforts to get help, returning to the doctor to say she was still depressed. She was sent to see a psychiatrist and she described how he

> was a young Chinese man and the first [thing] he asked was, was it ok to tape our conversation. I agreed but never told him what was bothering me as this was the last thing I wanted to happen. No one ever checked why I never went to any more appointments...

Although she claimed that she disengaged from the therapy because the doctor wanted to record the session, the manner in which she specified his ethnicity and gender implies that these were relevant to her as well. Her discomfort may have been related to racism and/or the increased discomfort of discussing intimate matters with someone she perceived as culturally 'different' to her. She may have preferred to receive health services from a woman or at least to be offered a choice of gender. The psychiatrist had prioritised recording the session over making his patient feel comfortable and exploring why she was seeing him. His lack of sensitivity alienated her from services for many more years. She described finally getting access to appropriate help through her GP in 1992, by which time she was in her thirties. Her letter described the type of response that might have been helpful two decades earlier. A 'lady doctor' gave her 'time, understanding and sympathy' and discussed with her in 'a long talk' what would be best

[50] Nigel Parton and Corinne Wattam, eds., *Child Sexual Abuse: Responding to the Experiences of Children*, Wiley Series in Child Protection and Policy (Chichester: Wiley, 1999).

for her. In talking to her about a referral for counselling, the GP asked if she objected to seeing a male therapist and she was able to discuss her fears about 'clamming' up again.

Even when a child had disclosed sexual abuse prior to being taken to a health practitioner, reactions could be negative. One letter writer told her mother that her uncle had sexually abused her. When her mother took her to the doctor, it was a bruising experience. She recalled in her letter that the doctor 'was a disgrace the way he treated me.' After undertaking a pelvic examination, he 'said I had been abused but what did we expect him to do about it.' She remembered leaving the doctors 'in a state' with a bottle of 'tablets for depression, I was just eleven years old'.[51]

A woman who had been 'mentally and physically' abused by her mother throughout her childhood described what happened when she was in her early teens and her father sexually assaulted her. After a second incident, she actively sought help, telling a friend of her mother's, who encouraged her to approach her local Rape Crisis Centre. They, in turn, supported her to think about what to do next and how to go about it. Her mother did not believe that her father had raped her until he admitted the abuse. Even then, like other survivors discussed above, she was sent away to her grandmother's house even though 'my nan was away and I had to fend for myself.' She described how her mother left her brother at home with her father and went to live at a boyfriend's. After a few weeks, she was allowed to return home and, she recalled, when she went back to her convent school, one of the nuns asked, 'what the matter was and I blurted out the whole story.' The school referred the case to social services who visited the family home and arranged for a GP visit.

She thought that the male GP's attitude was 'hopeless.' He treated her very badly. She had undergone a gynaecological operation at age eleven, and 'on my notes it said that my hymen was already broken, so my GP assumed I was already having intercourse with boyfriends.' She felt that the GP treated her mother as his patient and his primary responsibility, telling her mother that 'I probably encouraged my dad' and counselling her in his office for over an hour while she (the daughter) sat outside the closed door.[52] Social services recommended family therapy; they attended two or three sessions before her mother 'stopped us from going again.'

[51] Letter to NCIPCA, LL0007a.
[52] Letter to NCIPCA, LL0007b.

Her letter detailed the difficulties she encountered mentally and physically during the years that followed and the challenges she faced in trying to get the right support. Although she reported that her current GP had been 'patient, understanding and supportive to my condition,' she was still left with very strong feelings 'about the way in which I and also my family was treated in the early days.'[53]

It felt to many survivors that their GPs would have preferred not to know or wished that the whole matter could be forgotten as quickly as possible. One child's GP told her mother that explicitly. Her letter described how, in the late 1970s, her stepfather had begun to sexually abuse her. She was about nine years old. She did not remember how long it went on for because she had blocked it out of her mind but she stated that 'I only remember what he done to me which I cannot write down in nice words (I still can't say it out loud). I don't know what kinds of words can describe it.' Having discovered that her stepfather had also tried to molest her sister, both girls managed to get their mother to believe them and move them away to stay at their grandmother's home. When her mother sought help from the GP, he advised her to 'start again in a new home and forget about it, not to speak of it again so that I would forget it.' But writing to the Inquiry, aged twenty five, she reported that she had not forgotten it. Her mother had followed the GP's advice and 'still feels guilty for not doing anything about it at the time.'[54]

One of the letter writers reported a contrasting experience of empathy and reassurance when she went to her GP to have an internal examination and 'finally told someone in authority.' She had been worried about 'whether or not I'd be able to have children' but the female GP reassured her, telling her that she 'was fine and that she couldn't foresee any future problems.' The doctor also referred her to a child psychologist at the local hospital. She found it terrifying, remembering 'wanting to just run out of his room,' but by the time she wrote to the Inquiry, she felt 'so glad. By letting out every detail, emotion and memory I've felt drained but as though the whole burden had been lifted off me in one swoop.'[55] This doctor carefully considered what sort of worries and anxieties a child who had experienced sexual abuse might have had, including very real fears

[53] Letter to NCIPCA, LL0007b.
[54] Letter to NCIPCA, LL0006.
[55] Letter to NCIPCA, LL0001.

about whether her body would function 'normally' as she developed. This response, unlike many of the other reactions described, centred the child's embodied needs and emotional wellbeing.

In summary, the letter writers to NCIPCA described long periods during their childhood during which doctors and mental health practitioners failed to create the conditions that felt safe for them to disclose and, in most cases, failed to exhibit any curiosity about what had happened to them.[56] Behavioural signs of distress were treated punitively rather than seen as a means for obtaining help. Survivors felt health practitioners were quick to label them with medical terms rather than asking questions about what had happened to them. Negative experiences with health practitioners discouraged survivors from asking for help with mental and physical problems for long periods of time into adulthood. Even when the abuse was out in the open, health practitioners preferred to ignore it. Survivors had few positive examples of their local health service staff helping them to speak out about sexual abuse in order to end it.

## Part 3: Beyond the Inquiry

Even though anti-racist practice was high on the agenda in social work by the late 1980s,[57] few of the survivors' letter to NCIPCA had made any mention of race, ethnicity or culture. Neither did the final report have much to say on the matter although a specific examination of how race and culture affected the prevention of child abuse had been commissioned from the Race Equality Unit and was included in the second volume alongside Wattam and Woodward's analysis of the letters.[58]

As Melba Wilson highlighted in the early 1990s, fear within Black communities about fuelling racist stereotypes relating to Black people's

[56] They were not hearing what was said to them and not 'listening with a feminist ear … to hear who is not heard, how we are not heard.' Sara Ahmed, *Complaint!* (North Carolina: Duke University Press, 2021).

[57] Bandana Ahmad and Race Equality Unit - Personal Social Services, *Black Perspectives in Social Work* (Birmingham: Venture Press, 1990); Lena Dominelli, *Anti-Racist Social Work : A Challenge for White Practitioners and Educators* (Basingstoke: Macmillan Education, 1988); Laura Penketh, 'Three: CCETSW's Anti-Racist Initiative,' in *Tackling Institutional Racism* (Bristol, UK: Policy Press, 2000).

[58] Ratna Dutt, Melanie Phillips, and Race Equality Unit, 'Race, Culture and the Prevention of Child Abuse,' in *Childhood Matters: Report of the National Commission of Inquiry into the Prevention of Child Abuse.* Vol. 2: Background Paprs. (London: The Stationery Office, 1996).

sexuality led to increased stigma and greater secrecy surrounding the abuse in those communities.[59] Wilson described herself as a Black woman and an incest survivor in her book *Crossing the Boundary: Black Women Survive Incest*. She was an American who had moved to London in the late 1970s, and at that time, she worked as a freelance journalist on health and social affairs and an activist in the women's movement.[60] She had been a member of the socialist feminist Brixton Black Women's Group (BBWG) which existed from 1973 to 1985.[61] She would go on to work in senior policy roles in the statutory and non-statutory sectors in the UK including with the voluntary mental health organisation Mind, a range of Black community groups, the healthcare think-tank The King's Fund, and St George's NHS Trust, as well as a range of government working groups on race and mental health.

At the time Wilson wrote *Crossing the Boundary*, there had been almost no research on the interface between race and child sexual abuse and what little had been published originated in the US.[62] Understandably, Wilson felt nervous about 'exposing the dirty linen' of Black communities where, she wrote, 'tacit approval is given to keeping incest ... under wraps.'[63] Marlene Bogle, another member of BBWG and a pioneer in terms of her counselling Black survivors of incest, noted that the myths that circulated portrayed incest as 'problematic only for white women and children' and it was 'seen and believed to be the norm within the black culture and way of life,' which was completely false.[64]

Crossing the Boundary was replete with survivor testimonies but, like other sources quoted later in this chapter, for the most part they had no provenance. Some were unnamed and undescribed; others came from survivor accounts already published in magazine articles, the feminist press or other publications. Although floating in time and space, they were an important source in their own right, because Black survivors' voices were

[59] Melba Wilson, *Crossing the Boundary: Black Women Survive Incest* (London: Virago, 1993).

[60] *Crossing the Boundary.*

[61] 'Undaunted: The Melba Wilson Archive Project,' Black Cultural Archives, accessed 18 Dec 2023 https://blackculturalarchives.org/melba-wilson.

[62] Diana E. H. Russell, 'The Long-Term Effects of Incestuous Abuse: A Comparison of Afro American and White American Victims,' in *Lasting Effects of Child Sexual Abuse*, ed. Gail Elizabeth Wyatt and Gloria Johnson Powell (Sage Publications Inc, 1988).

[63] Wilson, *Crossing the Boundary*, 1.

[64] Bogle died during the Covid-19 Pandemic in 2020. *Crossing the Boundary*, 7.

often not heard at all. Only one of the survivors who had written to NCIPCA about health-related issues mentioned her race. This was a thirty-four-year-old Black woman who wrote in to explain that she had an abortion in 1973 after abuse by multiple family members. None of the professionals asked any questions or assisted her. Twenty-one years later, she still lived with her parents, she 'had become suicidal' and didn't know where to get help. She felt extremely isolated because she was from a Black family, so had 'to keep [her] mouth shut pretending everything is fine.'[65]

Although the accounts in *Crossing the Boundary* did include adult recollections of childhood abuse similar to those sent to NCIPCA, those remembering said little about seeking to divulge the abuse to anyone outside the family. It seems that it simply had not been a possibility that they could have considered in their youth because of the complexities of being Black or Asian or mixed race in Britain at that time. There was no discussion of the GP, school nurse, health visitor or child psychologist. There was only the occasional glimpse of the signs of physical harm that could have been picked up by a vigilant health practitioner:

> I was sixteen or seventeen when it ended. I didn't start my period until I was seventeen and a half. I had pelvic inflammatory disease for years. My kidney was fucked up - scarred. I had migraines from my teens and before - constant headaches and tummy aches.[66]

Fears of being misinterpreted, not believed, being 'labelled promiscuous' or accused of 'exposing oneself to an unsympathetic white professional establishment' abounded amongst adult Black survivors.[67]

Their reluctance to speak out because of a sense that it would be disloyal to the community and would bolster racist stereotypes about Black women and men meant their voices were rarely heard. The notion that society's oppression of Black men drove them to sexually abuse children circulated within the community where some held the view that Black men strove to exert a powerful role in the home because they were denied agency and respect in the hostile hierarchies of white society that they met once they stepped out the door. Exposing child sexual abuse was even more complicated when one belonged to a community that was so maligned and ill-treated in a racist society.[68]

[65] Letter to NCIPCA, LL0012.
[66] Wilson, *Crossing the Boundary*, 188.
[67] *Crossing the Boundary*, 176.
[68] *Crossing the Boundary*.

If the survivor submissions to NCIPCA gave a picture of the experiences of those who were abused prior to the early 1980s, albeit limited and fragmented, what of those abused in subsequent years? Some answers can be found in another NSPCC-funded endeavour. In the late 2000s, researchers Debra Allnock and Pam Miller interviewed young adult survivors of child abuse when they were between the ages of eighteen and twenty-four. Sixty individuals participated, of whom forty-four had experienced sexual abuse. Whilst the themes addressed in the Inquiry letters were entirely at the discretion of each victim/survivor,[69] this later study focused specifically on disclosure.[70]

The researchers conceptualised disclosure as a complex process that could happen in a variety of ways, including 'verbal or non-verbal means, directly or indirectly, partially or fully and prompted or accidentally.' Thirty eight of the forty four young people who had experienced sexual abuse (86 per cent) said that they *had disclosed during childhood*, and a majority (66 per cent) had done so *when the abuse was happening*. Earlier research had given a very different picture. To take just one example, an analysis of eleven retrospective studies carried out by a group of researchers in the US found that two thirds of those who claimed to have been sexually abused as children did not tell anyone until they were adults.[71] This was similar to Wattam and Woodward's findings for NCIPCA, where less than a third of those who wrote in reported having disclosed *at all* as children.[72]

Why were the Allnock and Miller results so different? We should note that the young people they interviewed were a small group and had experienced much higher levels of violence at home and in their communities than has been reported within the UK general population. The authors also surmised that another reason might be their methodological approach.[73] They collected quantitative data through a computerised questionnaire, followed by an in-person interview. These interviews were far more sensitive to the nuances of 'telling' and 'showing' than a survey and enabled a more sophisticated understanding of the meaning of

[69] Wattam and Woodward, 'And Do I Abuse My Children? No!,' 50.

[70] Debra Allnock and Pam Miller, 'No One Noticed, No One Heard: A Study of Disclosures of Childhood Abuse,' (London: NSPCC, 2013).

[71] K. London et al, 'Disclosures of Sexual Abuse: What Does the Research Tell Us About the Ways That Children Tell?,' *Psychology, Public Policy, and Law* 11, no 1 (2005): 194–226.

[72] Wattam and Woodward, 'And Do I Abuse My Children? No!,' 74.

[73] Allnock and Miller, 'No One Noticed, No One Heard,' 12.

disclosure and the multiple ways that children could 'disclose.' This included directly telling someone about the abuse but could also incorporate displays of behaviour or the use of indirect language to convey their message. Researchers also distinguished between informal disclosures (to the child's mother, friend or counsellor, for example) and formal disclosures (for example, to a social worker, police officer or doctor). Disclosures were most often made to mothers and friends, with teachers coming in as the third preference. Only a quarter of initial disclosures (person first told) were to professionals. Young people had a range of reasons for disclosing; to stop the abuse, to protect another child, to get emotional support or to seek justice.[74]

Fifteen young people who experienced sexual abuse initially disclosed to their mothers. Nine mothers acted to stop the abuse, either by ensuring the perpetrator was removed from the child's environment or by informing the police. The remaining mothers ignored what their child told them or denied that the abuse had happened.[75] Like many of the NCIPCA letter writers, these young people had lived in homes where they were being abused in a range of ways and mothers were often implicated and/or were themselves subjected to and fearful of violent and abusive behaviour from their partners or husbands. No matter who they disclosed to, young people usually had to make more than one disclosure; of the 203 disclosures made in childhood, only 117 (58 per cent) were acted upon by recipients.

In terms of the role of health practitioners, only ten per cent of disclosures (eight out of eighty) were made to counsellors and healthcare workers. Overall, health practitioners barely featured at all in the published report or in the quotations by young people that were included. The low number of approaches to health practitioners was despite the fact that a number of the young people had reported that

> in their adolescence, they were coping with significant levels of emotional distress which manifested in depression, suicidal ideation and self-harm. As a result, these young people had engaged with professionals such as GPs, psychiatrists and counsellors for help.

[74] 'No One Noticed, No One Heard,' 16.
[75] 'No One Noticed, No One Heard,' 6, 37–28.

They did not feel that they were treated well, with most describing 'adverse experiences with these professionals whom they believe failed to recognise the signs and instead, blamed the young person.' The details of their 'adverse experiences' with health practitioners were not described in the report but their feedback suggests that there had not been great improvement for this younger generation of survivors. Nor is there much mention of other community health practitioners to whom a young person might turn in search of emotional support; school nurses and counsellors were only briefly mentioned.

These were the views of forty four young people who had been sexually abused and cannot be compared directly to those who wrote the 577 letters to NCIPCA. Nearly twenty years had passed since the Inquiry and attitudes to sexual abuse had changed. The methods of the researchers were different. The forty four subjects were younger at the point of their interviews, less time had passed since the abuse took place. The latter were adults, some remembering very distressing incidents across many decades. What can be said is that when Allnock and Miller's cohort mentioned health practitioners, the comments were as negative as those written nearly two decades earlier and that, overall, health practitioners were very rarely seen as a possible source of help by the early 2010s despite the fact that the young people exhibited 'significant levels of emotional distress.' The physical health needs emanating from sexual and other forms of maltreatment were not mentioned at all, even though survivors experience significantly higher levels of chronic illness than the general population.[76]

In 2015 and 2018, survivor-led organisation Survivors in Transition and University Campus Suffolk (now the University of Suffolk) produced two reports in partnership with adult survivors. The first was based on a large-scale survey which generated nearly 400 responses from survivors aged fifteen to 72 (ninety per cent were between twenty and 59 years old). The second publication drew on twenty-eight in-depth qualitative interviews.[77] Given that the profile of child sexual abuse as a social problem rose in the 1980s, it would be very helpful to be able to differentiate

[76] Nelson, 'Surviving Well.'

[77] Noel Smith, Cristian Dogaru, and Fiona Ellis, *Hear Me. Believe Me. Respect Me. A Survey of Adult Survivors of Child Sexual Abuse and Their Experiences of Support Services* (Suffolk: Survivors in Transition and University Campus Suffolk, 2015); Emma Bond, Fiona Ellis, and Jenny McCusker, 'I'll Be a Survivor for the Rest of My Days. Adult Survivors of Child Sexual Abuse and Their Experience of Support Services,' (Suffolk: Survivors in Transition and University Campus Suffolk, 2018).

between those abused in the periods before and after 1980 within these reports but that is not possible. A rough analysis suggests that probably about equal proportions of these survivors were abused in each time period.

An important finding was that eighty per cent of survivors had not been asked whether they had been abused. The researchers explored what support survivors had received from different types of services, including GPs, police and social services, specialist rape or sexual abuse services and a range of non-profit organisations. The published report shows which services were their 'first port of call,' but not what age they were when they (or a non-abusing parent or carer) tried to get help from those services. GPs were the most common first service respondents had contacted in relation to the abuse (for nearly fifty per cent of survivors), but we cannot establish from the report whether this refers to help-seeking as children or adults, although the latter is more likely. The reports have a lot to say about attempts at disclosure (verbally or through behaviour), however, and how people were treated. Consider the way in which Clare* was dismissed by the practitioner assigned to her. Clare remembered the doctor saying, 'I need to lower my caseload, so you're being discharged.' Clare asked, 'could I tell you something?' and she replied, 'don't tell me anything, I don't want to know, we're discharging.' 'So,' Clare said, 'I just left it.'[78]

'Surviving Well' was a report produced in Scotland for health professionals working with people who had been sexually abused. It aimed to provide useful information and guidance on how survivors could be treated with empathy. Edited by feminist researcher Sarah Nelson, it was produced by survivors from Wellbeing Scotland and the Kingdom Abuse survivors' projects. It drew on similar work that had been carried out in Canada in 2009.[79] Its key message was that for survivors what was most important was 'not complex training, paper qualifications or long specialist study, but human qualities of empathy, genuine care and respect—along with informed awareness about some effects of sexual abuse.'[80]

Unfortunately, there was no contextual information provided in this report. For example, we do not know when survivors' experiences of abuse

[78] 'I'll Be a Survivor for the Rest of My Days,' 21.

[79] C. L. Schachter et al, *Handbook on Sensitive Practice for Health Care Practitioners: Lessons from Adult Survivors of Childhood Sexual Abuse* (Ottawa: Public Health Agency of Canada, 2008).

[80] Nelson, 'Surviving Well,' 6.

or their attempts to get help happened. Furthermore, in this case, survivors preferred that their names were not attached to quotations, so the report merely distinguished between male and female individuals. Much of the survivors' commentary was similar to that given to Survivors in Transition. Its usefulness was in its emphasis on the particular reasons why the vigilance of healthcare practitioners and the manner in which they respond to survivors were so important, because sexual abuse in childhood was a precursor of many physical health problems in adulthood, including 'auto-immune conditions, diabetes, gynaecological and urinary infections and certain cancers' as well as syndromes that were 'medically unexplained' such as 'irritable bowel syndrome, chronic pelvic pain, chronic fatigue and non-epileptic seizures.' Indeed, this was a factor that sometimes contributed to survivors' poor experiences of consultations with health practitioners who could 'become frustrated by the often baffling and wide-ranging symptoms of CSA survivors.'[81] Survivors experienced illness, disability and pain at high rates, probably due to a range of experiences including long periods of high stress in childhood, the effects on the body of childhood injuries or STDs and of self-harm in childhood and beyond, addictions developed through using drugs or alcohol as a coping mechanism, avoidance of routine dental or other healthcare and the side effects of psychiatric medication. Furthermore, when practitioners 'find out you've been abused, they think it's all in your head,'[82] or make assumptions 'that any health problem must be psychogenic' without appropriate further investigation.[83]

It is disappointing that we cannot situate these various small-scale efforts to collect the views of younger and older adult survivors of child sexual abuse accurately in their historical context. Nevertheless, they do tell us something about children's experiences. Firstly, children do try and tell someone about the abuse, but it is difficult for them to find someone to trust, their disclosures are often received badly and they are not that likely to get what they wanted out of the interaction(s), whether that was to stop the abuse, get emotional comfort or to see that the perpetrator faces justice. Secondly, survivors experience significant levels of emotional distress and try to get support to deal with that from health practitioners

[81] 'Surviving Well,' 8, 20.
[82] 'Surviving Well,' 12.
[83] 'Surviving Well,' 11.

but they do not, on the whole, think of those health practitioners as possible sites of disclosure. This is despite the long-standing notion of the doctor's consulting room or the counsellor's office as a confidential space to which many personal problems can be taken by the patient. Thirdly, despite evidence of the long-standing effects of childhood sexual abuse on individuals' physical health, the body and its pain seem to be less evident in the research with younger survivors, with the emphasis being much more on mental health. And, lastly, telling, trusting, how disclosures are received, how survivors are treated were each more difficult for Black child and adult survivors due to racism, structural disadvantages, community taboos, mistrust of majority white services and fears of being disloyal to the community.

## Conclusion

In this chapter, I set out to explore survivors' encounters with doctors, nurses and mental health practitioners. I wanted to know whether they or a protective adult in their environment had tried to seek help from a health professional. I was interested in the body and the mind of the child and young person—survivors' views about the physical signs of abuse as well as the emotional and behavioural symptoms—and the extent to which health practitioners should be able to recognise them.

Although the sources available are partial, hard to situate chronologically and impossible to place geographically, survivors' feedback was broadly consistent across the period in relation to their mainly negative experiences with health practitioners. This was despite awareness-raising campaigns, training regimes and a growth in specialist child protection posts. The broad outline of what survivors wanted—someone to notice their distress, listen to what they had to say and believe them—did not seem to change across these different projects or across the time period. They wanted practitioners to manage their own emotions, mask their own shock and discomfort and concentrate on creating a safe space and building a trusting relationship with them.[84] Often they hoped someone would not just listen but also ask them direct questions about what had happened to them.

[84] Myriam S. Denov, 'The Myth of Innocence: Sexual Scripts and the Recognition of Child Sexual Abuse by Female Perpetrators,' *The Journal of Sex Research* 40, no 3 (2003).

Sociological research shows that disclosure can be a complex process of long duration.[85] To support it, practitioners could take a stance of empathy and think about how to create safe spaces for children in order to make opportunities for disclosure. There is little evidence that has happened. Neither have healthcare practitioners become more relevant to children, young people or protective parents as someone to turn to and disclose to in the period. Perhaps some of this can be related to wider societal changes that meant children, young people and protective adults in their networks could find advice or help elsewhere, through peer support or online forums, for example. It could also be because despite increased attention to early intervention and prevention in child protection, community health practitioners did not prioritise it, felt unsupported to tackle it or adopted a position of deliberate ignorance. The specialist posts that developed to assess and treat children once child sexual abuse was identified were only helpful to that small proportion of children who did disclose or for whom the signs of abuse were recognised and acted upon. But perhaps having specialist posts allowed generalists to abdicate some responsibility. Practitioners based in the community who might have built relationships with children and noticed their distress such as a school nurse or mental health practitioner, or for a protective parent, the GP or health visitor are absent, they are not perceived as people who can help.

The NCIPCA Inquiry report in 1996 concluded idealistically that 'nearly all forms of abuse can be prevented, provided the will to do so is there.' It also determined that there was 'widespread goodwill towards efforts to reduce it.'[86] The main reasons put forward as to why abuse was

[85] Ramona Alaggia, Delphine Collin-Vézina, and Rusan Lateef, 'Facilitators and Barriers to Child Sexual Abuse (CSA) Disclosures: A Research Update (2000–2016),' *Trauma, Violence & Abuse* 20, no 2 (2019); Maria Larsen Brattfjell and Anna Margrete Flåm, '"They Were the Ones That Saw Me and Listened." from Child Sexual Abuse to Disclosure: Adults' Recall of the Process Towards Final Disclosure,' *Child Abuse & Neglect* 89 (2019); Rosaleen McElvaney, 'Disclosure of Child Sexual Abuse: Delays, Non-Disclosure and Partial Disclosure. What the Research Tells Us and Implications for Practice,' *Child Abuse Review* 24, no 3 (2013); Delphine Collin-Vézina et al, 'A Preliminary Mapping of Individual, Relational, and Social Factors That Impede Disclosure of Childhood Sexual Abuse,' *Child Abuse & Neglect* 43 (2015); Sally V. Hunter, 'Disclosure of Child Sexual Abuse as a Life-Long Process: Implications for Health Professionals,' *Australian and New Zealand Journal of Family Therapy* 32, no 2 (2011).

[86] 'Childhood Matters. Vol I,' 120.

not being prevented included public uncertainty about intervening, agencies that were focused on crisis rather than prevention, under-funding, legal and juridical failures, a system that did not prioritise children and a poor evidence base. Another reason given was that:

> Busy people, such as GPs, health visitors, teachers, childcare workers and others professionally concerned with children, too often, through other pressures miss or fail to respond adequately to signs of abuse in children they meet during the course of their work.[87]

Undoubtedly, a lack of time and resources heightened the risk that professionals would miss what children were trying to tell them or fail to respond sensitively. It is also possible that the Inquiry's critique of health practitioners was deliberately mild in a strategic calculation to win them over to the cause of prevention and early intervention, rather than to alienate them through overt criticism. However, their theories about why health practitioners did not prioritise prevention or early intervention were false as we can see from the analysis of survivors' letters. In fact, although the Inquiry took pride in soliciting the views of the public and survivors of abuse, they ignored what survivors said on this matter. Their letters demonstrated that 'being too busy' was not at the root of the problem. Survivors believed that medics chose a stance of deliberate ignorance and silenced them. As a survivor in Scotland said, 'when you are told to be quiet, medical professionals are saying the same thing as abusers do.'[88] Health practitioners refused to accept that this aspect of child protection was part of their job. Attitudes to girls were extremely misogynistic. Boys who were abused were hardly noticed and, if seen, their abuse was minimised and sometimes linked in a confused and prejudiced way to fear of homosexuality.[89] These were only the most obvious barriers. This failure

[87] 'Childhood Matters. Vol I,' 121.

[88] Nelson, 'Surviving Well,' 26.

[89] Bill Watkins and Arnon Bentovim, 'The Sexual Abuse of Male Children and Adolescents: A Review of Current Research,' *Journal of Child Psychology and Psychiatry* 33, no 1 (1992): 201–209. Easton, using a large sample of 487 male survivors, found that on average men delayed telling for between 21 and 28 years. Older age and being abused by a family member were related to delays in disclosure. Most of those who did tell as a child did not receive emotionally supportive or protective responses. Scott D. Easton, 'Disclosure of Child Sexual Abuse among Adult Male Survivors,' *Clinical Social Work Journal* 41, no 4 (2013).

to take survivor evidence seriously had longer term implications. Survivors cited in later reports have barely mentioned health practitioners at all as people they might talk to, who might notice something was wrong, who could potentially help them.[90] Where they did speak of them, there was not a lot of evidence of positive change. Research shows that the early identification of child sexual abuse in the family is still rare, and disclosure is delayed for years with a terrible cost to survivors and to the British health service.[91]

[90] Smith, Dogaru, and Ellis, *Hear Me. Believe Me. Respect Me.*

[91] Delayed disclosure costs the UK an estimated £3.2 bn and the British health service £182 m every year. Olumide Adisa, Megan Hermolle, and Fiona Ellis, 'Denial, Disbelief and Delays: Examining the Costs on the NHS of Delayed Child Sexual Abuse Disclosures in England and Wales' (Suffolk: Survivors in Transition and University of Suffolk, 2023).

[illegible]

[illegible]

CHAPTER 3

# 'Bring it out from the shadows.' Encouraging Health Visitors and Family Doctors to Respond

## Introduction

Whether written by historians or practitioners working with families, attempts to interpret responses to child abuse have tended to gravitate towards the idea of stages of awareness. The 1970s was seen as the decade when recognition that parents physically injured their children became widespread in Britain; the 1980s as a period when practitioners working with families and the wider public became increasingly cognisant that sexual abuse was not uncommon. This awareness—initially portrayed as necessary in order to 'fight the good fight' to protect children—was depicted as subsequently warping and distorting professional judgement. Awareness apparently developed into professional hypervigilance to possible cases of 'incest' and to fears that practitioners would 'see it everywhere.'

From the late 1970s, practitioners and researchers thought about why and how the social problem of child abuse was emerging and how responses to it might develop. In America, paediatrician C. Henry Kempe described the various stages of awareness that individuals, professional groups or whole societies might go through in relation to different forms of child maltreatment. First came a position of complete denial in which abuse was individualised and 'othered'—parents were depicted as psychotic, corrupted by drug use or perhaps violent to their children because they were 'foreign.' In stage two, there was an awareness of the 'battered child'; in stage three, there were better responses to physical cruelty and attention



R. Beecher, *Community Health Practitioners and Child Sexual Abuse in the Family, 1970s–2010s*, Genders and Sexualities in History, https://doi.org/10.1007/978-3-031-80052-8_3

to the infant who 'fails to thrive'; emotional abuse and neglect were noticed in stage four. The subject of this book, the 'serious plight of the sexually abused child,' was addressed in stage five. The sixth and final stage presented a utopian vision of a world in which all children were 'truly wanted,' loved and cared for.[1] Kempe reified these different forms of child abuse into a very particular configuration, which was embraced particularly by medics (more of this in the Chap. 4). However, what is important here is that Kempe sequenced these responses in a linear way and, within that, he portrayed sexual abuse as the phenomena that communities were least ready to tackle.[2]

Writing in the early 1990s (and hence without the benefit of much critical distance from the events he examined), historian Philip Jenkins set out his own chronology of awareness. His stage one ran from 1972 to 1979. During this time, there was an acknowledgement that 'baby battering' was common, affected families of 'all social strata' and could be 'lethal.' Stage two ran from 1979 to 1984. In these years, it was recognised that sexual abuse, commonly perpetrated by fathers or other male relatives, was a problem as 'widespread' as physical abuse. During stage three from 1985 to 1988, there was consensus that one in ten children was a victim of sexual abuse, that children's accounts of abuse should be believed because they did not lie, and that the criminal justice system must pay heed to the expertise of practitioners in adjudicating on sexual abuse cases.[3] The implication was that in the late 1980s, practitioners moved into a position of credulity in relation to child sexual abuse and that there was a self-aggrandising motive, which was to gain greater authority and status for themselves.

British professionals used Kempe's framework as a kind of yardstick by which to measure progress in raising awareness and responding to abuse.

[1] C. Henry Kempe, 'Recent Developments in the Field of Child Abuse,' *Child Abuse & Neglect* 2, no 4 (1978).

[2] Around the same time, UK social worker Nigel Parton traced the 'natural history' of physical abuse using sociologist Howard Becker's framework of discovery: (identify the problem), diffusion (convince others), consolidation (state takes responsibility) and reification (consensus that the problem is real and requires ongoing intervention from specific agencies). Nigel Parton, 'The Natural History of Child Abuse: A Study in Social Problem Definition,' *British Journal of Social Work* 9, no 4 (1979).

[3] Philip Jenkins, *Intimate Enemies: Moral Panics in Contemporary Great Britain* (New York: Aldine de Gruyter, 1992), 101–102.

By the early 1980s, they assessed Britain as being at 'stage three.' Physical abuse was better handled, and professionals were taking notice of infants who failed to thrive or were neglected. But neither emotional abuse nor sexual abuse were widely recognised. Psychiatrist Arnon Bentovim established a specialist team at Great Ormond Street Hospital (1981) and teams also formed in other parts of the country. Bentovim remembered this as a period in which there was a 'rapid process of community recognition,' followed by a backlash at the end of the decade.[4] Jenkins' and Bentovim's accounts had much in common, but the implications of each were different. Where Jenkins implied duplicity and untethered ambition on the part of at least some professionals, Bentovim depicted a practitioner journey that would help families by 'breaking through the barrier of silence' and providing appropriate treatment.

This chapter revises the claim that there was a neat linear progression in terms of awareness of different forms of abuse in this period. The chronology is more complicated than has been suggested by Jenkins or by the British doctors, psychiatrists and charity personnel who were involved in early evangelising to create greater awareness, develop services and influence policy in relation to sexual abuse.

Before discussing the messages designed to raise practitioners' awareness in the 1970s and 1980s, it is useful to travel back in time and gain an understanding of the tenor of the dialogue about 'incest' in the preceding decades. In the first part of this chapter, I examine two very different depictions of sexual violence against children that appeared in the *British Medical Journal (BMJ)*. Published ten years apart (1961 and 1972), they signalled a potential shift in terms of which professional groups could 'speak' with accepted authority on child sexual abuse (from police surgeons to psychiatrists) but also a change in relation to how the phenomenon was understood in terms of context, prevalence and impact. There was a hint too that the family doctor and their colleagues in the community would in the future need to play a greater role.

Part two moves from the *BMJ* to the trade newspapers commonly read by GPs and health visitors.[5] A close examination of these sources shows

[4] Arnon Bentovim, 'Commentary on Kempe C.H. 1978 Sexual Abuse, Another Hidden Pediatric Problem: 1977 C. Anderson Aldrich Lecture,' in *C. Henry Kempe: A 50 Year Legacy to the Field of Child Abuse and Neglect*, ed. Richard D. Krugman and Jill E. Korbin (Netherlands: Springer, 2013).

[5] See Chap. 6 for child and adolescent mental health practitioners.

that child abuse was just one 'social problem' that these professionals were encouraged to tackle. But not everyone was eager to do so; professionals bickered about whether these matters should fall within the scope of their professional responsibilities. Gender dynamics are scrutinised more closely in part three, in relation to general practice, which had been a male stronghold up until the 1960s, but was changing rapidly.

Health visitors' responses to these issues are explored in part four. The health visitor had a long history of outreach to family homes and had been seen by local and central government as well placed to 'detect' problems in families. Given the decline in infectious diseases, the profession sought a new central mission.

The final part of this chapter examines a selection of articles targeted at practitioners during the 1980s and designed to increase their awareness and encourage them to intervene in sexual abuse. They were not published as frequently as one might assume from the accounts of historians or medics. Nor was their content neatly packaged into stages of awareness with sexual abuse usurping other forms of maltreatment during the 1980s. This challenges the idea that public and practitioner recognition of sexual abuse was a 'rapid process,' an all-consuming preoccupation, or that a consensus was swiftly reached about its prevalence, impact or how neighbourhood nurses and doctors should respond.

## Part 1: Sexual Abuse in the *British Medical Journal* (*BMJ*)

In May 1972, the *BMJ* published an article about incest.[6] It appeared without fanfare, sandwiched between items on knee replacement surgery and thyroid cancers, but it anticipated the emergence of a medical and psychiatrist interest in this issue in Britain. The unnamed *BMJ* author observed that although incest had 'generally been considered rare,' a new 'comprehensive' study published by psychiatrist Narcyz Lukianowicz in the *British Journal of Psychiatry* had found otherwise. The author also recognised (in a slightly oblique way) that paternal incest might be harmful to the child, noting that only six out of the 26 daughters in the study showed 'no apparent ill effects from their incestuous relationship.' These acknowledgements of prevalence and impact, although slight, marked a change.

[6] 'Incest and Family Disorder,' *British Medical Journal* 2, no 5810 (1972): 364–365.

The psychiatrist in question (Lukianowicz) was sixty-five years old and an immigrant to the UK from Lvov, close to the Polish border in western Ukraine. A surviving photograph shows a man with a high forehead, soft white hair, narrow eyes and a sharply pointed nose.[7] An obituary in a psychiatric publication celebrated his 'congenial spirits, wide-ranging knowledge and brilliant presence,' but we have no sense of whether those qualities would have been evident to the children he saw on a daily basis. He was an experienced psychiatrist who had held posts in Lvov, Vienna and Austrian Carinthia. After time in a displaced persons' camp, he moved to Brighton on the south coast of England, where he set up a neuropsychiatric unit to rehabilitate Polish soldiers. He joined the NHS as a registrar in Bristol in 1952. His particular interests were in juvenile delinquency, parent-child relationships, sexual deviation and parahallucinations.[8] When appointed as consultant psychiatrist to the Holywell Psychiatric Hospital in Antrim, Northern Ireland, in 1962, he established a range of new services. These included postgraduate teaching, family therapy and a child guidance clinic at Whiteabbey Hospital, psychiatric services for a Remand Home and Training School for girls and psychiatric outpatients clinics at two general hospitals.[9]

For this study, Lukianowicz had collected data from admissions to these services and discovered a four per cent prevalence rate for paternal incest among the female psychiatric patients (26 out of 650 girls), as well as an identical rate for other forms of incest amongst a mixed gender cohort of 29 out of 700.[10] There were no special selection criteria, each consecutive admission to the services was included in the data analysed.[11] The girls had apparently 'quite casually' and 'rather unexpectedly and quite

[7] 'Lukianowicz, Narcyz,' Ukranians in the UK Online Encyclopedia. https://www.ukrainiansintheuk.info/eng/02/lukianowicz-e.htm. Accessed 24 Sep 2024.

[8] Parahallucinations are those due to 'an injury or abnormality to the peripheral nervous system.' Presumably Lukianowicz's interest came from his work with traumatised soldiers, but it is fascinating given that the notion of what was 'real' or 'not real' would become so central and divisive in debates about child sexual abuse two decades later. Rif El-Mallakh and K. L. Walker, 'Hallucinations, Pseudohallucinations, and Parahallucinations,' *Psychiatry* 73, no 1 (2010).

[9] Narcyz Lukianowicz, 'Incest,' *British Journal of Psychiatry* 120, no 556 (1972): 310.

[10] 'Incest,' 308.

[11] In other words, every girl admitted to any of the services in a set period of time was included in the study.

spontaneously' spoken about having 'incestuous experiences' with their fathers, 'without any questioning or prompting' by the researchers.[12]

Lukianowicz assessed eleven of the 26 girls as 'promiscuous [with] psychopathic traits such as drug abuse or delinquency.' He noted that five developed 'frigidity after marriage,' and that three gave other evidence of 'hysterical personality disorder.' One girl had an 'acute anxiety neurosis' reportedly brought about by her father's threats of violence if she spoke out, while a further three were depressed and had attempted suicide. The contemporary reader might consider the girls' lives subsequent to the abuse to be disrupted and damaged, but Lukianowicz was more interested in categories of mental disorder or illness, concluding that 'incest in a girl's early life may cause in some cases personality disorders, very rarely a neurosis, never a psychosis.'[13] The *BMJ* author, summarising Lukianowicz's research for the journal's readers, thought it was important to discourage any direct correlation between the girls' subsequent problems and the abuse, judging that in the 'presence of such gross family pathology,' the girls' 'abnormalities' could not be linked directly to the incest.[14] Nevertheless, both the original research article and the *BMJ* synopsis conveyed the sense that paternal incest was more common and more damaging than had been previously believed. The detail provided implied that the girls were seriously harmed by their fathers' actions. Furthermore, the very fact that the prevalence of incest in this cohort of psychiatric patients was higher than doctors had previously imagined undermined the *BMJ* rationalisation that generalised family pathology rather than incest might be the cause of the girls' distress.

An acknowledgement of harm, however hesitant, was noteworthy, particularly when compared to a major article published in the *BMJ* a decade earlier that had barely acknowledged the existence of incest.[15] It was commissioned following correspondence in *The Times* about the way children who had been sexually assaulted were treated within the criminal justice system. Claiming that 'the public conscience [was] uneasy' and judging the problem to be at least 'in part medical,' the *BMJ* published three articles; one from Basil Henriques (a magistrate who had initiated the letters

[12] Lukianowicz, 'Incest,' 301.

[13] 'Incest,' 308.

[14] 'Incest and Family Disorder,' 364.

[15] Basil Henriques and Nesta H. Wells, 'Sexual Assaults on Children,' *British Medical Journal* 2, no 5267 (1961).

to *The Times*' editor in May 1961), one from its own legal correspondent and one from Nesta Wells to represent the medical perspective.[16] In 1927, Wells had been the first (and for decades the only) woman appointed as a police surgeon in Britain. She was employed as 'Lady Doctor' to the police force in Manchester and she actively lobbied for improvements to sexual assault services. In her early days as a police surgeon, Wells was asked to examine those who had been sexually assaulted in unsuitable 'dark and inappropriate' rooms in police stations around Manchester. She insisted instead that girls and women who had been raped were brought to her own surgery at her home and that a woman police officer should be present. She also campaigned hard to recruit more woman officers and surgeons to the force.[17]

In this 1961 article, Wells described her experience in examining two thousand 'little girls' (and 'not more than a dozen' boys) who had been sexually assaulted. Eighty three per cent of this large cohort were children aged under sixteen. That Wells assumed those responsible for the sexual abuse were adults without close connections to the children, rather than members of their families, is evident from the language she used. For example, she claimed that not all parents reported assaults because they were afraid of publicity 'and the risk of increasing psychological trauma in an already disturbed child.' This stopped the police from 'tracking down' the men responsible, which was a shame because they had probably 'been assaulting other little girls.' She noted that very young girls (aged under seven years old) might be frightened following an assault, but could be

[16] The letters sent to *The Times* in early 1961 did not indicate that 'the public conscience [was] uneasy.' Henriques himself submitted the first letter asking, 'whether the general public is aware of the fearful ordeals of a girl [in court], perhaps of very tender age, who may have been sexually assaulted.' Arthur C. L. Paton, from the World Federation for Mental Health, wrote about improvements made in Israel. Esther Iwi warned that Henriques' suggestion that children's evidence should be given in an affidavit interfered with the 'rights of the accused.' Lastly, H. Marcus Bird, Chair of the Bury St Edmunds Juvenile Court and a doctor, congratulated Henriques for trying to 'ameliorate the appalling psychological damage to which children may be subjected by courts of law.' It was hardly a deluge of public support; Basil Henriques, 'Letter to the Editor, "Ordeal Prolonged,"' *The Times*, 31 May 1961; Arthur C. L. Paton, 3 Jun 1961; Esther Iwi, 5 Jun 1961; H. Marcus Bird, 6 Jun 1961. 'Sexual Assaults on Children.'

[17] Helen Meakin, 'How did Dr Nesta Wells fit into the professional, political and social networks which led to her medical appointments including that of Britain's first woman police surgeon in 1927, and what impact did her work have?' Masters dissertation, Edge Hill University, Jul 2022.

reassured by their parents and could begin to 'get over their fear of strange people.'[18] She described the men as 'usually perverts or mentally subnormal,' and noted that they were 'therefore apt to assault others if left unrestrained.'[19] The implication was that attacks were carried out by strangers who roamed around neighbourhoods in search of young girls to molest.

We have no information about the basis for Wells' assumptions that most assailants were strangers. We can surmise that attacks by unfamiliar men and boys were more likely to have been reported than those concerning members of the child's own family. It is also likely that there were more 'stranger' perpetrated offences prior to the 1970s because of the freedoms British children then had to move around in their streets, parks and neighbourhoods without adult supervision. They were more likely to encounter adult sexual advances in public spaces than most children of the 2020s who spend more time under adult supervision.[20] However, we know from survivors' testimonies that children were threatened by abusers (fathers or male relatives) to say that an attack was perpetrated by an unknown assailant, or were afraid that the family would be broken up if they told the truth.

Wells does not seem to have considered the possibility that abuse by fathers and male relatives might be common. She referred to incest in a single passing sentence, including it in within a small number of sexual offences categorised as 'miscellaneous'. She explained that when it did occur, it was usually carried out by a father or a brother with the 'extent of damage ranging from that in indecent assault to pregnancy.'[21] Her assumption that most of what she saw was stranger assault and not incest would be sharply contradicted by later data from the criminal justice system and by large-scale surveys with adult survivors (many of whom would have been abused in the period that Wells was examining children).[22] It seems

[18] Henriques and Wells, 'Sexual Assaults on Children,' 1631.

[19] 'Sexual Assaults on Children,' 1633.

[20] Mathew Thomson, *Lost Freedom: The Landscape of the Child and the British Post-War Settlement* (Oxford: Oxford University Press, 2013).

[21] Henriques and Wells, 'Sexual Assaults on Children,' 1631.

[22] ONS, 'Child sexual abuse in England and Wales, year ending Mar 2019. https://www.ons.gov.uk/peoplepopulationandcommunity/crimeandjustice/articles/childsexualabuseinenglandandwales/yearendingmarch2019. Accessed 24 Sep 2024; NSPCC, 'Child sexual abuse: statistics briefing,' March 2021. https://learning.nspcc.org.uk/research-resources/statistics-briefings/child-sexual-abuse. Accessed 24 Sep 2024; Noel Smith, Cristian Dogaru,

that during Wells' career, however, the idea that these crimes were actually carried out by fathers sexually abusing their children was unthinkable and unsayable.

Her denial was accompanied by a tendency to minimise any potentially harmful effects of the abuse. Most of the cases Wells examined were for indecent assaults on children aged under seven years old. She described the effects of 'handling of "the privates,"' causing redness and irritation 'up to tearing of the hymen by insertion of the finger with resulting hamorrhage.' Because 'a fair proportion' were as a result of 'pressure with the penis against the vulva or between the legs,' she was of the opinion that there was 'only slight damage' done to the very young girls' bodies. The impact on girls aged eight to twelve years old worried her more. Although she was not explicit, she implied that this was because penetration was attempted with this age group. She thought 'there may have been much physical pain, with tearing of the hymen and haemorrhage.' She believed that this group were more likely to have been emotionally damaged too, due to threats by the perpetrator to prevent them telling anyone and to their own feelings of shame.

Girls aged eleven years or over came to her attention as 'carnal knowledge' cases. In a growing proportion of these cases, she saw the girls as 'willing partners' in the sexual encounter or that, at the very least, they had not resisted their attacker strongly enough. They were 'sexually well-developed' girls who 'could and did respond to the man's advances.' Accordingly, 'partial or full penetration with the penis' had resulted in girls contracting gonorrhoea or other venereal infections. She saw girls from lower-class families where 'broken homes' were common as particularly prone to this. Girls 'with a better upbringing and higher moral standard' might, after getting 'a big shock ... manage to let the incident quietly recede.' Hopefully, they would recover. If, on the other hand, their 'whole emotional life' was 'thrown off balance,' they were deserving of assistance and swift psychiatric help. Lower-class girls, she thought, might require a stay in a remand home.[23]

and Fiona Ellis, *Hear Me. Believe Me. Respect Me. A Survey of Adult Survivors of Child Sexual Abuse and Their Experiences of Support Services* (Suffolk: Survivors in Transition and University Campus Suffolk, 2015).

[23] Henriques and Wells, 'Sexual Assaults on Children,' 1632–1633. Obstetrician and gynaecologist Josephine Barnes agreed that the harm done to children tended to be slight as most assaults 'amount[ed] to little more than fondling or handling the victim.' Although progressive in her activism for family planning and abortion legislation, she noted that it was

These articles, one by psychiatrist Lukianowicz and the other by police surgeon Wells, were published just over ten years apart, and they demonstrate changes in how doctors and psychiatrists understood sexual violence against children. The situation in which a doctor could not fathom fathers and male relatives being responsible for sexual assaulting their children gave way to a greater willingness to acknowledge that incest was perhaps not rare. The tendency to assume that sexual assaults were not damaging to many children (depending on assumptions about age, class and agency) had shifted to some recognition of harm, at least where paternal abuse was concerned. Multiple myths about rape and abuse were contained in these articles, and class prejudice and misogyny infused the texts. Some of these stereotypes had been around for decades and cast a long shadow,[24] while others were shifting and reforming in response to cultural and social changes that came into effect from the 1960s. They would play a prominent role in the developing discourses about child sexual abuse in both medical and psychiatric academic texts as well as in practice-focused writing.

There were hints too that community health practitioners might be called upon to take some responsibility for noticing and responding to child sexual abuse in the coming decades. Wells was conscious of the limits of the professional responsibility of police surgeons. Their roles were narrowly defined; they examined those who claimed to have been assaulted. Although she believed that most children in that category (and especially those from the lower classes) were not damaged severely, she was mindful that some children might need medical or welfare support in relation to the after-effects of abuse. The watchful parent might notice symptoms of venereal disease, changes in behaviour, restlessness, irritability or sleeplessness. Ideally, they would visit their GP, but she worried that families might be reluctant to do so because the child would not have an 'actual illness.' If the GP was not the right person, who was? Someone needed to 'watch developments and give advice as and when required' but at the time there was 'no one to take an overall view of the family'; it was 'nobody's job.' Wells thought a family welfare organisation, the health visitor or perhaps a child guidance clinic might be best placed to take on that role. Ultimately,

'easy for a woman to allege that she has been raped, and frequently the story of the circumstances is fabricated by a "victim" in order to account for facts which would otherwise be awkward to explain'; Josephine Barnes, 'Forensic Medicine and Toxicology: Rape and Other Sexual Offences,' *British Medical Journal* 2, no 5547 (1967): 293, 295.

[24] Joanna Bourke, *Rape: A History from 1860 to the Present Day* (London: Virago, 2012).

the child might need to see a psychiatrist 'and this help should be given early rather than late.' In Wells' mind, these practitioners would help after the assault.

By 1972, the *BMJ* article also made a tentative step towards community-based health practitioners but now there was a sense that perhaps they could step in early to prevent the abuse. Given that 'incest families' commonly made 'heavy demands' on medical and social services, the author thought that perhaps 'the doctor or his colleagues in the community may be the first to suspect incestuous behaviour.' There might be 'some prospect of prevention' to be achieved through 'early identification of families at risk and prompt intervention.' What suspicion, prevention, early identification or prompt intervention meant was not yet defined, nor was the role doctors or their community colleagues might take. It was also predicated on a number of specific assumptions, including the idea that sexually abused children were located in families operating outside the norm, defined as 'problem' or 'needy' families. Nevertheless, as a new wave of awareness about child sexual abuse began to stir in the UK, the GP and other community-based health practitioners were identified as potentially playing an important part in prevention and early identification.

## Part 2: The Trade Press

Interviewed for *GP* newspaper in 1971, Marjorie Proops, one of Britain's most recognisable 'agony aunts,' commented that when she received 'letters from girls of twelve or thirteen saying that their father or their uncle gets into bed with them and interferes with them,' she was 'compelled' to contact the police because if she 'failed to do this and the girl came to some harm,' she would be an accessory. She explained that she had a good working relationship with the police. She would ring up and instruct them not to send 'a great big flatfoot round to such and such an address, send one of your nice lady probation officers in a miniskirt to investigate.'[25] To the contemporary ear, it might seem that Proops was deliberately seeking to engage the prurient curiosity of a majority male GP workforce, but it was more likely that her turn of phrase was meant to explain that an adolescent girl might fear an intimidating male officer and be more likely to speak out to a young woman in fashionable clothes. Although Proops' matter-of-fact tone implied that such letters were not uncommon, hers

[25] 'Dear Marjorie,' *GP*, 4 Jun 1971, 17.

was a rare mention of incest or sexual assaults on children in the 1970s trade press for doctors and community-based nurses.[26]

Physical cruelty to infants and children did feature, however, from about 1968. Stories about 'battered babies' began to appear, along with a plethora of articles about the role of doctors in relation to other social problems journalists perceived as on the rise such as sexual promiscuity, mental illness, family violence and drug use.[27] Some GPs wished to retain a strict focus on medical matters and strongly resisted the push to what was referred to 'social medicine.'[28] The Bureau of Medical Practitioner Affairs voiced concerns about the 'numbers on national assistance, broken homes, problem families and many other of the social problems that impinge on general practice.'[29] Doctors were faced with a range of non-medical issues in the surgery, including mental illness, housing, legal troubles, drug abuse, 'wife battering,' 'baby battering' and other 'social problems.' In her interview, Proops told *GP*'s readers that the '[n]umber one problem is that of contraception and pregnancy among younger and younger girls. Number two is venereal disease, which is increasing all the time to a really frightening degree.'[30]

Stories about sexually transmitted diseases became more common and were skewed towards the corruption of the very young. In April 1970, hospital consultant William Fowler's report to Birmingham's Medical Officer for Health E. L. M. Millar was headlined 'Children catching VD.' Apparently 'more and more school-age children' were being diagnosed, including those as young as eight years old. Implying that their corruption could be ascribed to racial outsiders, the article highlighted the rising

[26] Crane highlights the work of agony aunts in publishing many letters about abuse in the period from the 1990s to about 2015. Jennifer Crane, *Child Protection in England, 1960–2000: Expertise, Experience, and Emotion* (Cham, Switzerland: Palgrave Macmillan, 2018), 164–166.

[27] 'New directions in venereal disease,' *GP*, 4 Sep 1970, 3; 'Is drug abuse a symptom of emotional delinquency?' *GP*, 19 Jan 1973, 18; 'Is the British girl more permissive?' *GP*, 1 Jun 1973, 17.

[28] The term had been around since the mid-nineteenth century in reference to bringing together clinical and preventive medicine, but it had a resurgence from the late 1960s in Britain in response to what were seen as the 'new' social problems stemming out of the permissive culture of that decade. W. Hobson, 'What Is Social Medicine,' *British Medical Journal* 4619, no 2 (1949).

[29] Bureau of Medical Practitioner Affairs, 'Group practice and community medical care,' *GP*, 4 Oct 1968, 13.

[30] 'Dear Marjorie,' *GP*, 4 Jun 1971, 16.

incidence of STDs among young immigrants although a Birmingham General Hospital 'spokesman' acknowledged that this was often due to factors such as overcrowding in sub-standard conditions.[31]

Later that year, *GP* provided a synopsis of an American article about the fight against venereal diseases, reprinting the warning that 'in today's permissive society it is as easy to catch gonorrhoea as it is to catch a cold.' The *New York Times* had reported 'a bizarre case in which a five-year-old boy was found to have contracted it from a nine-year-old girl with whom he'd had intercourse.' Although only nine years old herself, the female was depicted as the corrupter of the innocent male child, and this was accentuated by the fact that she apparently 'refused to name her contacts.'[32] The phrase was suggestive of tabloid stories of high-society prostitutes who refused to hand over their little black books containing clients' names to the police. Even putting aside the gender prejudice, the implication was that children were becoming infected by having sex with each other, without any mention of the possibility that adults were involved in any way. The flavour of these stories was sensationalist, and the emphasis was on the moral decline of the young in an increasingly permissive society. GPs were called upon, often in hyperbolic language, to get involved and offer sex education advice to the young, because the GP was often 'the only one the patient can turn to'; if these children were 'refused help because of the doctor's reticence, ignorance or differing moral ideas,' it could 'lead to tragedy.'[33]

Debates about the influence of more permissive attitudes to sex on young people's behaviour and health went hand-in-hand with discussions about the effects of social change on the institution of the family. Health visitor Patricia Scowen was attached to a practice run by two male GPs in Kingston-upon-Thames in the late 1960s. She could not remember them ever talking to her about child cruelty, but they 'worried sometimes about the contraceptive pill and what it was doing to families and young people....' Contraception, abortion, divorce, 'those sorts of things .... They were middle aged, the GPs, and for them, you see, this was new and threatening, a little bit.'[34] In *GP*, Dr Adrian Rogers bemoaned the

[31] 'Children catching VD,' *GP*, 10 Apr 1970, 1.

[32] 'New Directions in Venereal Disease,' *GP*, 4 Sep 1970, 3.

[33] Nathaniel Wagner and Raymond Goodman, 'How GPs can advise young people about sex and contraception,' *GP*, 23 Aug 1974, 13.

[34] Oral history interview with Pat Scowen by author, 19 Sep 2019.

breakdown of family life exemplified by rising divorce rates, alongside an 'unprecedented rise in sexuality' creating 'a massive need for State contraception and abortion facilities.' Rogers blamed the women's rights movement for attacking the family; in his opinion 'happy families have full-time mothers.'[35] In the subsequent issue of *GP*, Dr Peter Kandala dismissed Rogers and his ilk as Luddites. Changes to the way families were formed and behaved were 'as a result of inexorable social and economic changes' and no amount of pleading could return the family to 'its former mould' simply as a result of 'the exhortations of the reformers.'[36]

It was not only the institution of the family that came in for close scrutiny. Parents were also in the spotlight. Forensic doctors had published a number of articles about 'battered babies' in *Medicine, Science and Law* in the mid-1960s, so it is perhaps unsurprising that when the first extended exploration of the topic was published in *GP* in 1968, it was the work of a professor of forensic medicine, Frances E. Camps.[37] Having examined just over eight hundred cases of parents who injured or killed their babies in an attempt to understand their 'psychopathology,' Camps developed a crude typology; those parents who deliberately murdered their child, those who inflicted 'deliberate and persistent cruelty' and those who assaulted their children on 'the spur of the moment.' He situated the escalation of 'baby battering' within the general disintegration of society, alongside increased violence amongst adults and rising rates of drug dependency.

In terms of how it should be understood, he set out a series of random anecdotes in which he assigned the blame for assaults on children primarily to mothers. He argued, for example, that in cases of marriage breakdown and child cruelty, the father might want to reconcile with his wife and, because of this, take the blame for violence against the child that had actually been carried out by her. The wife, however, would be 'unrepentant' and rarely 'admit her own guilt to save him.' Other fathers, it seemed, were driven to child abuse because of their wives' promiscuity. Camps described a father who 'absolutely adored his baby.' Left at home to look after her

[35] Adrian Rogers, 'Happy Families: the game all must play,' *Pulse*, 15 Aug 1981, 11.

[36] Peter Kandala, 'Moral code,' *Pulse*, 5 Sep 1981, 16.

[37] G E Parker, 'The Battered Child Syndrome,' *Medicine, Science and Law* 5, no 3 (1965); J. M. Cameron, H. R. Johnson, and F. E. Camps, 'The Battered Child Syndrome,' *Medicine, Science and Law*, no 6 (1966): 2–21; A. C. Fairburn a nd A. C. Hunt, 'Caffey's "Third Syndrome:" a Critical Evaluation ("the Battered Baby"),' *Medicine, Science and Law*, no 4 (1964): 123–126; Francis E. Camps, 'Battered Baby Syndrome' *GP*, 20 Sep 1968, 8–11.

while his 'not terribly faithful' wife went out with another man, he could not concentrate because 'all the time he was wondering what his wife was doing with her "boyfriend."' Unable to soothe the crying infant, he threw her into the cot. He was 'terribly sorry the next minute,' but it was too late for the baby who could not be roused the next morning and died in hospital later that day. Sending the man to prison for ten years 'for loss of self control' was not, in Camps' mind, 'the right answer.'[38] Thus, GPs were introduced to the idea that 'mother was to blame' in relation to baby battering, a notion that would loom large in theories of child sexual abuse.

In the UK, it was the NSPCC's 1969 report '78 Battered Children: A Retrospective Study' that animated debates about baby battering in the trade journals read by practitioners on the ground. The report incorporated a sense of context and the influence of wider societal factors that was in contrast to Camps' singular focus on blaming individual parents (and particularly women). The NSPCC saw the families' social worlds as important too, with 'social, biological and intrapsychic stress' creating the backdrop for violence against children. The report was not applauded in *GP*, where editorial commentary criticised the potential introduction of mandatory reporting of non-accidental injuries.[39]

Perhaps because they had worked within the hierarchical structures of the local authority for decades, health visitors were less fixated on the obligation to report. Although the NSPCC emphasised context and structural barriers, *Health Visitor* judged the report's most significant finding to be that 'battering was not confined to any one economic class, nor to the mentally ill, but was due to a defect in the parents' character.' Parents were labelled as having a 'character disorder but no definable mental illness.' The 'character disorders' were evident in their violent responses to irritation, 'stormy' personal relationships and hostility against 'those in authority,' including doctors, nurses and health visitors. Some parents were 'emotionally impoverished' and expected their babies to provide them with attention and affection. Others were 'rigid and controlling' and 'became distraught by babyish behaviour.' In other words, parental violence came out of the adults' unmet needs. They had unrealistic expectations that their dependent babies and children could fulfil those needs and were frustrated and violent to find that they could not.[40]

[38] Camps, 'Battered Baby Syndrome,' 8–11.

[39] 'Sanctions will not protect battered babies,' *GP*, 3 Oct 1969, 13.

[40] 'Battered Babies,' *Health Visitor*, 42, 10, Oct 1969, 373–374.

These findings echoed those of a group of clinicians at the University of Colorado Medical School in Denver, who would become highly influential on both sides of the Atlantic.[41] They first deployed the terminology of 'battered child syndrome' in 1962 in an article in the *Journal of the American Medical Association* (JAMA). The group—paediatricians Kempe and Henry Silver, psychiatrist Brandt Steele, obstetrician William Drogemueller and radiologist Frederic Silverman—aimed to focus medics' attention on non-accidental injuries. Kempe was a consultant at the University of Colorado Hospital in Denver and had established the National Center for the Prevention and Treatment of Child Abuse and Neglect (later renamed the Kempe Center). Since the 1940s, paediatric radiologists in the US had published occasional research showing that children's injuries were 'traumatic in origin,' and yet no one had paid much attention to their findings.[42] Kempe claimed that he had made numerous unsuccessful attempts to publicise 'child abuse, non-accidental, or inflicted injury' over the previous decade, but they did not garner attention until he consciously rebranded the phenomena with a provocative label.[43]

The NSPCC researchers' descriptions of abusive parents' characteristics and behaviours were virtually identical to those reported on by psychiatrists Steele and Carl B. Pollock in a study of sixty families they had treated in Denver. The parents demanded 'a great deal' from their babies and children, acting like 'a frightened, unloved child' and treating their own child as if 'he were an adult capable of providing comfort and love.' Indeed, there was

> a high expectation and demand by the parent for the infant's performance and a corresponding parental disregard of the infant's own needs, limited abilities, and helplessness…[44]

[41] C. Henry Kempe et al, 'The Battered-Child Syndrome,' *JAMA* 181, no 1 (1962).

[42] Parton, 'The Natural History of Child Abuse.'; Crane, *Child Protection in England*, 27–44.

[43] Kempe et al, 'The Battered-Child Syndrome.' As Crane pointed out, the x-ray was important in making injuries visible, but it also displaced the child's testimony about their injuries. Crane, *Child Protection in England*, 29.

[44] Brandt F. Steele and Carl B. Pollock, 'A Psychiatric Study of Parents Who Abuse Infants and Small Children,' in *The Battered Child*, ed. Ray E. Helfer and C. Henry Kempe (Chicago, London: University of Chicago Press, 1968), 109–110.

Camps had located physical maltreatment in families where violence and addiction proliferated, where parents were said to be of low intelligence and from the lower social classes, or in the homes of supposedly promiscuous women with illegitimate children. Both the NSPCC and the Denver group insisted that child abuse could be found across the social classes. As commentator Ian Hacking has pointed out, if maltreatment crossed all social classes,[45] it could be defined not as a 'social' problem but as a 'welfare' problem which brought it under the jurisdiction of medics who must take 'responsibility' for it. This was the view of the Denver clinicians. This is borne out by paediatrician Ray Helfer's insistence that medics must 'assume the leadership in this field.'[46]

It was perhaps unsurprising that these UK researchers echoed the Denver clinicians' findings. The NSPCC found itself on uncertain footing, referrals had decreased, casework had shifted to local authority teams and the charity's finances were in a perilous state. It was seeking to update its vision and purpose. Leading the drive to protect British 'battered babies' could re-energise the organisation.[47] The NSPCC leadership, including director Arthur Morton, assistant director Ray Castle and research unit director Joan Court, visited Denver in the mid-1960s. Kempe reciprocated, visiting the UK on a number of occasions and in 1969 he spent a sabbatical year in London with the NSPCC for research, lecturing and training. He was very impressed with the British health visiting model and tried to encourage its uptake in the US.[48]

The NSPCC invested considerable energy and resources into campaigning for the prevention of 'battering' and encouraging practitioners to respond. Court, in particular, was prolific. She wrote many articles to raise awareness in nursing, medical and social work audiences in the research unit's early years.[49] She called attention to 'battering' as 'a potentially lethal

[45] Ian Hacking, 'The Making and Moulding of Child Sexual Abuse, *Critical Inquiry* 17 (1991): 268.

[46] Ray E. Helfer, 'The Responsibility and Role of the Physician,' in *The Battered Child*, ed. Ray E. Helfer and C. Henry Kempe (Chicago, London: University of Chicago Press, 1968), 25.

[47] Parton, 'The Natural History of Child Abuse,' 438–439.

[48] Kempe and Janet Dean, another member of the Denver group, visited Aberdeen because of their interest in the potential of health visiting in preventing child abuse. Janet G. Dean et al, 'Health Visitor's Role in Prediction of Early Childhood Injuries and Failure to Thrive,' *Child Abuse & Neglect* 2, no 1 (1978).

[49] These included social work, childcare, medical, nursing and health visiting publications. See footnotes 42 and 43, 449 in Parton, 'The Natural History of Child Abuse.'

disease and a significant cause of infant deaths and morbidity in many countries.'[50] As a trained nurse, midwife, health visitor and social worker who had worked in impoverished regions of India, Turkey and the US prior to becoming the research unit director at the NSPCC, Court was a convincing advocate for children. She also had direct experience of distressing events in her own childhood. Her father had committed suicide, her mother was dependent on alcohol and she had many disruptions and dislocations as a child and adolescent. [51] The NSPCC (along with a select group of paediatricians and psychiatrists that we will return to in the next chapter) made extensive efforts to proselytise about prevention and treatment to the community health professions. But beyond their direct outreach to doctors and nurses, they influenced national policy through strong links to senior figures in the government. Court herself joined the civil service directly after leaving the NSPCC in 1972 and worked with Sir Keith Joseph on legislation related to abuse.[52] However, the practitioners to whom the NSPCC and others reached out were distracted by changes within and across their professions that deeply affected how much attention they would pay to the abused child. Next, I will consider some of these contentious issues and how they affected responses to child abuse.

## Part 3: GPs

Many GPs baulked at the idea that any 'social problems' (including 'battered babies') should become part of their core remit. Marjorie Proops denounced the attitude of 'a good many' doctors who told her they 'regard the problems people take to them as trivial.' In this context 'people' meant 'women,' and this became obvious when she went on to say that if doctors gave some time to listen to these 'allegedly trivial problems,' they would find 'far fewer neurotic middle-aged women in their waiting rooms.' GPs complained to her that they were too busy to deal with 'people with matrimonial or sexual problems,' but, Proops asked, 'where else can people go?'[53] Proops's interview was a double page spread with her photograph in a central position looking straight into the camera,

[50] Jean Renvoize, *Children in Danger: The Causes and Prevention of Baby Battering*, Third edition (Penguin Books, 1976), 40.

[51] Andrew Taylor, 'Other lives. Joan Court obituary,' *The Guardian*, 22 Dec 2016.

[52] Nigel Parton, 'Child Abuse, Social Anxiety and Welfare,' *British Journal of Social Work* 11, no 1 (1981): 394.

[53] 'Dear Marjorie,' *GP*, 4 Jun 1971, 16.

as if challenging readers. The large print caption alongside it announced that she sometimes wished she had formal qualifications to help her respond to the 500 letters she received every week, but 'her compassion and human approach, which are vital for the job, might have been lost with a formal training.' To her, 'any problem related to human happiness' was important, 'however trivial it might seem on the surface.' It was a stinging reproach to GPs.

Part of the problem was that in 1970 nine out of ten GPs were men. And although rarely made explicit, gender dynamics were at play in GPs' reluctance to take on 'social medicine.' Misogyny undoubtedly played a part. Alongside the usual physical complaints and conditions, these mainly female and/or young patients brought practical, emotional and psychological problems to the doctor's surgery. Not only were women increasingly taking up GPs' time with their 'trivial problems,' they were also infiltrating the professional world of the family doctor. The patriarchal model of general practice was under threat. By 1982, one in five GPs and forty per cent of medical students were women. It was expected that by the 1990s, over half of GPs would be women.[54] *Pulse* noted the 'sharp rise in numbers' from 2,975 women GPs in 1974 to 4,876 in 1983; in community health and medicine there were 2,228 in 1974 increasing to 3,511 in 1983.[55] Male doctors were not happy with the incursion. Dr Margaret Ghilchik, herself a rare female consultant in the male-dominated specialty of surgery, contended that 'the power in the medical profession lies in the hands of men and they are hostile to allowing women into any of the major places in our NHS structure.'[56] The picture was not very different in general practice where there were clear signs that the 'old guard' was on the defensive.

Articles claiming to celebrate a 'new breed' of young female doctors in general practice were often patronising. There was an emphasis on feminine good looks, charm and naïveté. In an article about Dr Alison Hill (whose own piece on 'Making Equality into a Reality' had appeared in *Pulse* the previous year), Nick Wood declared that 'general practice has got its pin-up girl.' He claimed to see 'fresh hope for the future of general practice in [her] enchanting eyes' due to her 'intoxicating mixture of

[54] 'What is general practice?' *Pulse*, 27 Nov 1982, 41.
[55] 'Sharp rise in number of women doctors,' *Pulse*, 31 Mar 1984, 1.
[56] Ken Cooper, 'Women doctors on march,' *Pulse*, 30 Apr 1983, 14.

girlish charm and youthful idealism.'[57] In an opinion piece debating 'A Woman's Place - Surgery or Home?' Dr Ian McKee asserted that women were exploiting 'a chink of uncertainty in our masculine armour.' He objected to 'some female agitators' who said they would 'not be happy until over fifty per cent of our medical students are female' and that 'female doctors are more sympathetic and understanding of the needs of women patients.' McKee believed that a small group practice should not be blamed for 'often [choosing] a bright young man, perhaps in preference to an even brighter young woman.' After all, the 'average woman' was a less reliable 'member of medical society than a man...She might give up her career to run coffee mornings or because of childcare or to follow her husband's career.'[58]

The increasing proportion of women GPs seemed a positive move towards greater equality, but conditions worsened in some ways as more women entered general practice. For example, the women GPs working in the early 1970s were likely to be unrestricted principals,[59] but by 1983 about sixty per cent of women were in non-career posts as assistants in general practice or community health.[60] And like the health visitors and other community nursing 'ancillaries,' the female GP was often referred all the 'lady' problems. Health visitor Jane Bramwell worked out of a group practice in the early 1970s where there were four GPs. She remembered, 'I worked mainly with the young female GP. That's very traditional, isn't it, but she was the one who ran the baby clinic and so on.'[61]

Judith Trowell's experience was similar. She had left paediatrics to have her first child. She could not return while her baby was young as the shift patterns were unmanageable so she briefly worked part time as a medical officer doing infant welfare clinics and school medicals, which she found boring. In 1967, she joined a GP practice as a salaried partner where she worked for four half-days each week. It felt absurd to refer children to hospital for the procedures she had done herself as a highly skilled hospital paediatrician. But the main frustration was that she was the only woman working alongside five male GPs and they referred all the 'women's problems' to her. She had seriously considered specialising in psychiatry during

[57] Nick Wood, 'A political heart's delight,' *Pulse*, 14 Mar 1981, 13.
[58] Ian McKee, 'A Woman's Place - surgery or home?' *Pulse*, 9 Aug 1980, 9.
[59] 'Making equality into a reality,' *Pulse*, 19 Apr 1980, 22.
[60] 'Sharp rise in number of women doctors,' *Pulse*, 31 Mar 1984, 1.
[61] Oral history interview with Jane Bramwell by author, 4 Jul 2019.

her clinical training. After five years working part time as a GP and feeling that she 'couldn't cope with… peering up numerous vaginas and doing smears and doing all the other things that you had to do for gynae problems or unhappy women,' she left to begin training in psychiatry.[62]

GPs' reluctance to practise 'social medicine' extended to the 'battered baby syndrome.' In Camps' 1968 article, he concluded that doctors were just too nice; they didn't 'like to think the worst of anybody' and they could not believe that anyone could 'be so cruel to a small child.' This was especially the case, he thought, when you had 'a sweet young mother and the suggestibility of the average young [presumably male] doctor.'[63] Other reasons cited in the trade press as to why doctors did not often detect abuse included a fear of breaching the duty of confidentiality to the patient,[64] *GP* wondered whether an alternative process they used in the Netherlands might be a solution; doctors could report to a 'go-between' doctor rather than directly to social services or the police.[65] There was a specific anxiety too that other professionals could not be trusted with sensitive information about 'their' patient.[66] The latter, of course, could also be described as a fear of 'losing control' once they had shared information or referred them on.

Despite doctors' reluctance to identify child abuse, the Standing Medical Advisory Committee of the Central Health Service Council issued a memo to all GPs, paediatricians and relevant hospital doctors in 1970. It also went to the soon-to-be extinct Medical Officers of Health (MOH) and Children's Officers (CO) who were employed by local authorities. It described 'battered baby syndrome' and what action should be taken. Medics should consult with the local MOH and the CO before considering a case complete.[67] But it was the Inquiry into the murder of seven-year-old Maria Colwell by her stepfather in 1973 that really stimulated

[62] Oral history interview with Judith Trowell by author, 20 Apr 2021.

[63] Francis E. Camps, 'Battered Baby Syndrome,' *GP*, 20 Sep 1968, 1–2.

[64] The Association of Directors of Social Services claimed that doctors were afraid to breach confidentiality and therefore would not come forward; it wanted 'at risk' registers to have 'legislative backing with proper protection for informants.' Vivien Goldsmith, 'Loopholes appear in the Children Bill,' *GP*, 30 May 1975, 5.

[65] '"Go-Betweens" to fight child abuse,' *GP*, 1 Oct 1976, 8.

[66] A study at King's College Hospital showed that hospitals were also missing cases: eighteen out of 100 cases reviewed were likely to have been child abuse. Graham Jackson, 'Child Abuse Syndrome: The Cases We Miss,' *British Medical Journal* 2, no 5816 (1972).

[67] The NHS reorganisation of 1973–1974 led to the abolition of the MOH role. 'Battered Baby Syndrome Memo to GPs' *GP*, 7 Aug 1970, 1.

action. The report recommended a two-way flow of information between health and social services.[68] To support this, peers approved an amendment to the 1975 Children Bill to ensure that 'medical authorities' were notified when children were subject to court orders in care proceedings. The GP was seen as an essential figure who, along with the teacher and the police officer, 'shall be aware when a child or young person is at risk in this way.'[69]

By 1975, many local authorities had registers holding details of children known or suspected of being 'battered' by their parents. Some areas, such as Cambridgeshire, were proactively encouraging local residents to contact social services or the police 'if they fear a child is at risk.'[70] By the following year, 83 of 102 Area Review Committees had established child abuse registers and the Social Services Secretary Barbara Castle urged the remaining Area Health Authorities to do so.[71] When the Department of Health issued a circular requiring each area to set up 'at risk' registers in 1980, it did not meet with criticism in the GPs' trade press, perhaps indicating increasing acceptance by doctors of the need to participate in arrangements to protect children. The Association of Metropolitan Authorities (precursor to the Local Government Association) reassured readers that doctors were co-operative and that only 'diehards will complain.'[72]

The NSPCC's '78 Battered Children' report had appeared on the front pages of both *Health Visitor* and *GP*, but *GP's* commentary was defensive from the outset, leading with the news that 'general practitioners may be forced into reporting cases involving children who have been injured by "other than accidental means" to a designated child protective service.'[73] In October, their preoccupation with mandatory reporting was evident from the headline 'Sanctions will not protect battered babies.' NSPCC researchers had concluded that the medical profession was reluctant 'to

[68] 'Report of the Committee of Inquiry into the Care and Supervision Provided in Relation to Maria Colwell,' (London: HMSO, 1974).

[69] 'Children at risk will be known to GPs,' *GP*, 14 Mar 1975, 5.

[70] 'Child register scheme,' *GP*, 26 Sep 1975, 4.

[71] 'AHA child abuse registers urged,' *GP*, 13 Feb 1976, 3.

[72] Alison Hyde, 'Register on child abuse criticised,' *Pulse*, 8 Mar 1980, 52.

[73] 'Battered Baby Law Change,' *GP*, 19 Sep 1969, 1. *Health Visitor* had only mentioned the reporting recommendation briefly, noting the 'grave risk' that the relationship with the family would be damaged if 'notification' was required. 'Battered Babies,' *Health Visitor*, 42, 10 (10 Oct 1969): 373–374.

initiate measures to protect the child and treat the child batterers.' GPs Norell and Ashworth in Islington and Widnes respectively shifted responsibility away from general practice, claiming that they had only had 'two known cases in our practice in the past ten years' and that it was 'really a problem that confronts casualty officers and paediatricians.' The GP should not have to report, according to Ashworth, as it would further damage 'the already deteriorating patient/ doctor relationship.' Perhaps if a hospital consultant was 'only suspicious,' he could send a confidential letter asking the GP to 'keep an eye on the child.' This seemed to imply (somewhat paradoxically) that if oversight of the family could be enacted in a furtive manner, the trusting doctor/patient relationship would not be breached.[74]

Camden-based GP Dr Donald Grant disagreed with Norell and Ashworth, noting that there were 'two patients to be considered' and that when 'somebody comes to you for advice about a baby it is the baby in essence who is the patient, although somebody else is complaining for it.… The patient who most needs your help at that moment … is the baby.'[75] The author admitted that those 'required to treat or assist the families of battered children' (medics, lawyers, social workers and nurses) should be given information to assist with early identification and should be educated 'in a more understanding approach to problems of stress and crisis in people with character disorders.' But they were strongly against any plans to introduce a duty to report child abuse and their resistance did not break down swiftly.[76]

Just over ten years later, the dramatic headline, 'Doctors as "Informers" in Child Neglect Cases' demonstrated that the notion of 'professional secrecy' had not gone away. An 1899 law had stated that if a parent neglected a child and caused them 'suffering' or 'ill health,' they were guilty of 'wilful neglect.' The Lords of Appeal overturned that, ruling that parents who were 'feckless' and failed to obtain medical attention for their

[74] This behind-the-scenes information-sharing about families where there were suspicions of abuse is hard to document historically. But in a similar vein, Scowen recalled that she and other health visitors used to vet people who had applied to be registered childminders. If they were worried about the person's suitability, they checked with the local NSPCC Inspector. They could then reject the applicant, noting 'I cannot recommend this person to be a childminder… known to Inspector Buchanan.' Interview with Scowen.

[75] 'Sanctions will not protect battered babies,' *GP*, 3 Oct 1969, 12–13.

[76] Ibid.

child through 'ignorance' or a 'lack of intelligence,' might not be guilty of neglect. The *Pulse* commentator feared that doctors would have to assess how obvious a child's symptoms were and whether parents had deliberately or recklessly ignored them. Ultimately, they might have to 'inform' on the parents to social services and/or the police.[77]

The situation did not change quickly. Even in the mid-1990s, research on child protection cases found that doctors were reluctant to disclose concerns about child abuse to other practitioners for fear of damaging their relationship with their (adult) patients.[78] Jane Hutcheson recalled working in Manchester when she qualified as a health visitor in 1991 where rather than being seen as a referral that would protect a child, it was considered 'terribly serious to "report" a child or family.' 'Plus,' Hutcheson remembered, 'if a doctor said "there was no abuse," then that was it, there was no abuse.'[79]

The NSPCC regularly raised concerns about the persistently low rates of GP referrals, querying whether doctors were failing to identify children or were reluctant to make referrals when they spotted abuse.[80] When former GP Dr Alan Gilmour took up the role of Director of the NSPCC in 1981, he went on the offensive. Interviewed in *Pulse*, he took aim at GPs whom he believed 'may be among [his] worst enemies in identifying and tackling the problem of child abuse.' He claimed that they were often 'prepared to turn a blind eye to the causes when faced with a child with obvious symptoms of physical abuse.' Worse still, he accused some GPs of 'suffer[ing] from … the Goldilocks syndrome…Too often they have the attitude—who's been seeing my patient? They won't talk to social workers about a patient and they won't come to a case conference.'[81]

Two weeks after the Gilmour interview, an anonymous GP responded in *Pulse*. He believed that many of the increasing number of case conferences called by social services 'served no useful purpose' and that the presence at these meetings of 'non-professionals like home helps, housing welfare officers and on occasions the police,' meant that he could not share the information he held, which was 'too confidential to broadcast to

[77] 'Doctors as 'informers' in child neglect cases,' *Pulse*, 13 Dec 1980, 2.
[78] Corinne Wattam, *Making a Case in Child Protection* (Longman Group UK, 1992), 7.
[79] Oral history interview with Jane Hutcheson by author, 7 Jan 2019.
[80] 'Battered Babies,' *Health Visitor*, 46, 7 (Jul 1973): 243.
[81] Andrew Lycett, 'Ex-GP brings child abuse from shadows,' *Pulse*, 6 Jun 1981, 29.

such a large [and one might assume from the phrase "non-professionals," low status] audience.' Articles appeared fairly regularly judging case conferences to be futile, unnecessarily bureaucratic and a waste of the GP's precious time.[82]

Nevertheless, the case conference was emerging as the setting for important discussions about protecting children, and doctors often wanted to have the last say on decisions about a child's welfare. Indeed, some doctors claimed that was what the other attendees expected of them. A Yorkshire paediatrician remarked that he was

> relied upon to make the decisions. If I say 'yes, abuse' then it all follows on and if I say 'no' then there is often relief. I don't want to sound vain, but I do find I often lead them. They look to me to arbitrate and make the decision.[83]

As social worker Olive Stevenson observed, many doctors considered themselves to be the 'top dogs' trained to 'exercise authority' even in 'matters which have little to do with medicine.'[84] But their position was eroding as child protection procedures were formalised. Leadership and decision making gradually shifted to social services. Perhaps as a consequence of their declining power and/or the common opinion that the meetings 'served no useful purpose,' group practices made up primarily of men (as most still were) increasingly tended to 'delegate' responsibility for child protection to female GPs, along with other problems seen to affect primarily women and children. Trowell recalled that when child abuse cases came up in her practice, she was put forward to deal with them and go to the case conference: 'the men didn't want to go so I went to all of them.'[85]

[82] 'Can all this hot air save lives?' *Pulse*, 26 Jun 1981, 27. See also 'Give up on the case conference,' *Pulse*, 5 Sep 1981, 27; 'Case conferences face boycott,' *Pulse*, 23 Jul 1983, 2.

[83] Interview with Dr Brown,* paediatrician, Barnsley General Hospital, 19 Oct 1979, GC/225 Professor Robert Dingwall, ESRC QUALIDATA Study: 'The Protection of Children,' Wellcome.

[84] Olive Stevenson, ed. *Child Abuse: Public Policy and Professional Practice* (Herts: Harvester Wheatsheaf, 1989), 185–187. Another example of the gender dynamics comes from Constance Lee and Bill Roberts, Newcastle Polytechnic, who note that the 'health visitor, accustomed to regarding doctors as her professional superiors, might find it difficult to differ with a doctor over the judgement of a risk situation,' in Vida Carver, ed. *Child Abuse: A Study Text* (Milton Keynes and New York: The Open University Press, 1978), 85.

[85] Interview with Trowell.

## Part 4: Health Visitors

Concerns about social issues such as addiction, promiscuity and mental health played out in *Health Visitor* just as they had in the GP trade press.[86] As we will see below, it would be wrong to suggest that health visitors were in complete accord about their role in relation to personal welfare matters. But they did not disown these issues as beyond the scope of their profession. Most accepted that social problems fell within their remit. Their core functions were to do with prevention, early detection and identification of mental, physical and emotional ill-health. But they were divided in terms of how exactly to prioritise which families to serve and where they should sit in the structures of health and social care. They were aware that there were seismic changes afoot in health and local authority structures and delivery models. The health visitor was perched unobtrusively at the centre of them, often feeling overlooked by the 'changemakers' yet vulnerable to the changes that were coming. Nursing management structures, nursing education, child welfare centres, GP attachment, integration between community, school and hospital—all affected the health visitor.[87] The Seebohm report (1968) and its proposed structural changes would create major upheaval for health visitors and a heightened sense of insecurity in terms of their relationship to a new breed of social workers.[88]

Some GPs were of the view that perhaps health visiting was becoming obsolete.[89] Improvements in home hygiene, health education and the administration of childhood immunisations meant that preventing infectious diseases was no longer the mainstay of the role. Health visitors had previously delivered a 'life-saving service' fighting diseases like tuberculosis; now there was palpable anxiety as to whether they were redundant. In 1965, the Sheldon Committee began a review of the medical functions and staffing of Child Welfare Centres in England and Wales. These were

[86] 'Fighting Addiction,' 'Mental Health – The New Crusade,' *Health Visitor*, 41, 11 (Nov 1968): 486, 512; 'Smoking, VD and Drugs,' *Health Visitor,* 42, 8 (Aug 1969): 320–21.

[87] 'Working Party on Management Structure in the Local Authority Nursing Services,' (London: DHSS, 1969); 'Report of the Committee on Nursing. Chairman: Professor Asa Briggs', (London: HMSO, 1972); 'Child Welfare Centres: Report of the Subcommittee,' Ministry of Health and the Central Health Services Council Standing Medical Advisory Committee (London: HMSO, 1967); S. D. M. Court, 'Fit for the Future: The Report of the Committee on Child Health Services,' (London: HMSO, 1976).

[88] Audrey Leathard, *Health Care Provision: Past, Present and into the 21st Century*, Second edition ed. (Stanley Thornes, 2000), 1, 10, 22, 30.

[89] J. C. Arthur, 'A possible "new look,"' *Health Visitor,* 40, 12 (Dec 1968).

the buildings where community doctors and health visitors worked under the direction of their local Medical Officer of Health (MOH). Mothers brought babies to be weighed and health visitors could monitor risk of malnutrition, infection and poor hygiene. They sold baby milk and food. They provided advice and health education (often through ante-natal, post-natal and 'mothercraft' classes). Health visitors also used the buildings as a base for home visiting families across their 'patch,' an assigned geographical footprint. Local authorities were responsible for the centres, most of which were delivered from church and community halls.[90]

Responses to the review highlighted competition between the MOHs and GPs over the territory of the child and family and how services to them should be provided, with health visitors situated as a pawn between them. The Society of Medical Officers of Health wanted the centres (and their own positions at the helm) to be maintained and foresaw them playing an important role in tackling the 'problems of family relationships' and the 'disturbed behaviour of the pre-school child.' With the right training, medical staff in the centres could identify difficulties and prevent family break up. The health visitor in particular had 'a unique opportunity to observe any signs of stress.' The Sheldon Committee ultimately wanted such services delivered by family doctors in group practices operating out of purpose-built health centres.

At the beginning of the 1960s, sixty per cent of GPs worked alone. By 1980, that had decreased to fourteen per cent. Nearly seventy per cent had shifted into practices of three to six GPs.[91] The government was encouraging them to move in this direction, but many had already voluntarily joined other colleagues in shared premises, having seen some advantages in coming together. They could reduce excessive workloads, obtain more modern premises and individual GPs would have more opportunities to develop their special interests.[92] For the GP who saw the benefits of working more closely with a range of professionals with diverse skills (or put more cynically, the GP who did not want to dedicate himself to 'social medicine'), the group practice was an environment that could expand

[90] Health centres (though far fewer in number) had also been established through the National Health Act 1946; providing medical, dental and pharmaceutical services. A. D. Law, 'Welfare Centres and the Sheldon Report,' *Health Visitor*, 41, 6 (Jun, 1968), 276–280.

[91] 'Pulse Reference: The growth of group practice,' *Pulse*, 27 Nov 1982, 39–43.

[92] 'Changing role of the family doctor,' *GP*, 2 Aug 1968, 1–2.

beyond doctors. Health visitors, district nurses, midwives and other staff were encouraged to co-locate,[93] and by 1969, there were over 2,300 so-called 'ancillaries' attached to practices.[94]

The advantages of this arrangement for the GP were frequently repeated in the trade press.[95] Doctors, according to an anonymous GP, were in business with 'a commodity to sell to the public, and that consists of his expert advice.' Rather than being valued and respected like 'all other highly trained professional men,' they were instead 'required to fritter away' their valuable time on 'trivialities and tiresome repetitive para-medical activities of the sort that could be performed by a clerk or other ancillary worker.'[96] Based in the group practice, nurses and health visitors could undertake a range of functions that did not require medical expertise but would otherwise fall to the GP.[97] They were promoted as 'often far better able to deal with medico-social problems than is the doctor himself.'[98]

While doctors were quick to point out the benefits of the proposed co-location, not all health visitors shared their enthusiasm. Some were reluctant to lose their professional independence and feared being at the local GP's beck and call. Many had not up to that point had much contact with GPs and felt that they looked down on the local authority health services. Xavier recalled that in Leeds in the late 1960s, the health visitors

> had no communication with the GPs, none whatsoever, it was as if they were against us and we were against them… They did their own thing and I think they really rather denigrated the—the clinic. They'd rather their patients came to them for their immunisations and this, that and the other.[99]

What Xavier highlighted was that some GPs did not value public health work or those who practised it, which is one reason health visitors worried about being expected to defer to their authority. If their work was not respected, they might be expected to do menial tasks for the doctors. An article in *GP* seemed to reinforce this. It scolded doctors, instructing them

[93] Ibid.
[94] Eileen Forgacs, 'The visitor who's coming to stay,' *GP*, 6 Jun 1969, 6.
[95] I. A. McDougall, 'Community medical care,' *GP*, 16 Aug 1968.
[96] 'Return to Sanity,' *GP*, 26 Feb 1968, 7–8.
[97] 'Group practice and community medical care,' *GP*, 10 Apr 1968, 16.
[98] McDougall, 'Community medical care.'
[99] Oral history interview with Jennifer Xavier by author, 2 Aug 2019.

that the health visitor 'cannot, should not and must not be thought of or used as a secretary, chaperone, telephonist, receptionist, or filing clerk.'[100] Many health visitors felt this was exactly how they would be used if they were transferred from their specific geographical 'patch' and instead 'attached' to the local GP practice. There were practical considerations too. GP patients could be spread across a wide geographical area. The health visitor would have to travel further and might struggle to build and sustain relationships with families.

Health visitors' main concern was the loss of their autonomy. Scowen remembered the imposing figure of the MOH who 'ruled the community health services' in the outer London borough where she worked; she did not have much contact with him. 'He was in Tolworth Tower which was a huge tower block and he had a whole floor [laughs] and that's where the bosses were,' she recalled.[101] She and her colleagues operated at quite a remove from the MOH and often from his assistants as well. They had a great deal of control over their caseload, their daily activities and decision-making. The debate persisted into the 1980s with a significant number of health visitors reluctant to surrender that professional autonomy to GPs.[102] The push to convince GPs that preventive medicine should be a priority was also galling, particularly when the Royal College of General Practitioners suggested that the doctor should plan and coordinate this work, delegating its tasks to health visitors: 'a profession which has been practising preventive healthcare in their own right for over a hundred years.'[103]

Policy makers positioned the health visitor as well placed to notice potential problems in families. Those 'attached' to GP practices could have a crucial role in 'detecting' physical, mental and emotional 'defects' at the earliest opportunity. Parent counselling, health education and registering 'handicapped' children would be key functions.[104] They could be on the alert to potential mental health problems. As consultant psychiatrist, Dr S. Horsley, noted in *Medical Officer*, the health visitor was the

[100] C. D. Baker, 'General practice and ancillaries,' GP, 19 Apr 1968, 10.

[101] Interview with Scowen.

[102] See *Health Visitor*, 41, 3 (Mar 1968); 41, 6 (Jun 1968); 42, 3 (Mar 1969); 47, 8 (Aug 1974); 52, 8 (Aug 1979).

[103] Royal College of General Practitioners, 'Health and Prevention in Primary Care,' 1981; 'General Practitioners and Prevention,' *Health Visitor*, 54, 3 (Mar 1981): 81; 'HVA Policy on Health Surveillance,' *Health Visitor*, 58, 3 (Mar 1985): 81.

[104] 'Children's Health' *Health Visitor*, 41, 2 (Feb 1968): 57.

'only person in the right place at the right time to spot hazards in the family before these have led to psychiatric changes in young children.'[105] But once they had 'detected' difficulties, what was their role? In many areas, the health visitors reporting to the MOH had a track record of working with local families of concern in conjunction with other personal social services departments (such as Children's, Welfare, Education, Housing), as well as with voluntary organisations. As early as 1954, the Ministry of Health had issued a circular pointing to the health visitor as the 'official best suited to identify and intervene in "problem families."'[106]

But not all health visitors believed this should be their central purpose. Just before Christmas 1967, Evelyn Leahy, Superintendent of Health Visiting in Northampton, was incensed enough to take time out from her holiday preparations to write a letter to her trade journal. She was unhappy with the way the BBC Light radio programme, 'The Dales,' had portrayed her profession in a recent episode. She felt that by creating a fictional portrait of a health visitor as a 'Welfare Worker,' the BBC confirmed a misconception held by the public. In her view, the health visitor was 'not … primarily concerned with needy people, or people in distress, but with people living their ordinary everyday lives.' The role was to provide 'expert advice' on family matters from baby feeding to 'social problems.'[107] In the case of complex social needs, the health visitor would refer the family on to a caseworker in another agency.

Leahy's letter appeared in the Feb 1968 edition of the journal and provoked a debate in its pages. Tutor Margaret Willis felt that the health visitor's remit should include advice and education, but she believed that care for the 'needy' or 'distressed' should be a central aim. It was essential because of the high morbidity and mortality rates of illegitimate babies, the large proportion of babies injured in home accidents and the growing concern caused by 'battered baby syndrome.' The health visitor could also help with 'primary prevention of mental disorder' for children.[108]

In situating health visiting as a service for the 'normal' rather than the 'needy,' Leahy might be seen to represent the 'old guard,' clinging to an

[105] 'Letter to the editor,' *Health Visitor*, 41, 2 (Feb 1968): 89, 91, 93.

[106] 'Health of Children: Prevention of Break-up of Families,' (Ministry of Health, 1954); Michael Lambert, '"Problem Families" and the Post-War Welfare State in the North West of England, 1943–74; Volume One' (Lancaster University, 2017), 72; See also Crane, *Child Protection in England*, 36.

[107] Letter to the editor, *Health Visitor*, 41, 2 (Feb 1968): 91.

[108] Letter to the editor, *Health Visitor*, 41, 2 (Feb 1968): 89, 91, 93.

increasingly outdated notion of the profession's core practice. This was not strictly the case. The push and pull between 'needy' families and more universal prevention and advice work had been a perennial tension growing out of health visiting's roots in two mid-nineteenth century developments. The first was the 'lady-visitor' who dispensed charity and advice to poor families in their homes (serving the needy).[109] The second came out of the Manchester and Salford Ladies' Sanitary Reform Association (later Ladies' Health Society) formed in 1860, which was much more focused on advice about child-rearing and the cleanliness of the home (to those living their 'ordinary everyday lives').[110]

Structural changes in the NHS and local authorities also brought a new interprofessional tension—this time between health visitors and social workers. The Seebohm Committee's 1968 recommendations that there should be 'one door on which to knock' meant the creation of new Social Service Departments that would deal with local families and communities and which replaced local authority children's departments, home help, mental health and social work.[111] The idea of the 'one door' may have made a great deal of sense for families and communities, but it was an irritating metaphor for health visitors who believed they were often 'the only person with knowledge of existing family problems' as well as being 'the most constant visitor to the home.'[112] Some felt this was not appreciated in the Seebohm discussions and subsequent recommendations. These would group all of the relevant local authority social services together, but the health visitor would be transferred into the health authority thus creating a new and 'potentially divisive boundary line' between health services in the NHS and community-based social care under local government.[113]

Health visitors felt undervalued and excluded by this decision. They wanted to continue in 'prolonged supportive roles to families in need.'[114] While Leahy preferred to concentrate on giving 'expert advice,' passing

[109] Jennifer Smith, 'Illustrations from the Wellcome Institute Library: The Archive of the Health Visitors' Association in the Contemporary Medical Archives Centre,' *Medical History* 39, no 3 (July 1995): 358–360.

[110] Robert Dingwall, "In the Beginning Was the Work:' Reflections on the Genesis of Occupations,' *The Sociological Review* 31, no 4 (1983): 605–624.

[111] David Gladstone, ed. *British Social Welfare: Past, Present and Future* (London: UCL Press, 1995), 196.

[112] Book Review, *Health Visitor*, 41, 9 (Sep 1968): 413.

[113] Leathard, *Health Care Provision: Past, Present and into the 21st Century*, 1, 10, 22, 30.

[114] *Health Visitor*, 45, 12 (Dec 1972): 391.

the more needy families on to local authority children's officers or charities like the NSPCC or Family Service Unit (FSU), other health visitors were involved in ongoing support work to 'problem families.'[115] Health visitor research published in 1968 divided 'problem family' work into those affected by problems such as physical and mental illnesses, 'subnormality' and marital breakdown as well as those whose 'personal features' might 'cause instability.' This included, for example, poor housing, difficulty making friends, poverty, an unhygienic home, little education or an 'inadequate personality,' excessive drinking, gambling, being unreconciled to having a 'handicapped' child or difficulties in managing their children's behaviour. There might be 'language difficulties' in the family (presumably a coded reference to immigrants and race, neither of which were mentioned directly).[116] In Birmingham, Mrs. Whitehouse, centre superintendent at Nechells Green Health Centre, included the health visitor under the broad definition of 'social worker' alongside 'other social workers attending the centre.' For her, the category incorporated the children's officer and 'all the social workers who are also interested in [the health visitor's] cases' as well as the school welfare officers, the NSPCC inspector and the Mental Health officer. She believed that a primary objective of health visiting was dealing with 'social problems, the unmarried girls, the old people, the neglected child, the post-surgery cases,' and called for 'recognition of the social work content of our job.'[117]

Other health visitors had more practical grievances about the new definitions of who was in fact a 'social worker.' I. R. Dorset from Hertfordshire knew of health visitors who were failing to obtain posts as social workers because they didn't have the Social Workers' Certificate. Dorset

[115] Pat Starkey highlighted the 'problem family' work, or as the pro-eugenic MOH called it, 'medico-social work,' done by health visitors in Bristol from the late 1940s. She noted support to 'so-called problem families had moved from the orbit of MOHs to that of Children's Officers' much earlier than Seebohm due to the increased powers given to the latter via the 1963 Children Act. Despite that, the nature and number of problem families that health visitors worked with continued to grow, with immigrant families and those affected by parental mental health problems increasingly stigmatised as 'problem families' in the 1960s. Pat Starkey, 'The Medical Officer of Health, the Social Worker, and the Problem Family, 1943 to 1968: The Case of Family Service Units,' *Social History of Medicine* 11, no 3 (1998): 439–440.

[116] The pilot study was supported by the Christian Economic and Social Research Foundation who also published the report 'Families with Problems' (1968). H. D. Chalke, 'Social Enquiry - A New Look?' *Health Visitor,* 41, 7 (Jul 1968), 325.

[117] 'Nechells Green Health Centre,' *Health Visitor,* 41, 3 (March 1968): 132–133.

complained that 'some Medical Officers of Health recognize us as Social Workers, but Social Workers do not accept us as their equals.' She believed that the aim of social workers and health visitors was the same:

> to assist those who are unable to cope on their own with their problems, to encourage parents to bring up their children in a congenial and settled environment, so that they in turn will grow up to become stable parents, able to manage the problems of everyday life.

She was interested in the views of other health visitors on 'what we can do to let authorities know that we are highly trained professional women.'[118] It was a sentiment echoed by columnist 'Iduna' who asked the readership whether they had spent four or five years training only to be 'regarded—and paid—as a second-class social worker.' 'Iduna' suggested that the profession should use the Association to emphasise 'that we want proper definition and recognition of the social work content of our job.'[119]

Although the aim of Seebohm was to 'secure an effective family service,' once the new social services departments were activated, the emphasis shifted from family to community and 'the child was virtually subsumed.'[120] The Health Visitor Association was one of the few professional associations to object to the Seebohm recommendations, advocating instead for Family Health and Welfare departments. Health visitors 'remain[ed] firmly convinced of the impossibility of divorcing personal health and personal welfare.'[121] By 1972, the Association shifted its stance to a 'glass half full' position in relation to what was anyway a foregone conclusion. At the AGM, the Honorary Secretary voiced her hope that once Social Services departments were fully established,

> the health visitor would be freed from some social work functions to concentrate on health visiting… early detection and prevention of physical and psychological disorder, support to the family and group and health teaching.[122]

[118] 'Letters to the Editor,' *Health Visitor*, 41, 8 (Aug 1968): 366.

[119] 'Definitions,' *Health Visitor*, 47, 8 (Aug 1974): 253.

[120] Baroness Brooke of Ystradfellte, speech to House of Lords, 29 Jan 1969. Parliamentary Debates, Lords, vol 298 (1969), col 1168; Harry D. Hendrick, *Child Welfare: England: 1872–1989* (London: Routledge, 1994), 236.

[121] 'The Seebohm Report.' *Health Visitor*, 42, 1 (Jan 1969): 7.

[122] 'Hon Secretary's report to AGM,' *Health Visitor*, 45, 8 (Aug 1972): 260.

Columnist 'Iduna,' who had lobbied for recognition of the social work content of the job, now argued that health visiting was 'about routine visiting of normal families… prevention. I don't believe it is primarily about handicapped children, child abuse, or urgent referrals from GPs or hospitals.'[123] A 1978 editorial noted that 'health visitors can do social work but that social workers cannot do health visiting. If this is true, shouldn't we be doing health visiting with all our families and not just social work with some of them.'[124] Clearly there was a fear that preventative work would become unachievable in the face of intensive support to the 'needy,' which included disabled children and child abuse.

These debates insinuated themselves into discussions about 'battered babies'. When Marjorie Turner, Chief Nurse in the London Borough of Ealing and a trained health visitor, set up the first UK conference on 'battered babies' in 1973, she emphasised the preventative aspect of the health visitor and her potential as 'the antennae of the caring professions.' With her access to the family home, she could be an asset in 'identifying the signs, detecting the flaws' and referring families on to others for whatever specialist help was required.[125] The metaphor was apt. After all, antennae are the main sense organs of most insects. The image conjures up some sense of the degree to which health visitors were to attune themselves to the families they visited. It also connects to ideas of surveillance with all the implications of state supervision and intrusion. The health visitor could also listen in, as the minority report from the Maria Colwell Inquiry stated, 'Few people hear more than a health visitor!'[126] It was something that worried health visitors: as they told researchers in 1987, they sometimes felt more like 'health police' engaged in 'checking up' or 'spying on families.'[127] Despite attempts at clarity about the differences in the roles of

[123]'Health Visiting in the Seventies,' *Health Visitor*, 48, 11 (Nov 1975): 428. The arguments about the respective roles of health visitors and social workers continued into the 1980s, for example, there was little agreement between the HVA and the British Association of Social Workers on key working, confidentiality, or court appearances at a joint meeting in 1980 and no firm date was made to reconvene. 'Association News' *Health Visitor* 53, 12 (Dec 1980): 539.

[124]*Health Visitor*, 41, 12 (Dec 1978): 461.

[125]*The Ealing Battered Baby Conference: Proceedings of a One Day Conference Organised by the Health Department of the London Borough of Ealing*, (London: Edsall and Co. Ltd., 1975).

[126]Cited in Department of Health and Social Security, *Child Abuse: A Study of Inquiry Reports 1973–1981* (London: HMSO, 1982), 15.

[127]Steve Taylor and Debby James, 'Children at risk: the changing role of the health visitor,' *Health Visitor*, 60, 10 (Oct 1987): 330.

health visiting and social work, the lines remained blurred, particularly in relation to who would be the 'keyworker' liaising with or watching over the abused child and their family.[128]

## Part 5: 'Deal with it'

As noted above, the traditional 'story' told about the 1980s is that from its earliest days, British practitioners were 'flooded' with information about child sexual abuse which had replaced other forms of abuse in terms of awareness raising. The reality was less clear cut. Although information about child sexual abuse began to circulate through books and articles, items about other forms of maltreatment also continued to be published in the trade press. This section of the chapter looks at the legacy of earlier misogynistic representations of sexual violence against women and girls which lingered in the trade press (seduction, mendacity and false accusations), and how the 'new' problem of child sexual abuse was presented to health practitioners.

While training as a health visitor in 1980, Gill Abramovich bought a book called *Child Abuse* by Ruth and Henry Kempe. She remembered the 'horrible picture ... the picture on the front is quite distressing. You don't particularly want to open the page and go there.'[129] The cover was monochromatic with a photograph of a young boy with severe facial bruising. The only colour came from a stark red banner across the bottom on which was printed in capitals: 'THIS YEAR 2 CHILDREN A WEEK WILL DIE AT THEIR PARENTS' HANDS—NSPCC REPORT.' The book described different types of abuse, including 'incest.' It reached many British practitioners, and its language became familiar to the wider public. It was reviewed in *The Guardian* and *The Daily Mail.* Psychiatrist, psychoanalyst and frequent media commentator Anthony Storr provided a recommendation on the cover, noting that the book would be useful to 'physicians, social workers, health visitors as well as intelligent mothers.' Although Abramovich didn't want to 'go there,' many practitioners did

[128] 'BASW/HVA Joint Statement: The Role of the Health Visitor in Child Abuse,' (London: Health Visitors' Association, 1982); Health Visitors Association 'BASW policy on child abuse,' *Health Visitor,* 59, 1 (Jan 1986): 8.

[129] Oral history interview Gill Abramovich with author, 22 May 2019.

read the Kempes' thinking on how practitioners could contribute to prevention, prediction and treatment.[130]

*Child Abuse* was published in 1978.[131] By then, Ruth and Henry Kempe had been married and working as a team for thirty years, having met whilst training as doctors at Yale University. Ruth was an Associate Professor of Paediatrics and Psychiatry at the University of Colorado and one of the founding members of the multidisciplinary child protection team established in the late 1950s at what was then called Colorado General Hospital.[132] That same year, Henry Kempe gave a rousing speech at the Second International Congress of Child Abuse and Neglect in London. He told the audience that sexual abuse was 'as numerous and, in many ways, as serious as physical abuse' and denounced the complacency of those who denied its harmful effects for they 'fail to take into account the enormous emotional costs paid by many of these children and the scars they bear for a lifetime.'[133] Six years after publishing *Child Abuse*, the Kempes followed up with *The Common Secret* (1984), which focused entirely on the prevention, treatment and legal ramifications of sexual abuse.[134] Reviewing it for the *American Journal of Nursing*, Linda Ledray, Director of the Sexual Assault Resource Service in Hennepin County, Minneapolis, praised its 'easy-to-understand information.' In the US at least, she believed that the increase in reporting and treating abused children was

> to a great extent, the result of teachers' and nurses' willingness to come to terms with their own disbelief, denial, and uneasiness with this issue. These professionals increasingly are making efforts to identify symptoms of abuse, to credit the victim's story, and to intervene.[135]

[130] Adrian Bingham, "'It Would Be Better for the Newspapers to Call a Spade a Spade': The British Press and Child Sexual Abuse, C. 1918–90,' *History Workshop Journal* 88 (2019): 102.

[131] Ruth S. Kempe and C. Henry Kempe, *Child Abuse*, ed. Jerome Bruner, Michael Cole, and Barbara Lloyd, The Developing Child (London: Fontana/Open Books, 1978).

[132] Virginia Culver, 'Ruth Kempe healed child-abuse victims,' *The Denver Post*, 1 Aug 2009. https://www.denverpost.com/2009/08/01/ruth-kempe-healed-child-abuse-victims/. Accessed 24 Sep 2024.

[133] Kempe, 'Recent Developments in the Field of Child Abuse,' 262–264.

[134] Ruth S. Kempe and C. Henry Kempe, *The Common Secret: Sexual Abuse of Children and Adolescents* (New York: W. H. Freeman, 1984).

[135] Linda E. Ledray, 'Review of the Common Secret: Sexual Abuse of Children and Adolescents, Ruth S. Kempe, Henry Kempe,' *The American Journal of Nursing* 85, no 8 (1985): 930.

In Britain, GPs and health visitors began to read stories exhorting them to do something about child sexual abuse. They were urged to 'bring it out from the shadows,' to 'deal with it,' to 'be on guard against it' and to assist in dismantling 'the last taboo.'[136]

Initially though, there was some ambivalence about the extent of the problem and its effects were downplayed, especially in items targeted at GPs. Writing in *Pulse*, Tom Smith described the different phases of sexual abuse, taken from an article in the *New England Journal of Medicine*. Although rape-counselling and rape-prevention centres for adolescents were proliferating in the US, Smith was not sure that they were needed in Britain.[137] His scepticism was perhaps unsurprising given that only a few years' earlier, articles in the GPs' trade press propagated extremely negative stereotypes about girls and women in relation to rape. The lines between adult women and under-age girls as well as between consenting sex and assault were often blurred.

In 1974, Dr Ralph Lawrence suggested that there were 'varying motives for a false allegation, such as blackmail, establishment of an alibi in the case of a girl coming home late, fear of discovered adultery, fear of pregnancy or VD [venereal disease], and revenge.' Perhaps complainants had inflicted the injuries on themselves 'in order to produce misleading evidence.' In most of the sixteen cases he had dealt with in his time as a police surgeon, there was 'little or no evidence of putting up a struggle.' Only three of the girls, who were aged six, thirteen and fourteen, were 'virgo intacta.' The others, he noted, in very sexualised language, 'were attempting to test the temperature of the water and found that it was hotter and deeper than they had expected.' Lawrence blamed advertising for 'hot pants' and 'mini skirts' which, he claimed, was 'all calculated to make us mere males succumb to their blandishments.' This, he concluded, made 'these teenie and weenie boppers arriv[e] to be examined … looking like miniature versions of their big sisters and displaying their charms with gay abandon.'[138] The

[136] Tom Smith, 'Child sexual abuse swept under the carpet,' *Pulse*, 21 Feb 1981, 54; Tony Whitehead, 'Dealing with incest and its aftermath, *Pulse*, 7 May 1983, 68; Andrew Lycett, 'GPs urged to be on guard against child sexual abuse,' *Pulse*, 6 Aug 1983, 10; Jean Moore, 'The last taboo: child sexual abuse – its causes and effects,' *Health Visitor*, 54, 7 (Jul 1981): 279–281; Rosalind Meek and Gabrielle Markes, 'Sexual abuse of children,' *Health Visitor*, 55, 7 (Jul 1982): 366; Eileen Vizard, 'The sexual abuse of children,' *Health Visitor*, 57, 8 (Aug 1984): 234–236.

[137] Tom Smith, 'Child sexual abuse swept under the carpet,' *Pulse*, 21 Feb 1981, 54.

[138] Ralph Lawrence, 'When rape is only a word,' *GP*, 4 Oct 1974, 21.

insinuation was that even if these were not false allegations of rape or sexual assault, rapists were not to blame because young girls were behaving seductively and dressing provocatively.

GP David Samuel Filer put across similar views. He was a part-time police surgeon for Hammersmith and Fulham Police Stations.[139] Although he did not see 'many cases of rape,' because the women usually requested a woman doctor, this did not prevent him from giving forthright opinions on why male doctors were better suited to the task of forensic examination. He implied that he and [male] police officers were experienced and justifiably cynical (claiming that the police 'can pretty well smell out a genuine rape') in contrast to gullible women doctors who had to deal with a mendacious 'girl' in a 'diaphanous pair of panties.'[140] Men (doctors or police officers) were properly sceptical about sexual crimes; women (whether doctors or victims) were naive or dishonest.

Such insinuations were less often made in the 1980s. Overt misogyny was in decline. Articles on sexual abuse featured more frequently. The format varied from short reviews of discussion papers (often by the NSPCC), synopses of articles from journals such as *Child Abuse and Neglect* or *The Lancet* and longer articles written specifically for the trade press by psychiatrists, social workers or others working in the child abuse field.[141]

The messages could be confusing and conflicting. Police surgeon Hugh de la Haye Davies urged GPs to 'always be suspicious about the possibility of sexual abuse, particularly if a child has behavioural problems.' He argued that GPs' knowledge of the families they treated meant they ought to 'be able to spot it quickly,' but provided no guidance as to how a GP might 'spot it.'[142] Tony Whitehead, a consultant psychiatrist at Bevenden Hospital in Brighton, emphasised how common incest was, that it far outweighed assaults by strangers and that it usually involved father or stepfather and daughter 'relationships.' He explained that each child might react

[139] 'Obituaries – David Samuel Filer,' *BMJ* 2022; 376: o65.

[140] 'Four hundred weeks in the surgery,' *GP*, 10 Jan 1975.

[141] Summary of an NSPCC report in 'Developing a child-centred response to sexual abuse,' *Health Visitor* 58, 1 (Jan 1985); summary of research by Dr Geoffrey Lealman published in *The Lancet* in 'Child abuse - detecting the at risk families,' *Pulse*, 16 Jul 1983, 15; summary of article by A H Tyler and M R Brassard in *Child Abuse and Neglect*, 'The effect of incest on the family,' *Health Visitor* 57, 8 (Aug 1984).

[142] Lycett, 'GPs urged to be on guard,' 10.

differently. Because 'sexual stimulation is usually pleasurable, regardless of who is involved with who,' children may 'enjoy the experience' or it may be 'terrifying, disturbing, or downright painful or disgusting.' While Kempe and his British followers claimed the abuse caused long-lasting harm, Whitehead was less categorical, stating that it was difficult to assess the impact. He did, however, describe high rates of incest amongst runaway girls and the greater likelihood that adults abused as children might experience depression, attempt suicide or abuse their own children physically and sexually. Turning to what the GP should do, Whitehead warned GPs that the child's or their relative's 'accusation' might be false and recommended Jean Goodwin's *Sexual Abuse* for her chapter on how to investigate in situations where a 'false accusation' was suspected.[143] It was a classic basket of mixed messages: 'incest' was common but perhaps not that harmful to children who anyway might be making the whole thing up.

Other articles encouraged practitioners to believe the child victim. In *Health Visitor*, April 1985's 'Recent Papers' summarised an article explaining why children's 'stories about being sexually abused' were unlikely to be lies. The consequences—family rejection, foster care, separation or divorce of the parents and the ordeal of testifying to numerous professionals and to a court of law—were too daunting.[144] The same year, *Pulse* published a feature on a conference at Manchester's Booth Hall Hospital at which Leeds paediatrician Chris Hobbs provided detailed information about the physical and behavioural signs of abuse. He asserted that 'my first rule is to believe the child,' explaining that it was extremely rare for children, especially pre-pubertal children, to make up stories of molestation. Most children did not have the language to describe such sexual activities.[145]

Should doctors involve themselves in the criminal justice system? Dr Paul Griffiths at the NSPCC advised doctors that a legal approach was best taken given the proclivity of perpetrators to silence their daughters and encourage them to say 'I made it all up.'[146] Whitehead seemed to argue against this view. He acknowledged that incest was a criminal offence but questioned whether reporting it to the authorities was always 'the best

[143] Whitehead, 'Dealing with incest and its aftermath,' 68; Jean Goodwin, *Sexual Abuse: Incest Victims and Their Families* (Boston: J Wright, 1982).

[144] 'Recent Papers: Sexual Abuse,' *Health Visitor* 58, 4 (Apr 1985): 104.

[145] Mark Pownall, 'Helping victims of child sex abuse,' *Pulse*, 20 Apr 1985, 56.

[146] Lycett, 'GPs urged to be on guard:' 10.

solution.' It might, he felt, be 'unethical,' because to 'simply report or not report' suspicions of incest without offering help and support breached professional standards. It was essential to ensure that 'expert counselling and advice' was 'offered and provided' to the family. The practical pitfalls of offering such expert services to a 'family' that included both the perpetrator and the victim were not explored.[147]

Most of the content practitioners encountered in their trade journals failed to provide any concrete information about what, if anything, the family doctor or community-based nurse should do if they suspected sexual abuse. Writing in *Health Visitor*, Jean Moore, a senior tutor at the NSPCC's School of Social Work, set out definitions, causes, possible signs of abuse and its effects on the child. She debunked some myths including that this was a crime committed by strangers, that the 'primary sexual orientation' of the adult was 'towards children' and that sexual abuse was more prevalent in poor families or overcrowded homes. Although articles published alongside Moore's on other forms of child abuse set out concrete actions health visitors and school nurses could take when faced with possible deliberate *physical* harm, Moore had nothing practical to offer in relation to action on *sexual* harm, merely concluding that 'a great deal of working through one's feelings has to be done before it is possible to handle these cases with the skill and sensitivity that is required.'[148] Psychiatrist Judith Trowell also called attention to the emotions. She had encountered her first sexual abuse case in London in 1979. By 1985, she had dealt with many abused children and their families. She identified the feelings provoked in the professionals as 'the main problem' in such cases, pointing out that practitioners must be at ease with their own sexuality. She noted that the 'pressures to apportion blame, to take sides, to deny what has happened or to act in a precipitate way were difficult to resist.'[149]

Eileen Vizard, also a psychiatrist, called on practitioners to act. Using a rather didactic tone, she entreated practitioners to respond to child sexual abuse 'in a serious and concentrated way.' They could make a real difference to a child's future by intervening early and thereby helping to prevent mental illness and maladjustment. She also believed that they could 'bring many *more* cases of sexual abuse to public notice and hence

[147] Whitehead, 'Dealing with incest and its aftermath,' 68.

[148] Jean Moore, 'The last taboo: child sexual abuse – its causes and effects,' *Health Visitor*, 54, 7 (July 1981): 279–281

[149] Judith Trowell, 'Working with Families where Incest is Actual or Feared,' *Health Visitor* 58, 7 (July 1985): 191.

stimulate further pressure for guidelines.' She warned that if health visitors and GPs took a passive stance and waited for clear national guidance, 'many young children [would] continue to be sexually abused, often within their own family circles.'[150]

Although sexual abuse increasingly featured in the trade press in the 1980s, it in no way eclipsed articles about other forms of child abuse, including non-accidental injury and neglect. The deaths of Darryn Clark and Paul Steven Brown led to calls for greater investment in earlier intervention; as the Brown Inquiry report stated, 'money spent wisely on the provision of dedicated qualified social workers and health visitors ... is money saved on hospitals, the police, the law and prisons.' There were fears that health visitors would be blamed when children died and regular calls for more training and support.[151] GPs' behaviour was scrutinised. There were a handful of articles in *Pulse* about the death of Maria Mehmedagi who was killed by her father when she was just under a year old. She had previously been removed from the family and was on a full care order. The health visitor was concerned that the baby was being physically assaulted, but the GP she asked to visit the family refused.[152] Many aspects of child abuse continued to be explored, including the principles of confidentiality, the importance of good record keeping, debates over who should be a keyworker for particular children or families, whether it was possible to predict child abuse, how decisions were made about which parents might be abusing their children and video surveillance in cases where mothers were suspected of fabricating their children's illnesses.[153] Sexual abuse featured occasionally across the publications, but practitioners were by no means bombarded with messages about it.

[150] Eileen Vizard, 'The sexual abuse of children - Part 2,' *Health Visitor*, 57, 9 (Sep 1984): 279–280.

[151] *Health Visitor* 53, 1 (Jan 1980); 54, 2 (Feb 1981); 56, 1 (Jan 1983); 58, 6 (Jun 1985); 58, 11 (Nov 1985); 59, 1 (Jan 1986); 59, 5 (May 1986); 59, 11 (Nov 1986); 60, 7 (Jul 1987).

[152] 'GP could face inquiry,' *Pulse*, 20 Jun 1981; 'GP - case conference probe held up,' *Pulse*, 12 Sep 1981.

[153] 'Confidentiality: duty or danger?' *Health Visitor* 60, 7 (Jul 1987): 213; 'Child Abuse and Neglect,' *Health Visitor* 57, 10 (Oct 1984); Keyworker articles, *Health Visitor* 54, 8 (Aug 1981); 54, 10 (Oct 1981); 54, 11 (Nov 1981). 'Predicting child abuse,' *Health Visitor* 54, 10 (Oct 1981); 'Child abuse - detecting the at risk families,' *Pulse*, 16 July 1983; Robert Dingwall, 'Defining child maltreatment,' *Health Visitor* 56, 7 (Jul 1983): 249–251; 'Video recording and child abuse,' *Health Visitor* 60, 10 (Oct 1987): 343; Hugh Mackenzie, 'Tackling child abuse and battering,' *Pulse*, 16 Jul 1983; Steve Taylor and Debby James, 'Children at Risk,' *Health Visitor* 60, 10 (Oct 1987): 329–330.

## Conclusion

The notion that there was a 'rapid process of community recognition' about child sexual abuse in the 1980s, followed by a swift retreat in the face of a backlash at the end of the decade, is overly simplistic. It was certainly not the case for community health practitioners. As coverage in the medical and trade journals demonstrates, messages about the prevalence of sexual abuse and its negative effects on children were broadcast only gradually and unevenly to these professional groups.

From the 1970s, the NSPCC, influenced by US paediatricians and psychiatrists, pushed hard to promote 'baby battering' as a phenomenon that should be taken on by doctors and nurses. However, this was just one of a host of social problems practitioners were encouraged to tackle as part of their role in administering 'social medicine.' Wider social and cultural changes affected not only how individual professionals thought and felt about children, young people and families, but also how each professional group responded to these seemingly new and highly challenging social problems related to sex, abortion, mental illness, drug use and family violence. Features in the trade press were often infused with misogyny, with heavy hints that these societal problems were escalating because of women's increasing insistence on greater independence.

GPs and health visitors were preoccupied with inter- and intra-professional insecurities, and arguments about their roles in relation to child abuse were enmeshed in wider debates about disciplinary boundaries, as well as each profession's relative status and authority. This had major implications for GPs' attitudes to the matters brought to their surgeries, often by women, which included violence and abuse against them or their children in the home. Many GPs operated as single-handed sole traders providing personal medical care and referring patients on to more specialist services. Now they were being drawn into 'social medicine' and broader welfare issues that required greater collaboration and information sharing. In comparison to GPs, health visitors were less resistant to absorbing 'child abuse' into their remit, as most accepted it as a new iteration of their traditional role with 'problem families.' But the profession had vacillated between nursing, medicine and social work for decades and struggled to achieve consensus on their core purpose and the nature and intensity of their engagement with families.

In the 1970s, it was very unusual to see any reference to incest, molestation or the sexual abuse of children. A close analysis of the 1980s trade press reveals that although articles about sexual abuse began to appear, it was not the dominant topic in that decade, as all forms of abuse continued to feature. Furthermore, the underlying assumptions about how much practitioners knew about the phenomena and the extent to which they were involved in identifying it and responding to it on a day-to-day basis varied a great deal as is evident from the articles that appeared in print. This chapter was about the messages directed at practitioners; I will address practitioners' experiences on the ground in Chaps. 5 and 6. But first, in order to explore why certain historians and practitioners have portrayed the 1980s as a decade of 'rapid recognition' of child sexual abuse, the next chapter will investigate the activism of two groups that claimed to hold special expertise in relation to child sexual abuse: feminist/survivors and medics/psychiatrists.

[illegible]

CHAPTER 4

# 'Colonising the Field': Feminism vs Psychiatry

## Introduction

> I saw the field being colonised by professionals … I think 'colonisation' for me … is the right term … It became an industry … and if you were prepared to put your toe in the water … there was no competition so you could make a name for yourself, you could make a reputation.
>
> Gerrilyn Smith, *feminist and clinical psychologist*, 2021.[1]

The last chapter examined the messages targeted at doctors and nurses working in community settings from the 1970s and challenged the notion of a smooth, swift rise to a state of general awareness about sexual abuse by the end of the 1980s. It exposed ambivalent attitudes towards child protection, as well as changing gender dynamics, misogyny and professional boundary-disputes. These themes continue in this chapter. We remain in the same stretch of time but with a new set of characters. The focus shifts to two factions that formed in this period and that considered themselves to have specialist expertise and knowledge: firstly, feminist and/or survivor activists and, secondly, clinicians (doctors, psychiatrists and psychologists).[2]

[1] Oral history interview with Gerrilyn Smith by author, 12 May and 25 Jun 2021.

[2] The term is often used to denote religious or political groups, but here I mean 'a group of people united in maintaining a cause, policy, or opinion in opposition to others.' Oxford English Dictionary, s.v. 'faction, n.[1], sense 2.a,' July 2023. https://doi.org/10.1093/OED/9609369251.



R. Beecher, *Community Health Practitioners and Child Sexual Abuse in the Family, 1970s–2010s*, Genders and Sexualities in History, https://doi.org/10.1007/978-3-031-80052-8_4

For feminist/survivors, that sense of authority was often rooted in the sense they made of their own personal experiences of sexual violence, their political critique of cultural misogyny and systemic failures to protect women and children and the practical expertise they gained through involvement in Rape Crisis work.[3] Psychiatric practitioners felt their training and clinical experience gave them insight and influence. To be clinical was to be detached and analytical, and many perceived themselves as operating in a politically neutral space, whilst building an evidence base that drew on their observations of the sexually abused 'patients' they assessed and treated. Before long, relationships between the two factions became fraught. Each had specific understandings of the causes and dynamics of child sexual abuse and what action should be taken to prevent it or, failing that, to intervene to stop it as soon as possible.

Is it careless for an historian to depict those on different 'sides' of a debate as completely polarised? There were undoubtedly survivors and feminists at work in medicine and psychiatry. The discourses, however, were particularly dichotomised. There was very little common ground in terms of theory and practice about prevention, early intervention or treatment, at least in what was articulated publicly in this decade. This chapter seeks to understand what each faction thought they were setting out to achieve, how they arrived at certain stances and why their different perspectives and actions were so divisive. Unpacking these schisms provides a deeper understanding, not just of events and reactions in these years, but also of their legacy for sexually abused children and adult survivors.

I begin with a concrete encounter between survivors of sexual abuse and medical professionals as an example of the friction between the two groups. I go on to examine how ideas from American paediatricians and psychiatrists on the one hand and feminists and survivors on the other translated to the UK. Survivors of abuse had grave objections to the models and opinions voiced by psychiatric 'experts' and sensed that victim-survivors were being objectified and exploited under the guise of impartial assessment and treatment. Medics and psychiatrists believed that their own efforts were worthwhile; they aimed to improve responses to abused children by shifting the emphasis away from a purely criminal justice

[3] The survivor activists and feminists in this chapter are in the majority women; and the children are mostly girls. This does not imply that boys are not victims of sexual abuse or that men cannot be feminists, survivors and activists.

approach to a model that offered all family members a chance to heal and to repair their relationships. The chapter explores why there was a deep schism between these two factions; a schism which had long-lasting implications for the early recognition and intervention in child sexual abuse in community settings.

## Part 1: London, Spring 1982

In May 1982, the London-based Incest Survivors' Campaign used their newsletter to share 'one woman's report on what she got for her twenty pounds registration fee' at a conference about child sexual abuse held the previous month.[4] Organised by the British Association for the Study and Prevention of Child Abuse and Neglect (BASPCAN), the attendees included survivors of abuse from the Incest Survivors' Campaign itself and from Nottingham's Organisation for Parents Under Stress (OPUS). Whilst BASPCAN was led by and directed at professionals including doctors, psychiatrists, social workers, lawyers and the police, the Incest Survivors' Campaign and OPUS functioned as support groups and campaigning organisations by and for survivors of incest.

Angela Young,* the woman writing in the newsletter, was deeply dissatisfied with what she had witnessed at the conference.[5] 'The morning,' she wrote, 'was taken up with an Expert from America.' He was psychiatrist David Corwin and as part of his presentation, he showed a film in which he and a female therapist asked a group of girls 'about the pleasure they had derived from the incest.' Providing a live commentary on the visuals as the conference attendees watched the screen, one victim, Corwin stated, was 'leading men on' because she 'stroked her thighs and pushed her hair back.' After the film, he played an audio recording of a woman being raped, telling the audience that a Rape Crisis service had advised her to record the assault in order to get a conviction against the perpetrator. Young wondered, 'what point he was trying to make' by replaying certain parts of the recording 'over and over again.' His presentation continued with an account of a girl he had treated. After being assaulted by a stranger in a fast-food restaurant, she was left 'frozen' and 'unable to react.' Corwin

[4] The conference took place on 6 Apr 1982. *Incest Survivors' Campaign Newsletter*, 2 May 1982.

[5] The woman in the newsletter is anonymised. I call her 'Angela Young' in this chapter.

explained to the audience that the man had pressed his groin against the girl. In order to 'make her more assertive,' Corwin described a roleplay he initiated in which he 'pressed against her too,' but 'without the pelvic thrust.' This statement was met with laughter from the conference audience. The archival source does not tell us whether they found the girl's humiliation genuinely comical or whether they laughed out of anxiety or embarrassment.

Young was not critical of all the sessions at the conference; she felt that a talk by a Black female American child therapist about using anatomically correct dolls was 'very well done.' But the afternoon's talk by Arnon Bentovim, consultant psychiatrist at the Hospital for Sick Children at Great Ormond Street in London (referenced as Great Ormond Street hereafter), presented her with 'the worst shock I have ever had about psychiatry.' Young was horrified by the videos he showed of therapy sessions, in which, she felt, he 'harangued' and 'bullied' the child victims. In the newsletter, she wrote:

> We saw a video of a six-year-old child who had been raped by an older boy … For the ten or so minutes of this video - I'm not kidding - Bentovim harangued her solidly. He would ask a leading question, she would not answer, he would nag, (all this in a raised voice), patronise, bully and finally turn to the grandmother and ask questions about the girl referring to her as 'she' and 'her' right in her presence. The poor kid was by now trying to cover her grandmother's mouth with her hand, so Arnon froze the video and pointed at a detail on the screen: 'Look now she's pulling down her skirt.' (It had ridden up over her thighs). All his questions consisted of was the physical details of the event and the size of the cock. I am not joking. He kept saying, 'It was big wasn't it? Too big for a little girl like you. That's what big people do, big people like me.' … Etc etc etc, terrible even from a straight Freudian point of view. But the worst was to come. The poor child was utterly bemused and picked up the dolls Arnon thrust into her hands … She was just about to start playing with them when he cried 'Aha! You're making them DO IT aren't you? They're DOING IT!!! YOU MADE HIM DO IT!'[6]

Bentovim then showed a video of a different girl aged ten, who cried in her therapy session. While he 'hailed [this] as a major breakthrough because she had been unable to express her trauma before,' Young felt that 'he had bullied her into tears.'

[6] 'Incest Survivors' Campaign Newsletter,' 2 May 1982. The Feminist Library Archive, London.

Young's account highlights stereotypes about child sexual abuse that permeated the psychiatrists' descriptions of their therapeutic interventions. The implication was that girls enjoyed the sexual encounter and that they were deliberately seductive towards adult men. There was also an uncomfortable voyeurism in the material presented. Some of it was blatant, such as playing an audio recording of a man raping a woman. Some was more subtle in the way the distress and confusion of the girls in treatment were put on display like a performance for the audience. Corwin, in particular, seemed to deliberately draw the audience into a state of collusion with him and this reached a pinnacle in the 'role play' in which he, an adult male, re-enacted a sexualised assault on a child and seemed to encourage audience laughter.

Young's criticisms of Bentovim's behaviour were similar; in the first film, she felt that he was 'haranguing' the young girl to provoke some sort of reaction; he drew attention to details that seemed eroticised, '[l]ook now she's pulling down her skirt'; and he concentrated heavily on the physical aspects of the male body and the sexual act. Young implied that he had attempted to lead this six-year-old to disclose sexual abuse by 'nagging,' that he then jumped too quickly to conclusions about what the girl was enacting when she picked up the dolls when he exclaimed, 'Aha! You're making them DO IT aren't you?' And that he concluded with a victim-blaming statement, 'YOU MADE HIM DO IT!' Her criticisms here foreshadowed later criticism of the Great Ormond Street team's interviewing techniques.[7]

When Bentovim went on to introduce a documentary film, the survivors present immediately objected, pointing out that he did not have the creators' permission to show it and that there was an injunction in place because it had previously been screened 'against the wishes of the women who had participated.' The film had been made as part of a short-lived music and arts series on London Weekend Television called 20th Century Box, produced by Janet Street-Porter. The activists saw Bentovim's attempt to show the film as a male professional misappropriating women's work to further his own agenda and career. Women had 'made that programme to speak out to other women suffering in isolation, to show that you could get over the pain etc, and now they were being used as further MATERIAL!' When Bentovim claimed that he had not intended to show

[7] Eileen Vizard, Arnon Bentovim and Marianne Tranter, 'Interviewing Sexually Abused Children,' *Adoption & Fostering* 11, no 1 (1987).

the film but was merely describing it, Young interpreted his response as 'the revolting authoritarian have-to-be-right-always way that is the prime characteristic of abusing men!'[8]

After a series of workshops, the conference participants reassembled as a large group to review the proceedings. Young spoke up to protest against the psychiatric theories that had been presented, and the way the models put forward ignored power relations within the family. Even though the conference organisers had taken some steps to be inclusive of survivors, and had incorporated a workshop by OPUS and Parents Anonymous about their self-help group in Nottingham, survivors felt peripheral. More than that, they felt unwelcome and pathologised. In the newsletter, Young explained what happened next:

> But this the [sic] worst bit for us as survivors. The president settled back to his notes and said, 'Ah, what workshop came next... where were we... Ah yes, 'Effects on victims in adult life'... Well, we've all seen a good example of that just now, so I think we can pass on to the next topic...' And I realised clearly that whatever we do, it will always be material, we will always be sick, disturbed, our opinions invalid. Mine were extreme, obviously I lacked 'Ego defences' or suffered from some kind of pathological hysteria and aggression etc, I'm not so worried about that, as the fact that if we had even behaved coolly and calmly, then we would have been 'Introverted,' 'withdrawn,' 'cataleptic,' or something always to deny us.[9]

[8] Although LWT's Head of Legal Services warned Bentovim in writing not to use the segment again, he continued to do so. *ISC Newsletter*, Jul 1982; Oct 1982. Emily Driver later described a family therapy session shown at a conference in Birmingham in 1984 without the permission of the girl who featured in the film. She and her siblings had been sexually abused by their father. The girl had been told that the video would only be used for training purposes within Great Ormond Street and was not given a contract to sign even after she complained. Driver's organisation CSAPEP contacted the Royal College of Psychiatrists to seek reassurance that clients' rights would be respected in relation to audio and video recordings of therapy sessions but received no response. Family Rights Group, 'Child Sexual Abuse after Cleveland – Alternative Strategies: Practice Reader 1' (1988): 45–46.

[9] Other statements made that day that the survivors found offensive were recorded in the newsletter. For example, Young described a woman who told her to 'remember that [the abusers] have been abused themselves' and that if Young had children she would be 'at a very high risk' of abusing them and have to be watched carefully. *ISC Newsletter*, 2 May 1982. This was a lasting myth. At the Inquiry into Child Abuse in Cleveland in 1987, Counsel asked a witness whether they had heard that 'victims... sometimes find as they get older that they either become a perpetrator themselves or marry people who become or are perpetrators?' TNA, BN 68/15 Day 13 hearing – Rev Michael Wright 01.09.1987, 59.

Survivors were only too aware that their lived experience was not valued in the conference space and that any display of emotion would invalidate their views. In fact, they had planned in advance how they would behave on the day. They intended to keep their emotions under strict control and present their case dispassionately. This, they believed, would help them to gain maximum positive exposure for their own aims, which were to publicise to attendees how fast the survivor movement was growing and to garner support to set up a refuge for sexually abused girls. Young, however, was unable to adhere to that approach in the face of what had been said about victims, survivors and perpetrators by those she called the 'Experts' on the day. She acknowledged this after the fact in her piece for the newsletter: 'Oh God I know I behaved too angrily for our advantage, but can you imagine how I felt?'

The Incest Survivors' Campaign and BASPCAN were each established around the same time in the early 1980s.[10] BASPCAN's remit was to protect children and educate adults in relation to child abuse. They aimed:

> To protect the physical and psychological health and relieve the distress and disturbance (whether physical or mental) of children whose development and participation in society is being or is likely to be impaired by neglect, cruelty or physical or mental abuse including sexual abuse.
>
> To educate the public and especially those persons concerned with the care of children, whether professionally qualified or not, about the incidence and effect of such neglect, cruelty or abuse.[11]

The Incest Survivors' Campaign was an advocacy group of and for survivors of child sexual abuse. On first glance, these organisations seemed to share similar goals: to increase public understanding of the causes of child sexual abuse and to lobby for better responses to child (and in the case of Incest Survivors' Campaign, adult) survivors.[12] Both groups sought ways of effectively tackling the phenomenon. And yet, this activist's account of the BASPCAN event demonstrates the deep discord between survivors

[10] BASPCAN had an 'inaugural' meeting chaired by Dr Alfred White Franklin on 23 June 1978 and another meeting a year later on 27 June 1979, also titled 'inaugural' in the minutes. BASPCAN files, York. The first ISC report in the Feminist Library, Peckham is dated 1 Dec 1981, but they may have been operational before that.

[11] BASPCAN Constitution, undated, filed with inaugural meeting minutes.

[12] Sarah Nelson, *Incest: Fact and Myth*. 2nd edition (Edinburgh: Stramullion, 1987), 107; John Pickett, 'The BASPCAN Founders,' *Child Abuse Review* 1, no 1 (1992): 2–4.

and professional elites. Survivors experienced the conference as a hostile space, dominated particularly by psychiatric 'Experts' from both the US and the UK. Young's report about the proceedings conveyed a deep revulsion at the content and tone of their talks. The 'Experts' showed video recordings of their therapy sessions with children as examples of innovation and good practice, but the survivors perceived them as victim-blaming, bullying and re-traumatising for the children themselves and for the adult survivors watching them at a remove. Survivors were explicitly labelled as 'damaged' and at high risk of abusing the next generation of children.[13]

Although Young's description of what she saw on the therapy video implied that clinicians lacked empathy for children, this is contradicted by other evidence of the care they took in the planning and execution of interviews and in their consideration of their methods of working and the impact of those methods on children. At times, clinicians showed an awareness of the historical and cultural stereotypes that painted women and children as untruthful. They could admit that misogynistic 'Freudian notions' of fantasy and the Oedipal complex had a continuing impact on themselves as practitioners. They also had the capacity to reflect on their own emotions, noting in an article about interviewing that having worked with several hundred children, 'we still experience feelings of disbelief, disgust and dismay when, for instance, four-year-old children talk about willies put into their bottoms.' However, they did not seem able to apply the same degree of empathy to their encounters with adult survivors.[14]

BASPCAN invited survivor organisations to contribute to the conference but by establishing the event as a space in which displays of emotion were signalled as inappropriate and where lived experience was discounted as 'evidence,' these figures of authority marginalised what survivors had to

[13] *ISC Newsletter* referred to the event as a 'conference' held on 6 Apr 1982, location not stated. *Health Visitor* provided a review of a BASPCAN 'study day' held in Apr 1982 where the speakers included David Corwin, paediatrician Margaret Lynch, psychiatrist Sydney Brandon and barrister Helena Kennedy. Bentovim was not mentioned. The synopses of Corwin's talk mentioned the 'serious effects' of child sexual abuse, noting that 'responses can vary from self-hate and self-destructive behaviour, prostitution and sexual dysfunction to severe mental disorders. The more immediate effect was guilt at taking part in these activities, especially if they enjoyed them.' Rosalind Meek and Gabrielle Markes, 'Sexual abuse of children,' *Health Visitor* 55, 7 (Jul 1982). Papers from the early 1980s have not survived in the BASPCAN (now the Association of Child Protection Professionals) archive.

[14] Vizard, Bentovim, and Tranter, 'Interviewing Sexually Abused Children,' 109.

contribute. These 'rules of engagement' were not perceived by survivors as neutral or objective. Furthermore, survivors sensed professional voyeurism both in the way psychiatrists applied new methodologies to children and their female caregivers, and the way they treated those individuals as material through video demonstrations of treatment sessions at conferences. Professionals were understood as exploitative in their readiness to appropriate material made by and for survivors for their own advancement, whilst refusing to involve activists in any meaningful way in developing theories about the causes of the abuse and possible approaches to prevention and treatment.

## Part 2: Psychiatric 'Experts'

Survivors' criticisms implied that ambitious and insensitive psychiatrists were colonising the field of child sexual abuse and becoming the 'expert' authorities to whom practitioners in the field and the media turned for opinions. It was certainly the case that this was a new field of endeavour for professionals and until the early 1980s there were very few doctors, psychologists or psychiatrists involved in studying this new 'syndrome' of child sexual abuse. Even in the US, which was ahead of Britain in recognising this form of abuse, there were only a handful of treatment services in operation. Dr Suzanne Sgroi, who led one such programme in Hartford, Connecticut, commented that in 1978 it had been possible to bring most of the 'notable professionals' involved 'together in one room and have fewer than thirty persons present.'[15] There were even fewer in Britain. But by the early 1980s, the number of medical and psychiatric 'experts' was expanding rapidly in both countries. Sgroi also pointed out that because very little had been written about sexual abuse, 'it was possible to secure national attention by the publication of a single paper or article.'[16] In other words, one did not have to have significant clinical experience in order to become an acclaimed member of this emerging elite. Below I explore how the 'expert' psychiatrists at the BASPCAN conference came to be involved in child sexual abuse research and practice and how their ideas (ideas that alienated and offended survivors) coalesced.

[15] Suzanne M. Sgroi, ed. *Handbook of Clinical Intervention in Child Sexual Abuse* (Lexington, MA: Lexington Books, 1982), 4.

[16] *Handbook of Clinical Intervention in Child Sexual Abuse*, 4.

Corwin first worked with sexually abused children in the late 1970s when he held a fellowship in child psychiatry under Dr Gloria Powell's supervision at the University of California Los Angeles (UCLA) Neuropsychiatric Institute where Powell had established the UCLA Family Support programme. Its name was generic, but it delivered specialist treatment to children who had been sexually abused within their families. Corwin was appointed co-director.[17] He completed his psychiatric training in 1981 and went into private practice.[18] Although he did not have years of clinical experience with abused children, he quickly developed a national profile.[19] Following a family violence conference held in Durham, North Carolina in 1981, Corwin and Kathleen J. Tierney co-authored a chapter about 'intrafamilial child sexual abuse' for a book called *The Dark Side of Families.* Sociologist Murray Strauss had posited that family violence was 'so common as to be almost universal' and that it was a 'systemic product rather than a product of individual pathological behaviour.' Corwin and Tierney took Strauss's systems theory thinking and applied it as a mechanism to understand 'incest.'[20] They portrayed 'incest' as the product of the 'socioecological'; 'aspects of family structure; predisposing factors in the perpetrator, victim, and spouse,' as well as 'situational factors.'[21]

[17] The National Resource Center on Child Sexual Abuse, *Think Tank Report: Allegations of Sexual Abuse in Child Custody & Visitation Situations* (Huntsville, Alabama: National Children's Advocacy Center, 1989). Powell was the first African American full professor of psychiatry in the UCLA system although the collection she edited with Gail Wyatt did not pay particular attention to race and culture. Gail Elizabeth Wyatt and Gloria Johnson Powell, eds., *Lasting Effects of Child Sexual Abuse* (Sage Publications Inc, 1988).

[18] Sylvia Paull, 'ACEs Champion: Child psychiatrist David Corwin's campaign against spanking rooted in ACEs science.' PACES Connection. 26 Jan 2021. www.pacesconnection.com/blog/aces-champion-child-psychiatrist-david-corwin-s-campaign-against-spanking-rooted-in-aces-science. Accessed 24 Sep 2024.

[19] His profile rose in the succeeding years as an 'expert witness' in custody disputes involving sexual abuse allegations and in the so-called 'memory wars.' David L. Corwin and Erna Olafson, 'Videotaped Discovery of a Reportedly Unrecallable Memory of Child Sexual Abuse: Comparison with a Childhood Interview Videotaped 11 Years Before,' *Child Maltreatment* 2 (1997); Nicole S. Kluemper, 'Published Case Reports: One Woman's Account of Having Her Confidentiality Violated,' *Journal of Interpersonal Violence* 29, no 18 (2014).

[20] The authors acknowledged that it followed Gerald T. Hotaling et al, eds., *Coping with Family Violence: Research and Policy Perspectives* (Newbury Park, Beverly Hills, London, New Delhi: Sage Publications, 1988).

[21] Kathleen J. Tierney and David L. Corwin, 'Exploring Intrafamilial Child Sexual Abuse,' in *The Dark Side of Families: Current Family Violence Research*, ed. David Finkelhor, et al (Beverly Hills: Sage, 1983), 106.

Corwin was a presenter at the British conference simply because he had volunteered his services to the organisation. He wrote to them in March 1981 to say that he was planning to travel to the Third International Congress in Amsterdam the following month and could deliver a workshop for them.[22] It is not clear whether Corwin did deliver any lectures in 1981 but he returned the following Spring. Such visits from US 'experts' in child abuse were not unusual. Key medical names in child abuse such as Denver doctors Ruth and Henry Kempe visited the UK, as did psychiatric social worker Patricia and psychiatrist David Mrazek. Similarly, family counsellor Anna and psychologist Henry Giarretto came and described the Child Sexual Abuse Treatment Programme they ran in California to a small gathering of BASPCAN members and representatives of the Department of Health and Social Security and the Home Office in 1979.[23] We will return to these clinicians below.

Bentovim had more clinical experience than the US 'Expert.' Like a number of his peers, he was a qualified child psychoanalyst as well as a psychiatrist. After his clinical training at the Maudsley in south London, he obtained a position at Great Ormond Street in 1968. He was also employed to deliver a weekly reflective practice session at the Tavistock Clinic. Like Corwin, he was interested in 'family systems thinking,' which he had arrived at through the work of Ronnie Laing who brought many ideas about it from the US. Bentovim recalled the excitement of these different influences converging to inform his own approach.

> I was fortunate that I was training at an exciting time when a number of influences, the traditional psychodynamic interest in Freudian ideas of development, the way the child develops, superego; the developmental processes which Anna Freud described; the systemic ideas about the interaction between relationships, those elements [were circulating].[24]

Child abuse did not feature in Bentovim's psychiatric or psychoanalytical training, but once he got to Great Ormond Street, he was quickly drawn into thinking about child maltreatment. Social worker Jan Carter chaired a 'high level' group alongside Bentovim, neurosurgeon Kenneth Till and paediatrician John Wilson. Till examined the records of children who had been admitted with serious head injuries and they realised 'there was a

[22] Minutes of BASPCAN Executive Committee, 19 Mar 1981.
[23] Minutes of BASPCAN Executive Committee, 14 Sep 1979.
[24] Oral history interview with Arnon Bentovim by author, 15 Jun 2021.

denial of the possibilities that head injuries might have been caused by … parents.' To encourage identifications of abuse, they established a child maltreatment group and it was agreed that Bentovim and Carter would be called if there was a concern about a child in the hospital at which point they would facilitate a case conference.[25]

Initially, the focus at Great Ormond Street was on physical and emotional abuse, babies who were 'failing to thrive' and a small number of poisoning cases.[26] But Bentovim was in the London audience of the second International Congress of Child Abuse and Neglect in 1978 and his interest was piqued by a galvanising speech about sexual abuse delivered by Kempe. His first reaction was incredulity; he thought that this did not happen in Britain.[27] However, when Kempe's colleague Patricia Beezley Mrazek (a psychiatric social worker who had been Assistant Director of the Kempe Centre in Denver) approached him about sending out a survey to gauge the extent of professional recognition of incest in Britain, Bentovim and paediatrician Margaret Lynch saw it as an opportunity to gain some sense of the scale of the problem. It was to be an important initiative since, in Britain, no data was available at the national level about incidence or prevalence rates and only a handful of small-scale research studies had been carried out.

They sent the questionnaire to 1,619 GPs, police surgeons, paediatricians, forensic psychiatrists, child psychiatrists and Area Child Protection Committee (ACPC) chairpersons. It asked for basic details about sexually abused children seen between June 1977 and May 1978, with more detailed data requested on the children most recently seen. ACPCs were asked about policies and procedures.[28] Forty-two per cent of the professionals responded with reports of over a thousand cases; from which Mrazek, Lynch and Bentovim extrapolated an incidence of approximately three per 1,000 children reporting some form of sexual abuse during their childhood.[29]

An important finding of the survey was that most of the professionals who responded did not recognise sexual abuse in the way that Kempe's

[25] Interview with Bentovim.

[26] David Rogers et al, 'Non-Accidental Poisoning: An Extended Syndrome of Child Abuse,' *BMJ* (3 April 1976): 793–796.

[27] Interview with Bentovim.

[28] Patricia Beezley Mrazek and C. Henry Kempe, eds., *Sexually Abused Children and Their Families* (Oxford: Pergamon, 1981), 35–49.

[29] Arnon Bentovim, Letter, 'Special doctors for rape victims.' *BMJ* (Clin Res Ed) 1982: 284.

team had, as a type of child maltreatment. Instead, Bentovim realised, they 'were seeing it as part of a sexual crime' rather than as 'part of a family pathology, family processes, they were seeing it as the individualised action of a perpetrator with a psychopathology which included a sexual interest in children.' When he spoke to 'colleagues at the [National Society for the Prevention of Cruelty to Children] and in government' he discovered that they also 'found it very difficult to think about sexual abuse as a form of maltreatment.'[30] Prosecution and punishment of the 'sex criminal' was the focus, rather than any form of treatment for perpetrator or child.[31] This was a legacy of the oversight and 'ownership' that police surgeons like Nesta Wells had held in relation to sexual assaults against children.[32]

Mrazek, Lynch and Bentovim were interested in how the family system operated and in how each member of the family could be 'healed.' The survey confirmed their perception of themselves as being at the forefront in terms of the recognition of sexual abuse and its 'life-long' impact, as well as in the new and enlightened way they conceived of the abuse. Rather than destroying the family, leaving the children without help and punishing rather than rehabilitating the perpetrator, their systems approach offered the opportunity to heal the whole family. To some extent, it was this pushback against the criminal justice 'solution' to child sexual abuse that drove the dramatic language of adult disintegration that so irked survivors. In Kempe's speech to the 1978 Congress, he noted that recent studies had shown that 'a disproportionate number of prostitutes have been involved in incest in early years, and that most children involved in incest do not grow up to have happy lives.'[33] As late as 2013, Bentovim, reflecting back to the time of the Mrazek survey, remembered that their concerns were about long-term damage: this included 'years of self-sacrificial behaviour, suicidal attempts to escape intolerable situations, risk of antisocial activities, prostitution, or drug and alcohol abuse.'[34]

[30] Interview with Bentovim.

[31] Arnon Bentovim et al, eds., *Child Sexual Abuse within the Family: Assessment and Treatment* (London: Wright, 1988), 40.

[32] See Chap. 3.

[33] Kempe, 'Recent Developments in the Field of Child Abuse,' 262–264.

[34] Arnon Bentovim, 'Commentary on Kempe C.H. 1978 Sexual Abuse, Another Hidden Pediatric Problem: 1977 C. Anderson Aldrich Lecture,' in *C. Henry Kempe: A 50 Year Legacy to the Field of Child Abuse and Neglect*, ed. Richard D. Krugman and Jill E. Korbin (Netherlands: Springer, 2013).

A 1984 article by Furniss, Bingley-Miller and Bentovim described a 'sense of helplessness' among British professionals because their professional skills were under-developed and treatment facilities were sparse. Citing the Mrazek survey findings, they argued that 'the threat of criminal proceedings against the perpetrators, who are most frequently the child's father or stepfather, prevents disclosure.'[35] This was rather misleading because the survey did not prove that the threat of criminal prosecution *discouraged disclosure or reporting suspicions.* It merely found that criminal prosecution was, at the time, the most common outcome following identification of child sexual abuse.[36] The second reference provided in support of this claim was Roland C. Summit's groundbreaking article about the 'child sexual abuse accommodation syndrome.' This made no comment at all on the impact of criminal justice procedures on the likelihood of disclosure but did argue for 'the advocacy of an empathic clinician within a supportive treatment network' which could 'provide vital credibility and endorsement for the child.'[37] The research cited did not support the claim put forward by Furniss and his colleagues.

Other research was also used imprecisely. Members of the team claimed that one reason that professionals did not recognise the sexual abuse of children within the family was the difficulty in 'distinguishing between what is appropriate erotic physical contact between adult and child and what is abusive sexual behaviour.'[38] In support, they cited Deborah Anderson who was the Director of Sexual Assault Services in the Hennepin County Attorney's Office in Minneapolis. Anderson's 1979 article barely touched on any potential difficulties professionals might have in making that distinction. Rather, her research was about whether 800 elementary school children could distinguish 'between touch which they experience to be caring and touch which is exploitative.' Although she described the different stages of children's sexual development, she did not examine whether professionals struggled to differentiate along the 'continuum of

[35] Tilman Furniss, Liza Bingley-Miller, and Arnon Bentovim, 'Therapeutic Approach to Sexual Abuse,' *Archives of Disease in Childhood* 59, no 9 (1984): 865.

[36] Patricia J. Mrazek, Margaret A. Lynch, and Arnon Bentovim, 'Sexual Abuse of Children in the United Kingdom,' *Child Abuse & Neglect* 7, no 2 (1983): 152.

[37] Roland C. Summit, 'The Child Sexual Abuse Accomodation Syndrome,' *Child Abuse & Neglect* 7, no 2 (1983): 177.

[38] Furniss, Bingley-Miller, and Bentovim, 'Therapeutic Approach to Sexual Abuse,' 865.

touch.'[39] The knowledge and expertise claimed by this emerging elite of psychiatric professionals (which was what survivors felt was weaponised against them) were built on a shaky foundation. They deployed the research of others in questionable ways. This was very likely not a deliberate ploy, more an uncritical acceptance of what little research had been published to confirm their own thinking. Nevertheless, they were rarely challenged. They became 'Experts' whose views were accepted as balanced and fact-based, whilst (and I will return to this below) survivors felt their opinions were discounted as emotional and, consequently, unsound.

The team's observation that little was available in terms of treatment for the child or other members of the family was accurate. Neither was there much available to preserve the family (if that was a desired outcome). Their desire to rectify the dearth of support was shared by the BASPCAN Executive at this time. In September 1980, the Association's outgoing chair, paediatrician Alfred White Franklin, acknowledged that '[u]nfortunately the law, if applied, tends to be punitive, with a jail sentence while little is done to rehabilitate the family or treat affected children.'[40] The Executive established a sexual abuse sub-committee; they also prepared leaflets to encourage the children's workforce to be more aware of the signs and to develop assessment and treatment skills.[41] Bentovim lobbied other medics, stating in a 1982 letter to the *British Medical Journal* that there was an 'over-reliance on legal response and insufficient attention being given to diagnosis, assessment, and treatment.'[42] He believed that if sexual abuse was only thought about as a 'sexual crime,' practitioners would fail to confront the problem; they would deny the child's distress; and they would turn away from the possibility that the child was being harmed for fear that the criminal justice system would break up the family. Furthermore, professionals would not be able to develop the multi-agency liaison and protocols for assessment that were increasingly being established for other forms of abuse.

[39] Deborah Anderson, 'Touching: When Is It Caring and Norturing or When Is It Exploitative and Damaging?,' *Child Abuse & Neglect* 3, no 3 (1979): 793–794.

[40] Alfred White Franklin, 'British Association for the Study and Prevention of Child Abuse and Neglect,' *Child Abuse & Neglect* 5, no 1 (1981): 69–70.

[41] Three thousand leaflets were printed. BASPCAN Executive Committee minutes, 16 Jul 1981. 'Child Sexual Abuse,' (London: BASPCAN, 1981).

[42] Arnon Bentovim, Letter, 'Special doctors for rape victims.' BMJ (Clinical Research Edition) 1982: 284.

Publicity about the Mrazek survey established the Department of Psychological Medicine at Great Ormond Street as a centre of expertise in sexual abuse cases. Professionals contacted the team to say, 'would you like to see this child we've just seen … because you might like to see is there a mental health issue here?'[43] The number of referrals grew and, in 1981, psychiatric social workers Liza Miller and Marianne Tranter, along with trainee psychiatrist Tillman Furniss and Bentovim, set up a Child Sexual Abuse Team. They felt that they had to act fast to respond to these children and families. They developed an assessment and treatment programme, which they claimed as the first in Europe to use 'individual, group and family approaches with victims, protective family members, and abusing parents and young people.'[44]

They were influenced by changes that had happened over the previous score of years in Britain. During the 1960s, there had been increasing recognition that sick children could not be treated in isolation and that wider psychosocial factors must be addressed. To help facilitate this, members of the Department of Psychological Medicine were assigned to the various specialist medical units such as gastroenterology, general medicine and cardiology so that social, cultural, environmental and psychological factors could be considered. Play workers were introduced to run art, craft and other play activities on the wards to help manage children's distress on being separated from their families.[45] Visiting regimes had been liberalised and parents became increasingly visible at their child's bedside. This was in response to John Bowlby, James and Joyce Robertson's work on bonding, attachment and the impact of separation, and to wider debates in medical circles and the popular press about hospital visiting.[46] An unforeseen

[43] Interview with Bentovim.

[44] 'The Development of Child and Adolescent Psychiatry from 1960 until 1990,' (Witness Seminar Centre for the History of Medicine, University of Glasgow, 2009), 97.

[45] Interview with Bentovim.

[46] Frank C. P. van der Horst and René van der Veer, 'Changing Attitudes Towards the Care of Children in Hospital: A New Assessment of the Influence of the Work of Bowlby and Robertson in the UK, 1940–1970,' *Attachment & Human Development* 11, no 2 (2009): 119–142. Children had previously been seen without their parents in hospital as visiting hours were extremely limited. In 1959, the Platt Committee recommended liberalisation, but hospitals were slow to change. Mothers were often unable to find care for other children to enable them to visit more. Joanne B. Bluestone et al, 'Hospitals, Children and Their Families: The Report of a Pilot Study,' *Journal of Health and Social Behavior* 12 (1971): 180–182.

consequence of the relaxation of the rules was that where staff had previously observed the child in isolation, they now saw them interacting with their parents. As Bentovim remembered it, 'a whole set of phenomena came into awareness' because 'you bring in the parents … and you begin to see the pathology and the harmful relationships as well.'[47] The parents' presence was positive in maintaining attachment and comforting the child, but it also brought increased identification of parental abuse in the hospital and, in reaction, complaints about surveillance and control.[48]

The main influences on the model Great Ormond Street developed came from two directions: innovations in structural family therapy and the Kempe/Denver approach to child protection. Other forces also nudged the team towards treating the whole family. These included attachment theory and ideas about parent-child bonding, as well as groupwork models developed in Seattle and California.

Since the late 1970s, Bentovim and psychiatric social workers Miller, Tranter, Anne Elton and Judy Hildebrand had forged links with developments and personnel in North America: these included connections to Nathan Epstein and colleagues at McGill University in Canada who had developed the McMaster model of family functioning, as well as Salvador Minuchin and therapists at the Ackerman Institute in New York. They were particularly interested in the way the Ackerman clinicians used pioneering technology to record video and audio. This enabled retrospective reflection on ways of tackling problems within the family work.[49] Great Ormond Street practitioners met regularly with around a dozen London-based colleagues including Robin Skynner, John Byng-Hall, Michael Crowe and Margaret Robinson. In 1977, they founded the Institute of Family Therapy. Bentovim felt they were bringing together 'systemic thinking, understanding the whole [family], as well as trying to see the impact on the child and the young person.'[50] Looking back he saw the 'two elements' as having had 'a very powerful organising effect' on the ways they identified and treated sexual abuse.

> By not only working in identifying abuse as it occurred in the child or young person but looking at the context and working with the whole family includ-

[47] Interview with Bentovim.

[48] Rogers et al, 'Non-Accidental Poisoning'; Roy Meadow, 'Video Recording and Child Abuse,' *BMJ* (Clinical Research Edition) 294, no 6588 (1987).

[49] 'The Development of Child and Adolescent Psychiatry from 1960 until 1990,' 95.

[50] Interview with Bentovim.

ing—and this is an important factor—including the perpetrator as part of the process rather than being totally excluded, which was of course the field as I found it when I started my psychiatric training.[51]

The programme developed was based 'on a systemic view of incest as an expression of family dysfunction.'[52] Whenever feasible, the team saw the entire family together for the assessment. Therapeutic work could be carried out with them as a unit or with children and parents individually. As the number of referrals increased, they established therapeutic groups for both children and adults.[53] The way they designed the groupwork and the materials they used were influenced by US approaches pioneered by social worker Lucy Berliner at the Sexual Assault Center in Seattle, Washington and Giarretto in California.[54] The Giarretto approach was to treat the entire family, rather than the victim and the abuser alone. Protecting the child from further sexual assaults was prioritised, often by separating the father from the family home during the treatment programme. Nevertheless, unless the perpetrator refused to take responsibility for the abuse, the work was conceived and implemented with all family members. The idea was to bolster the family unit to enable both 'dynamic patterns preceding the abuse and the family's subsequent adjustment' to be tackled.

The Great Ormond Street team usually ran four groups simultaneously in the evenings, including one each for young children, early teens aged eleven to fourteen, older teenagers and a parents' group. Psychiatrist Eileen Vizard, for example, facilitated a group with sexually abused children aged five to eight with the aim of ensuring that they would be less vulnerable to further predation.[55] The content was designed to repair the children's self-esteem and re-educate them about 'basic sexual facts' as well as 'good and bad touches,' thus promoting assertiveness so that children could reject unwanted contact; placing responsibility on the perpetrator not the child, and helping children to tell an adult 'until they are

[51] Interview with Bentovim.

[52] Judy Hildebrand and Constanze Forbes, 'Group Work with Mothers Whose Children Have Been Sexually Abused,' *British Journal of Social Work* 17, no 3 (1987): 285.

[53] Eileen Vizard, 'Self Esteem and Personal Safety: Comments on Secondary Prevention Work with Young Sexually Abused Children,' *Newsletter of the Association for Child Psychology and Psychiatry* 9, no 2 (1987): 16.

[54] 'Self Esteem and Personal Safety,' 16.

[55] 'Self Esteem and Personal Safety,' 16–22.

*heard* [emphasis in original].' Vizard made a videotape and provided guidance for professionals interested in setting up groups elsewhere.[56]

There was also a sporadic group for fathers who acknowledged being abusers. That group was held in the hospital boardroom, located away from the main hospital building, because those identified as perpetrators of sexual abuse could not be permitted into the main hospital building for reasons of child protection.[57] Thus those responsible for abuse were greeted and treated in the most prestigious and formal setting within the hospital campus. There were other aspects of the treatment which implied that the perpetrator was controlling the family and the wider system. The Great Ormond Street team ran 'apology sessions' with prisons like Grendon that were offering a therapeutic environment.[58] Critics saw these as ignoring the family dynamics and putting the child into an uncomfortable and potentially abusive situation. In addition, the timing of the apologies seemed to relate more to the prisoner's programme of rehabilitation than the child's readiness. As clinical psychologist Gerrilyn Smith described it, a man undertaking a Sex Offender Treatment Programme in prison reaches the part of the course, which is about empathy and so,

> he's written a letter and he's ready to meet the child. We get, 'can we meet the child please, he needs to complete this block?' I'm simplifying but you are getting the idea. And it was a bit like 'well, no, actually,' [laughs]. The mum and the kid don't want to see him, they are not ready to see him, and he may be ready to make his apology but actually the child's not ready to hear it.

In Smith's view, this maintained the perpetrator's control over the child; the person who was 'driving the treatment programme [was] the same person who did the offending, which is it's his time to do his empathy block.'[59]

Neither Giarretto nor the Kempes were opposed to police or court involvement, but they were in favour of delaying prosecution of the perpetrator during the therapeutic process. If the programme was successful,

[56] *Self Esteem and Personal Safety: A Guide for Professionals Working with Sexually Abused Children* (London: Tavistock Publications, 1986).

[57] Interview with Bentovim.

[58] Interview with Bentovim.

[59] Interview with Smith.

proceedings could be avoided; if the treatment failed, the criminal process would resume.[60] A key difference between the California and London-based programmes was that British fathers or stepfathers were not mandated to attend individual or group therapy. When Bentovim and Tranter presented tentative results following the treatment of 120 sexually abused children and their families referred to Great Ormond Street between 1981 and 1984, they emphasised the 'need for the firm support of a statutory agency.'[61] In reality, this meant that parents responded best (or were more compliant) when a legal sanction or care order was in place to mandate their involvement in treatment. Where the child's situation had improved, this was often due to separation of the abused child from the perpetrator rather than 'major restructuring of relationships.'[62] In other words, despite their commitment to changing the dynamics of the family and treating the perpetrator, they achieved little success in this area.

Another important difference between the Great Ormond Street and the Giarrettos' model was the way services had developed. The Giarrettos' Child Sexual Abuse programme in California had been conceived by the Juvenile Probation Department of Santa Clara County. In their dealings with families, the practice was to arrest the father or male carer who had abused the child; subsequently, the mother was expected to 'choose' her daughter over her husband and to initiate divorce proceedings. The family were often subsequently left in a financially precarious situation. Alternatively, if the mother chose to support her husband over her child, her daughter would be placed in the care of the County and would feel 'abandoned, rejected and was left to deal with the shame and guilt by herself.' Probation workers often felt caught in the middle of a family trying furtively to reunite without official sanction. Giarretto was asked to volunteer a few hours to provide counselling to the families. This was well received, and funding was made available to pay for a full-time service which became the Child Sexual Abuse Treatment programme.[63]

[60] Patricia Beezley Mrazek, 'Sexual Abuse of Children,' *Journal of Child Psychology and Psychiatry* 21, no 1 (1980): 93.

[61] Later published in Bentovim et al, *Child Sexual Abuse within the Family*, 256–268.

[62] Helen Agathonos, 'Report of Meeting: First European Congress on Child Abuse and Neglect, Rhodes, Greece, April 6–10, 1987,' *Child Abuse & Neglect* 12 (1988): 124.

[63] Henry Giarretto, 'A Comprehensive Child Sexual Abuse Treatment Programme,' in *Sexually Abused Children and Their Families*, ed. Patricia Beezley Mrazek and C. Henry Kempe (Oxford: Pergamon, 1981), 179.

However, even with the programme's support, the mothers of these sexually abused children still felt isolated. Probably inspired by the self-help organisation Parents Anonymous,[64] Giarretto encouraged a small number of mothers to make telephone contact with each other. They decided to meet in person and began to seek funding for various practical family support needs. One of the fathers who was incarcerated at Elmwood Correctional Facility was allowed to speak to his family, but not to the daughter he had abused. Giarretto, the probation officer and the parents appealed to the court to allow the father (on day release) and the child to attend counselling together. Supported by the Probation Department, fathers from the prison began to meet with the mothers' group. They named themselves Parents United, registered as a non-profit organisation in 1975 and set up a children's section called Daughters and Sons United. By 1979, there were twenty-four other chapters in place in California and the Santa Clara County chapter alone had 400 members and an average of six new families joining per week.[65]

The narrative provided here is from Parents United material and is no doubt a romanticised origins story. Certainly, the organisation has been criticised, most recently by historian Mical Raz who has demonstrated how much their advocacy model drew attention away from the social, economic and racial inequalities that contribute to child abuse.[66] Nevertheless, Parents United was a very robust part of the model developed in Santa Clara county. This was partly due to how it had evolved, the parents' initiative drove its creation and expansion, and it was strongly supported by the local agencies who had intentionally and voluntarily come together in partnership to improve services. Its development had been organic, the parents saw themselves working together with the professionals, and the approach had the support of each of the parties involved. This was not replicated in the UK where the treatment model was established by one agency and type of personnel—psychiatric practitioners at Great Ormond Street. There was no grassroots parents' organisation in London, the team delivered therapy *to*, rather than *with*, the families. The team were experimenting, and they were quite open about that at times,

[64] Judith Reed, 'Working with Abusive Parents, a Parent's View. Interview with Jolly K,' *Children Today* 4, no 3 (1975): 6.

[65] Giarretto, 'A Comprehensive Child Sexual Abuse Treatment Programme,' 179–184; Suzanne Landig-Hevezi, 'Biological Mothers and Intrafamilial Sexual Abuse' (University of Arizona, 1982), 47–51.

[66] Mical Raz, 'Lessons from History: Parents Anonymous and Child Abuse Prevention Policy,' *Pediatrics* 140, no 6 (2017).

acknowledging that they were at the early stages of developing a treatment programme. Paradoxically, however, they also accepted their 'Expert' status and did not put any caveats around that.

The Giarrettos' programme was at that time the most long-standing in the US, in terms of an approach that sought to integrate the therapeutic and legal pathways.[67] By 1982, they boasted of a high success rate, claiming that their service had provided therapy to over 4,000 families with 'about ninety percent of the children … returned to their families; and the recidivism rate in the families who have completed the treatment program remain[ing] at less than one percent.'[68] However, this may have been unvalidated data, drawn from the service's own records. An anthropologist at Stanford University claimed that by 1987 the model had been 'used successfully' to treat over 4,000 families in the San Jose area. It is unclear whether they were merely repeating Giarretto's claims or had independently verified the results. Even though the outcomes did not seem to have been independently evaluated, the model was reportedly rolled out to 105 other treatment programs in the US, Canada and Australia.[69]

All of this points to the fact that the psychiatrists who appeared at the BASPCAN London event were not established 'experts.' They were in fact only embarking on the first stages of understanding, assessing and treating child sexual abuse in the spring of 1982. And yet by presenting themselves as holding all of the expertise and knowledge and by dismissing survivors' lived experience, it appeared that they were 'colonising the field.' To understand how this came about in Britain, we have to step back a little in time.

## Part 3: Building an Elite Group

A number of transatlantic alliances formed through the International Society for the Prevention of Child Abuse and Neglect. Its first International Congress in Geneva in September 1976 was where, for example, Lynch and Bentovim met Kempe and Mrazek for the first time. The second

[67] Giarretto, 'A Comprehensive Child Sexual Abuse Treatment Programme,' 179–198; A similar programme in St Paul, Minn is discussed in Lorna M. Anderson and Gretchen Shafer, 'The Character-Disordered Family: A Community Treatment Model for Family Sexual Abuse,' *American Journal of Orthopsychiatry* 49, no 3 (1978).

[68] Henry Giarretto, 'A Comprehensive Child Sexual Abuse Treatment Program,' *Child Abuse & Neglect* 6, no 3 (1982).

[69] M. Scott Brown, 'Father-Daughter Incest: A Model for Treatment,' in *Current Issues in Clinical Psychology: Volume 3*, ed. Eric Karas (Boston, MA: Springer US, 1987): 79–85.

International Congress was held in London in September 1978 and was organised by a British committee. That group went on to form BASPCAN and voted themselves in as the first Executive Committee in June 1979.[70] Bentovim hosted many of the Executive's early meetings at Great Ormond Street. Visits from US medics and psychiatrists (like that of the Giarrettos to London) were co-ordinated through the Executive. The 1981 Chairman's Report recorded that 195 individuals and 41 organisations were members of BASPCAN.[71]

That same year, Ruth and Henry Kempe visited the UK and lectured at the London headquarters of the CIBA Foundation, an international educational and scientific charity funded by a Swiss pharmaceutical company. This was the catalyst for a study group which met at CIBA between September 1981 and March 1984.[72] Half of the group's sixteen members were medics. There were four psychiatrists: Bentovim and Furniss (Great Ormond Street), Lionel A. Hersov (formerly Great Ormond Street, then the Maudsley)[73] and Sydney Brandon (University of Leicester). Paediatricians included Anthony Jackson (Royal London Hospital and Queen Elizabeth Hospital for Children), Lynch (Guy's) and Christine Cooper (Newcastle). Cooper had replaced White Franklin as Chair at BASPCAN. That the influence of police surgeons had waned was obvious; Hugh de la Haye Davies (Northampton) was the only forensic doctor. The group produced a book that would influence practice and policy across the country.[74] The text advocated the same sort of multidisciplinary

[70] There was great interest in the British Association to the point where there were 47 nominations for the Executive in June 1979. BASPCAN Executive Committee minutes, 27 Jun 1979.

[71] Chairman's Report, BASPCAN undated, c1980/1981.

[72] CIBA had a long history of sponsoring study groups on scientific and medical matters and had run seminars on child development. See, for example, 'Series of four seminars/study groups on 'Mother-infant interaction' organised by the Tavistock Institute of Human Relations in collaboration with the CIBA Foundation,' 'CIBA Study Group 1961,' Sep 1961, PP/BOW/E.3/2, Wellcome Collection.

[73] Sebastian Kraemer, 'Lionel Hersov obituary,' *The Guardian*, 24 Apr 2018, https://www.theguardian.com/society/2018/apr/24/lionel-hersov-obituary. Accessed 24 Sep 2024.

[74] Other members were Detective Chief Superintendent John Bissett from Devon and Cornwall Constabulary, Dennis Tunney from Probation, Paul Griffiths, NSPCC, solicitor Richard White, barrister Helena Kennedy, social workers Carolyn Okell Jones from the Child Guidance Training Centre at the Tavistock and R. James Christopherson at the University of Nottingham as well as Ruth Porter from CIBA. CIBA Foundation, *Child Sexual Abuse within the Family* (Cambridge: Tavistock Publications, 1984).

approach as that used for other forms of child abuse, but in addition, urged the police, the criminal justice system, health and social services to ensure that 'a therapeutic stance' was centred in 'thinking and planning.' The idea was, similar to the Giarretto model, to combine 'control with therapy' and hence create a 'fear of punishment,' contributing to the reduction of sexual abuse.[75]

This did not mean that the CIBA group subordinated their expertise to the unquestioned legitimacy of the criminal justice system, rather that they tried to shift policy away from its emphasis on the punishment of the perpetrator as the preferred solution to a model that combined control of the perpetrator with a 'therapeutic stance' that could potentially heal and replenish all family members. Although its instigators on both sides of that Atlantic saw the model as progressive, the CIBA text reiterated many older misogynistic stereotypes. Mothers were criticised as potentially putting children at risk or creating susceptibility by distancing themselves from their child. The authors surmised that this could be because they adopted a punitive attitude to sex or were absent for any reason (the examples of physical or mental illness, or because they used drugs or themselves been sexually abused as children were given). Because the mother retreated from the family, it was suggested that

> her children and her husband may turn to one another for support, practical assistance or comfort and the foundations of an incestuous relationship are laid. In other cases, a man deprived of his conjugal rights may turn to the nearest available source of gratification—a dependent child.[76]

This conceptual framework recalls some of the misogynistic commentary about working mothers causing family disintegration ('happy families have full-time mothers') and unfaithful wives driving their husbands to injure or kill their babies in some earlier 'theories' of 'baby battering.'[77] The Kempes had also found fault with mothers; a mother might collude in sexual abuse in order to 'hold on to her man for her own needs,' particularly if she was 'frigid, rejected sexually, or herself promiscuous.'[78]

[75] *Child Sexual Abuse within the Family*, xii.

[76] *Child Sexual Abuse within the Family*, 8–9.

[77] See Chap. 3, part two, Adrian Rogers and Francis E. Camps.

[78] Ruth S. Kempe and C. Henry Kempe, *Child Abuse*, ed. Jerome Bruner, Michael Cole, and Barbara Lloyd, The Developing Child (London: Fontana/ Open Books, 1978), 66.

The CIBA book's conceptual framework for understanding sexual abuse drew heavily on the theorising of Furniss, who was training as a child psychiatrist at Great Ormond Street. He promoted a crude typology of families. In the 'conflict-regulating' family, the mother was emotionally distant from her daughter, sex was not discussed within the environment and the mother dismissed any allegations made about sexual abuse. A second family 'type' was 'conflict-avoiding,' in which the child took on the maternal role to compensate for her mother's shortcomings and the child's abuse was used by the family to reduce parental conflict.[79] Bentovim found these classifications useful and believed that these scenarios 'certainly seemed to be the case in some of the cases we were seeing.'[80] The Great Ormond Street team's book would include a chapter that relied heavily on Furniss's typologies.[81]

Nor were children blameless according to the CIBA group: they indirectly contributed to their own 'vulnerability' to sexual abuse. After all, a man with unmet needs for affection or sexual gratification might 'misunderstand the adolescent's behaviour and be sexually aroused by it' or become over stimulated by 'physical chastisement'—'the excitement that blends into sexual activity.' Stepfathers were especially prone to this; they not only lacked the biological bond but often joined the family as the adolescent's sexuality was developing without having experienced the 'maturing effects' of earlier phases of child-rearing.[82] Here again, the evidence base was very limited. These statements were backed up by only two sources. The first was a study by psychologist Lindy Burton of 41 children known to the police as victims of a sexual assault. She argued that the children tended to be 'affection hungry' and therefore indiscriminate in whom they befriended. They could also gain emotional satisfaction from the assault, she claimed, and might in the long-term become perpetrators themselves.[83] The second source was a survey of 796 college students in New England undertaken by sociologist David Finkelhor in the late 1970s. He found that comparatively more girls from lower-income or socially isolated backgrounds were victimised, and girls from stepfather families were five times more vulnerable than the others. Girls were at higher risk if they had ever lived without their mothers, if their mothers had significantly less education than their fathers, or if their mothers were

[79] *Child Abuse*, 12–13.
[80] Interview with Bentovim.
[81] Bentovim et al, *Child Sexual Abuse within the Family*, 8–9.
[82] *Child Sexual Abuse within the Family*, 8–9.
[83] Lindy Burton, *Vulnerable Children: Three Studies of Children in Conflict* (London: Routledge and Kegan Paul, 1968).

particularly punitive about sexual matters. While Finkelhor cautioned readers not to interpret high risk or vulnerability as a justification for victim-blaming,[84] the CIBA group did not include any type of warning or caveat. The Great Ormond Street team's book provided a more detailed exposition than the CIBA publication in relation to how practitioners could manage disclosures, family assessments and treatment, but overall it covered much of the same ground as the CIBA publication on definitions, contributory factors, means of recognition and the legal context.[85]

One of the problems with the British interest in American ideas and models of practice relating to child sexual abuse in this period is that they were adopted uncritically. It seems that the individuals and groups involved in the UK programmes were unable to hold on to nuance and uncertainty. Was it anti-feminist conservatism that pushed Great Ormond Street practitioners to ignore the extent of a father or stepfather's control over women and children in the home? Although Great Ormond Street personnel at times paid lip service to the contribution of feminist/survivors in raising the profile of the problem, they were deeply uncomfortable with the feminist understanding of sexual abuse. There was a paradox in that they saw themselves as members of a politically neutral 'child abuse lobby' driven by reason and a growing evidence base, as opposed to the 'feminist movement… supported by sociological theorists' and yet they (as much as feminist activists) wished to exert political influence on national policy.[86]

In an article written for health visitors, Vizard noted that the subject of child sexual abuse 'could well be reframed by an extension of feminist thinking, as the old story of sexual exploitation of women (in this case little girls) by men.' This could, she posited,

> be seen as happening in a culture where men are traditionally viewed as more powerful and more able to affect decision-making processes than women, so that sexual exploitation (it could be said) is therefore made easy for them.[87]

The argument 'could be pursued into political realms in order to protect women … inside and outside the family unit, from sexual harassment.' It was a peculiar statement, phrased as if feminists had not already made these

[84] David Finkelhor, 'Risk Factors in the Sexual Victimization of Children,' *Child Abuse & Neglect* 4, no 4 (1980): 272–273.

[85] Bentovim et al, *Child Sexual Abuse within the Family.*

[86] *Child Sexual Abuse within the Family*, 1.

[87] Eileen Vizard, 'The sexual abuse of children—Part 2,' *Health Visitor* 57, 9, Sep 1984: 279–280.

arguments about male abuse of power forcefully in the public and political domains. By repeatedly using the phrase 'could be' and describing feminist thinking as a particular 'framing' of the issue, Vizard emphasised that categorising sexual violence by men against 'little girls' as sexual exploitation was only one way of looking at the problem. She felt it was 'more immediately productive' to view it as the result of a 'dysfunctional family system.' Why? Because psychiatry could 'break the mould' with therapy and might enable such families to 'become reintegrated and more functional.'[88] Noting that sociologist David G. Gil had defined child/woman abuse as a 'misuse of power' in a capitalist system; Vizard and Tranter implied that such opinions were slightly fanatical, stating that however 'extreme such an analysis may seem' it was important to remember feminists' impact on wider social awareness of rape and 'wife battering,' and that improvements in police interview techniques, for example, had 'stemmed from such sociopolitical pressures.'[89] In other words, feminists could make a difference by making noise, voicing 'extreme' views and applying 'pressure.' Professionals in psychiatry and medicine, on the other hand, made measured, discriminating theoretical contributions to the debate about child sexual abuse.

What are we to make of Vizard's dismissal of the feminist framing of sexual abuse and her preference for the 'dysfunctional family system' concept? Was this conservatism about the family or an insecurity related to the fact that women were only now entering psychiatry in significant numbers?[90] It had been very difficult for women to manage childcare and train in psychiatry up until the 1970s, but some women training in psychiatry found ways to do so. Danya Glaser had her first child at twenty-six in 1968; she took jobs that she found tedious at times while her children were young and trained part-time in adult and child psychiatry between 1973 and 1983. She chose positions with reduced hours until her youngest child was in secondary school and did not work full-time until she was forty-one. Beyond the lack of childcare, there was other blatant gender discrimination in the workplace. For example, part way through Glaser's psychiatric training, she was dismissed from a job on a Mother and Baby unit because they said 'that [because she was pregnant] she might fall

[88] Vizard, 'The sexual abuse of children - Part 2.

[89] Eileen Vizard and Marianne Tranter, 'Chapter 4 Recognition and Assessment of Child Sexual Abuse,' in *Child Sexual Abuse within the Family: Assessment and Treatment*, ed. Arnon Bentovim et al (London: Wright, 1988), 60.

[90] John M. Eagles and Sam Wilson, 'The Feminisation of Psychiatry: Changing Gender Balance in the Psychiatric Workforce,' *Psychiatric Bulletin* 30, no 9 (2006).

down the stairs and sue them and so [she] had better not continue.'[91] Trowell had complicated childcare arrangements involving a friend who was a retired paediatric nurse and her own father. This enabled her to train and develop her successful career as a psychiatrist, but she remembered it as 'not straightforward at all,' 'it was a balancing act.'[92]

Trowell's description of her first 'pivotal' case of sexual abuse, a case that she said had 'stayed with' her for over forty years, was strikingly similar to the family models described in the CIBA and Great Ormond Street publications. In 1979, a family visited her service. A woman with three children had married a younger man and they had two further children. The mother was exhausted and perhaps 'didn't have a lot of time for [the man].' The middle child in the family, a 'pretty girl' aged maybe seven, eight or nine, had been lonely and depressed and the stepfather had 'taken an interest in her… that led on to an intimate relationship with her….' He told his wife and the couple voluntarily sought therapeutic help to ensure the abuse did not happen again and to repair the damage to the family. The child, however, was 'heartbroken.' She felt

> was it her fault, you know, had she led him on? So, there was terrible guilt from her, and she'd broken up the family and she missed him but, you know, she was relieved [the abuse] wasn't going on.[93]

Trowell knew Bentovim well, they worked together at the Tavistock where he ran a monthly training workshop on sexual abuse.[94] She remembered the sorts of criticism Great Ormond Street had received for victim- and mother-blaming. She recalled that at one point, the team

> had the abuser, the man—father or whoever it was, older brother or whatever. They'd go—have them go down on their knees and apologize as kind of trying to do something about the family dynamics rather than just—these people just disappearing out of their lives, and whether there was any way of the family being able to sort of have some ongoing connection with this person…[95]

[91] Oral history interview with Danya Glaser by author, 20 Jul 2020.

[92] Interview with Trowell.

[93] Interview with Trowell.

[94] He ran the workshop with Carolyn Okell Jones, a social worker at the Tavistock Child Guidance Clinic who had also been on the CIBA group.

[95] Interview with Trowell.

Trowell remembered that 'the whole thing blew up about how appalling this was.' She (at the time and decades later) was not sure whether it was appalling, because she did not think that 'this man disappearing totally from this child's life was necessarily the right thing.'[96]

Glaser thought that it took time for those treating families to understand the levels of denial by the perpetrator and that 'the abuser, usually a man, would have to do quite a lot of work on his own ... before he was ready to really own up—in a genuine way.' She felt that the models in circulation in the 1980s were more sophisticated than feminist critiques of them allowed. This idea of 'the colluding mother or the mother who denied her husband sex and therefore he had to go for the daughter' was linked to a 'therapeutic hope that you'd be able to deal with it in a family-systems way, almost possibly bypassing the crisis' in the family. This, she believed, was flawed. But equally, the 'feminist line being entirely power—these men were only out for power' was too simplistic.[97]

Glaser and clinical psychologist Stephen Frosh worked together on a book about child sexual abuse which espoused an intermediate position.[98] It came out of their work together in a multidisciplinary child sexual abuse clinic established by Glaser in Lewisham in London.[99] The book was divided into two parts, a theoretical and a practical, with Frosh mainly writing the former and Glaser the latter. They acknowledged the feminist critique of the family systems model, arguing that it was important to distinguish between the immediate cause which was situated in 'the psychology of the abuser' and the 'constellation of relationships, social arrangements and values' that made the child more vulnerable. Their theory clarified that the abuser was responsible for the act of abuse when it happened, the blame could not be shifted to other family members.[100] As Glaser noted later, 'explanation is very useful and actually very dangerous because we have a tendency to say, if we understand why something happens, somehow that exonerates it.'[101] She and Frosh did not excuse perpetrators. Instead, they noted the significant theoretical, practical,

[96] Ibid.

[97] Interview with Glaser.

[98] Danya Glaser and Stephen Frosh, *Child Sexual Abuse* (Basingstoke: Macmillan Education, 1988).

[99] See Chap. 6 for a more detailed discussion of Frosh's early career and the Lewisham clinic.

[100] Glaser and Frosh, *Child Sexual Abuse*, 26–27.

[101] Interview with Glaser.

psychological and ethical differences between abusing a child and failing to protect a child against abuse.[102]

From 1988, Smith led a national sexual abuse training programme at the Institute of Child Health and delivered clinical sessions with the Great Ormond Street team.[103] Although she had extensive experience in working with the client group, as a feminist outsider she 'never felt that they incorporated any of the ideas that [she] brought into their presentations.' In her view, if the team embraced *theories* of 'conflict-regulating' and 'conflict-avoiding' families, they should address them in *practice* within their treatment programme. If a hypothesis was that men sexually abused their daughters because their wives were not 'giving them sex,' Smith felt that the team needed 'to be talking to the women about the sex.' What she found when she spoke to women attending the group she ran was that

> often the guy was asking for sex morning, noon and night, and what's shocking and disturbing … Often when women heard what their children said about what daddy asked them to do, many of them were horrified because what daddy asked the child to do, he had asked the mum to do and she had refused.[104]

Smith wanted the team to test their theories in the clinical setting, to 'integrate them into their practice.'[105] Exploring these issues with families would expose the combination of conjugal coercion and abuse that often co-existed alongside the man's sexual assaults on the child. Perhaps interrogating the rhetoric of the concepts against family members' testimonies would have enabled the team to update their theories.

There was a strong insinuation from the Incest Survivors' Campaign critique of the video presentations that male psychiatrists either failed to notice problematic perpetrator behaviour or did not want to enter into conflict with the perpetrators by challenging it. Smith and other psychiatric practitioners did challenge such behaviours. But these difficult dynamics and the complexities of the therapeutic work did not make it into the publications that became well known.

[102] Glaser and Frosh, *Child Sexual Abuse*, 27.

[103] See Chap. 5. Gerrilyn Smith, *Systemic Approaches to Training in Child Protection* (London: Routledge, 2018).

[104] Interview with Smith.

[105] Ibid.

## Part 4: Activism

Various forms of feminist writing encouraged activism against rape and sexual abuse in Britain. Both the medical/psychiatric and the feminist/survivor factions were paying careful attention to material from the US. Feminist authors Susan Brownmiller and Florence Rush were influential. Brownmiller's definition of rape, as 'nothing more or less than a conscious process of intimidation by which all men keep all women in a state of fear,'[106] was not controversial with British feminists who saw unfettered male power and control over women and children at the centre of virtually all sexual violence.[107] Rush's blending of her personal story alongside a blistering critique of five formative studies of sexual offence victims and offenders provided a model for feminist action.[108] Her articles were circulating in the UK long before her book *The Best Kept Secret* came out in 1980.[109] Diana Russell drew on interviews with more than twenty survivors to come up with ways of improving responses to rape.[110] Louise Armstrong's *Kiss Daddy Goodnight* (1978) was read in the UK, replete with a cover endorsement by Brownmiller claiming it as 'the first significant book on incest ever to appear in print.' Maya Angelou's autobiographical account of her own abuse in *I Know Why the Caged Bird Sings* (1984) crossed over to a wide British audience.[111] Other writings in circulation by Black feminists included novels by Alice Walker and Egyptian feminist Nawal El Saadawi's fictionalised account of abuse in her novel *Woman at Point Zero* and her analysis of sexual violence against Arab Women *The Hidden Face of Eve (1980)*.[112]

[106] Susan Brownmiller, *Against Our Will: Men, Women, and Rape* (New York: Bantam, 1975), 5.

[107] Christopher Lehmann-Haupt, 'Books of The Times: Rape as the Combat in a War.' *The New York Times*, 16 Oct 1975, Page 37.

[108] Joseph E. Davis, *Accounts of Innocence: Sexual Abuse, Trauma, and the Self* (Chicago, London: University of Chicago Press, 2005), 26, 29.

[109] Florence Rush, 'The Sexual Abuse of Children: A Feminist Point of View,' in *Rape: The First Sourcebook for Women*, ed. Noreen Connell and Cassandra Wilson (New York: New American Library, 1974).

[110] Diana E H Russell, *The Politics of Rape: The Victim's Perspective* (New York: Stein and Day, 1974).

[111] Maya Angelou, *I Know Why the Caged Bird Sings* (London: Virago, 1984); London Rape Crisis Centre, *Sexual Violence: The Reality for Women* (London: Women's Press, 1984), 133–135.

[112] Alice Walker, *The Color Purple* (London: The Women's Press, 1986); Nawal El Saadawi, *Woman at Point Zero* (London: Zed Books, 1983); Emily Driver and Audrey Droisen, eds.,

A book that attracted readers in both factions was Judith Herman's *Father Daughter Incest* (1981).[113] This became an important resource for survivor activists in Britain and was frequently cited. Born in New York in 1942, Herman became a civil rights activist, a feminist and a psychiatrist. She situated her work (patient treatment, research and writing) within a tradition of political awareness and activism, believing in the importance of embracing the 'murky, messy, social issue stuff.' Her mother's aspirations in research psychology were thwarted because she had briefly been a member of the Communist Party and hence was ostracised in the McCarthy era. She subsequently pursued a different career path via clinical training. Her 'righteous indignation and her sense of… a kind of an expectation of integrity and standing up for your beliefs' were formative for Herman who remembered her mother's 'really keen sense I think of irony and indignation about all the weaseling, all the kind of fancy excuses that people made to compromise with something that was morally reprehensible.' Herman's mother also provided a blueprint for a way of living and work. She was committed to 'bridg[ing] the divide between academia and activism' and this became a model for Herman's own approach to child sexual abuse.

She was engaged in the Civil Rights Movement and in protests against the Vietnam War. Whilst at Harvard Radcliffe Institute, she met Kathie Sarachild of the radical feminist New York Redstockings. In 1964, they went to Mississippi together to participate in the Freedom Summer voter registration drive. As Herman recalled in an interview in 2000, Sarachild had conceived of the term 'consciousness raising' and called it 'basically an empirical method of investigation.' Sarachild argued that

> for people whose experience was not articulated, not recognized, not visible in the 'theory class' so to speak, the only way to begin to make our experience known to ourselves was to start with the testimony about the concrete conditions of our lives. So it was a connect for me and many women of my generation, I think, to start to apply those methods not only to the social issues of racism and war but to the conditions of our own rather privileged lives and to recognize that oppression takes many forms.[114]

*Child Sexual Abuse: Feminist Perspectives* (London: Macmillan, 1989), 200–202. Incest Survivors' Campaign newsletter, Jul 1983.

[113] Judith Lewis Herman and Lisa Hirschman, *Father-Daughter Incest* (Cambridge, Mass: Harvard University Press, 1981).

[114] 'Conversations with History: Judith Herman interviewed by Harry Kreisler,' 20 Sep 2000. https://conversations.berkeley.edu/herman_2000. Accessed 24 Sep 2024.

Herman applied this knowledge to child sexual abuse. As she set out in *Father Daughter Incest* and in later interviews, she and Hirschmann were newly qualified as a psychiatrist and psychologist respectively. Whilst peer reviewing their cases together, they realised that they were seeing a high number of incest cases,[115] and wondered:

> What's going on here? Why are we seeing all these cases? Is there something about us that's attracting that, or is this something that everybody starting out as a therapist sees? And if so, why isn't anybody else saying anything about it?' And we kept waiting for someone else to say something about it, and we waited and waited and nobody did, so then we finally said well maybe we ought to.[116]

They were convinced that the histories the women told them were accurate because they 'had all the vividness, the accuracy of detail, and the internal coherence characteristic of real memories.' But in every case, 'the veracity of the patient's history was officially questioned' and their supervisors reminded them that 'women often fantasize or lie about childhood sexual encounters with adults, especially their fathers.'[117] Herman and Hirschman turned to the literature. Finding mainly suppression, silence, apologists and deniers, they decided to write about the problem themselves. Herman felt that feminism and specifically consciousness-raising gave them the courage to do that, 'having come out of feeling that we were part of a movement where it was okay to trust your own observations even if nobody else seemed to think that what you saw made any sense.'[118]

For Herman, there was not a hierarchy in which survivors' experiences were trivialised, while clinical information was posited as 'hard data.' She believed that psychology was 'a very soft science, putting it at its most charitable.'[119] As feminist researcher Sarah Nelson commented, such writing may have posed as neutral or apolitical, but it was not. Under its guise, 'experts' made 'numerous assumptions about human nature, male and female sexuality, class, the family and the social order' with 'profound consequences' for policy and children's lives.[120]

[115] Herman and Hirschman, *Father-Daughter Incest*, vii.
[116] 'Conversations with History.'
[117] Herman and Hirschman, *Father-Daughter Incest*, 8–9.
[118] 'Conversations with History.'
[119] 'Conversations with History.'
[120] Nelson, *Incest: Fact and Myth*, 7.

Herman appreciated the significance of social and political context. Observers of human behaviour and relationships could not avoid being affected by the context, no matter how much they espoused an official position of neutrality. How a professional attended to what a woman said depended entirely on

> what one thinks a woman ought to be saying, ought to be feeling, is legitimate to express, unless you have a political movement that says, 'Forget what everybody else thinks you ought to be feeling, what you ought to be saying. Get down to it, tell the truth. What did you actually think and feel and notice in your body?' You need a safe space to be able to do that. You need a political context to be able to do that.[121]

British activists appreciated Herman's commitment to listening to what children and adult survivors were telling her and her recognition that this was valuable data. The Incest Survivors' Campaign planned to use a similar format and ethos as *Father Daughter Incest* for its planned collection of survivors' accounts.[122] Activist Emily Driver opened a collection of feminist essays on child sexual abuse by juxtaposing Freud's early twentieth century denial of the extent of incest with Herman's recognition of the frequent suppression of the facts.[123]

Like Herman, Smith and Sam Warner bridged the factions of feminism and clinical practice. Each worked as part of a Rape Crisis collective, Smith in London and Warner in Manchester and they both joined the 'professional' world of clinical child psychology. Smith's experiences as a sixteen-year-old in Toronto affected her career path. In 1970, her parents divorced, and she moved in with her maternal grandmother in Toronto. Once a week, her great aunt Lily came to visit for dinner. Aunt Lily was a bit 'odd.' She 'mumbled a lot,' which made the conversation at the table rather difficult; Grandma was deaf and couldn't hear what was going on. Smith could tune in to her aunt though, she 'could hear everything' and she enjoyed mealtimes with the two old ladies. She found the pair pretty 'funny.' On 26 June 1972, her Aunt Lily was raped and murdered by a group of young men who had followed her home to her rooming house

[121] 'Conversations with History.'

[122] They were also interested in the way feminist and sex educator Shera Hite constructed *The Hite Report* (New York: Macmillan, 1976). *Incest Survivors' Campaign Report*, 7 Feb 1982.

[123] Driver and Droisen, *Child Sexual Abuse: Feminist Perspectives*, 1.

on Gloucester Street in Toronto. She was 77 years old. Smith recalled 'it was ... like a hole in my life.' She spent the next few months in a daze of sorrow and confusion. She was due to go to university in September and

> I don't really remember much about between May and September, it's like ... And I didn't—I certainly didn't—nobody talked to me, nobody in the family talked about what happened to Aunty Lily. Nobody.[124]

Warner was studying psychology in Manchester when her friend 'was raped at knifepoint leaving the pub opposite where [Sam] used to live.' Warner remembered that 'obviously that was a personal tragedy for her, but it also felt like an attack on us as a class of women….' In recounting their histories, both Smith and Warner recalled vicious acts of rape (and in Smith's case murder). But both also remembered sexual violence in their youth as pervasive, it was something that was always there in some way, it was all around them. Warner thought that it was 'fairly hard to get to eighteen without experiencing some form of sexual assault or unwanted sexual encounter as a woman in particular.'[125] Smith worked as a waitress at a local golf club where she had 'older men coming on to [her] perpetually.' She remembered 'inappropriate sexual touching as a little girl, being flashed at ... [it was] completely endemic.'[126]

In Manchester, Warner and her activist allies organised a Reclaim the Night march, a benefit to raise money and a training day with workshops from Rape Crisis and Women's Aid, as well as anti-deportation and anti-racism campaigners. In London, Smith inhabited two worlds, training as a clinical psychologist at the Maudsley and working as a volunteer with the London Rape Crisis Centre (LRCC). It had opened in 1976 and other centres soon followed.[127] Although sexual violence had not been one of the original demands articulated at the first Women's Liberation Movement conference in Oxford in 1970, it was added eight years later in Birmingham. That conference called for 'freedom for all women from intimidation by the threat or use of violence or sexual coercion regardless of marital status; and an end to the laws, assumptions and institutions which perpetuate

[124] Interview with Smith.

[125] Oral history interview with Sam Warner by author, 28 Jun 2021.

[126] Interview with Smith.

[127] Helen Jones and Kate Cook, *Rape Crisis: Responding to Sexual Violence* (Dorset, UK: Russell House Publishing Ltd, 2008).

male dominance and aggression to women.'[128] By 1983, there were eighteen Rape Crisis Centres in England, four in Scotland, one in Wales and three in Ireland.[129] To these collectives, society was engaged in an active refusal to acknowledge rape. Just as in the US, consciousness raising was a core value. Their activism on sexual violence was grounded in their experiences in the Women's Liberation Movement where they had 'learnt that talking and working together to break this silence can be enormously strengthening.' Rape Crisis helplines had women callers say again and again that the agencies they encountered did not believe them and they took the opposite stance which was to 'always believe any woman who calls us.'[130]

The work at Rape Crisis was varied. They offered practical advice and emotional support, including escorting women wherever they needed to go in the aftermath of an assault, such as to medical appointments or police stations. Answering calls to the helpline was a priority. Although most centres were staffed by unpaid workers and were open only a few hours a week, they introduced call-forwarding systems to ensure that they could provide a twenty-four-hour answering service to women. Smith recalled that often the calls coming in were from women who were ringing from telephone boxes in the immediate aftermath of having been raped. As well as providing immediate support to women in crisis, they intended from the outset to wield strategic influence in terms of public education and dismantling the myths 'which distort and deny women's experiences.' This was to be achieved through the delivery of training, talks at meetings and conferences and by writing articles for the feminist press and the mainstream media.[131]

Rape Crisis Centres had expected to deal with adult women, but Smith recalled that they 'also got a lot of—not surprisingly—adult survivors of incest and sexual abuse within their families.'[132] Because the London Rape Crisis Centre was fast realising how prevalent child sexual abuse was, Angela Hamblin and Romi Bowen decided to write an article about it for

[128] Anna Coote, 'Seven pillars of liberation,' *The Guardian*, 4 Apr 1978, 9.

[129] The list had grown from one and a half to three and half pages by the time the second edition of the book was published in 1988. London Rape Crisis Centre, *Sexual Violence: The Reality for Women*, 136–137.

[130] *Sexual Violence: The Reality for Women*, 136–137.

[131] *Sexual Violence: The Reality for Women*, 136–137, ix.

[132] Interview with Smith.

the British feminist magazine *Spare Rib* in May 1981.[133] Monica Hill of Bradford Rape Crisis recalled that they too quickly realised 'how many women hadn't just been abused as adults, they'd also experienced sexual violence much earlier in their lives, when they were children.'[134]

By the time the London centre put together a book *Sexual Violence: The Reality for Women*, the sexual assault of girls merited a whole chapter. Speaking directly to adult women, the authors urged them to take on a protective role, whilst remembering that if a girl was assaulted, 'it is not your fault or hers.' They stressed that 'any man no matter how trusted is capable of assaulting a girl.' There was a strong appeal to adult women to listen, both to girls who might be victimised and to their own feelings. Women readers were encouraged to use their intuition in order to protect girls because usually, 'our suspicions are based on concrete things and dismissing them as a "paranoia" or "neurosis" may well result in a girl being very badly hurt.' Like many medical and social workbooks about child sexual abuse, this book asked women to be vigilant and look out for a range of signs. The signs themselves differed from the medical model because feminists paid attention to the otherwise often invisible perpetrator.[135] While doctors and nurses were told to be vigilant to physical signs of abuse on the child's body, or behavioural indicators of distress, the authors of *Sexual Violence* advocated watching the behaviour of perpetrators: men touching girls who clearly did not want to be touched, adults inviting contact with children, men talking to girls in a sexualised way, men who said that girls tend to lie and men who asked girls to keep secrets.[136]

Alongside the growing numbers of Rape Crisis centres, new groups appeared for adult survivors of child sexual abuse. In 1987, Warner joined Taboo, formerly known as the Manchester Support Group for Incest Survivors. This was one of the first specialist services for 'women and children who have been sexually abused by any male member of their family or by any other male in a position of trust.' It had been set up in 1983 by probation officer Anne Bannister, by the end of that decade it was

[133] Angela Hamblin and Romi Bowen, 'The Sexual Abuse of Children,' in *Women against Violence against Women*, ed. Dusty Rhodes and Sandra McNeill (London: Onlywomen Press, 1985), 146–147.

[134] London Metropolitan University/ The UK Women's Liberation Movement UK/ Violence Against Women. Sat 31 Jan 2009 Hillside Leeds, 'Sexual Violence' panel, LSE.

[135] Lesley Macmillan and Deborah White, 'The Missing and Imagined Perpetrator in Rape Prevention Efforts,' *Women's History Review* 32, no 7 (2023).

[136] London Rape Crisis Centre, *Sexual Violence: The Reality for Women*, 87–96.

survivor-led.[137] Warner recalled that Taboo had been 'doing good things' including setting up a project for Black women and a refuge for young women. But, at some point, she recalled

> some of the people who were running it left and there was a— there was an open meeting in Moss Side saying, 'what do we want to do? Do we— As a community, do we want to support this organisation?' I went to that and argued for the service to stay open and then needed to put my money where my mouth was [laughs] and therefore that's when I joined Taboo. [Laughs]. Yeah.[138]

The London-based Incest Survivors' Campaign also emerged in the early 1980s. Their approach was similar to many small feminist collectives. By the end of 1981, they had two separate monthly groups running: one specifically for consciousness-raising and self-help therapy, the other co-ordinating their campaigning work. They produced a newsletter for their members and wrote articles for other feminist newsletters such as the *London Women's Liberation Newsletter* and the York-based *Women's Information and Referral Enquiry Service (WIRES) Newsletter*. They spoke at the 'Women Against Violence Against Women' (WAVAW) conference in London in Nov 1981,[139] the 'Male Power and the Sexual Abuse of Girls' event held in Manchester in Jan 1982 and 'Feminists Against Sexual Terrorism' (FAST) in Sheffield in March 1982. A key aim was countering negative messaging about survivors in the media. Some journalists were sympathetic, especially agony aunts in women's and 'teen-girl' magazines. Jill Nicholls, agony aunt at *Honey*, had started out at *Spare Rib* magazine. She printed a letter from a young adult survivor who had been abused by her father over a number of years and subsequently experienced sexual difficulties with her boyfriend. Nicholls emphasised the support available to overcome feelings of fear and guilt.[140] Survivor organisations actively pursued collaborations with reporters and media producers that appeared sympathetic to their aims.

But it seemed to the activists that many reporters were careless, ill-informed or misogynistic. After an 'appalling page and series of letters'

[137] John Christey-Casson, 'Anne Bannister obituary,' *The Guardian*, 6 Apr 2015.

[138] Interview with Warner.

[139] Sandra O'Neill recalled that there are about forty WAVAW groups all over the country. London Met/ The UK Women's Liberation Movement UK/ Violence Against Women. Sat 31 Jan 2009 Hillside Leeds, 'Campaigns and film panel.' LSE.

[140] *ISC Newsletter*, Sep-Oct 1983.

about the Incest Survivors' Campaign in *New Society* in 1981, the women were reluctant to 'lay ourselves open to further misrepresentation.'[141] An approach from Joyce Robins, a journalist at *Woman* magazine, stalled when they persistently questioned her about her stance. In February 1982, they were interviewed by Su Carroll for her 'Families' programme on Manchester's Radio Piccadilly, but after the broadcast she failed to send them the recording she had promised of the interview. She had also assured them that callers would be referred on to the Incest Survivors' Campaign. This did not happen. Even when they participated in producing media content with 'friendly' journalists, there were risks and frustrations in terms of how abuse was portrayed. For example, both Incest Survivors' Campaign and OPUS took part in the current affairs programme 'Brass Tacks' broadcast on 13 May 1982 on BBC 2 England. The all-female crew they were promised did not materialise. Instead, five men turned up. The sound engineer attached microphones to their chests and constantly touched them to adjust the sound. They felt manipulated and bullied by the producer Claire Walmsley. When the programme aired, they were disappointed to find that it was 'predictably family oriented,' meaning it promulgated the CIBA/ Great Ormond Street model that attributed some responsibility for the abuse across family members, rather than locating it with the perpetrator.[142]

The Campaign also directed its energies at combatting misrepresentations in newspapers, magazines, radio and television programmes. They campaigned against the film 'Butterfly,' an exploitative drama about a 'God-fearing Appalachian coal miner who had an incestuous relationship with his nymphet daughter,' which the *New York Times* described as 'a most entertainingly sleazy melodrama.' Pia Zadora played Kady, 'a trashy teenager whose mother is a prostitute … and who finds her father and seduces him so that she can get at the silver in the mine.'[143] Much was made in the American and British press of Zadora's reception as the new 'sex kitten' at the Cannes Film Festival, and of her marriage to the film's producer, thirty years her senior. Incest Survivors' Campaign described that as 'blaming the victim' as usual. They picketed cinemas and campaigned

[141] *ISC Newsletter*, Dec 1981.

[142] *ISC Newsletters*, 7 Feb and 2 May 1982.

[143] Vincent Canby, 'Pia Zadora in Cain's Butterfly,' *New York Times*, 5 Feb 1982; Alvin Klein, 'Pia Zadora relishes her stardom,' *New York Times*, 7 Mar 1982.

to have posters of 'what appears to be a preteen child with massive breasts being abused in the bath' removed under London's new obscenity laws.[144]

Closer to home, 'expert' psychiatrists' responses to readers' letters and their opinions in magazine articles proved frustrating to survivor activists; they were often inaccurate and misogynistic. For example, a mother wrote to *Company* magazine having 'glimpsed her 17-year-old daughter being abused in bondage gear.' The magazine cited an 'expert's' advice that 'young girls often want to test their budding sexuality on the nearest male, and some men are just too weak to resist their advances.' In a 1983 'Woman's Hour' radio programme, Jenny Bond let survivors 'do most of the talking,' but the 'expert,' consultant psychiatrist Brendan McCarthy (a member of the BASPCAN Sexual Abuse sub-committee), spoke about 'victims' and 'incestuous relationships,' rather than using terminology of 'survivors' and 'incest' favoured by the Incest Survivors' Campaign.[145] He remarked that children felt guilt 'about the aspects of the relationship that (were) rewarding, pleasurable and satisfying, *because there is always that.*' [Emphasis Incest Survivors' Campaign].[146] 'Behind Closed Doors,' a 'spicily sensationalised' article in teen magazine *19*, included Bentovim's statement that

> I would emphasise that everybody in the family has their own sense of responsibility, and it's not any one person's fault... very often the whole family plays a part in it... it's not easy for a mother who discover she's living under the same roof as her husband's mistress.[147]

*19* magazine had used the contents of a *New Society* article that presented survivors as 'a bunch of victims.'[148] That was a frequent problem, paired with stories that survivors were deeply damaged and put their 'own children at risk by marrying a man who's likely to behave in that way.'[149] The Campaign had a tape of Hilary Osborn's report on Capital Radio on 16 Mar 1983 in which Osborn said, 'it seems that many incest victims tend to marry other incest victims and continue to commit the offence with their

[144] *ISC Newsletter*, May 1982.

[145] Interestingly given the ISC commentary on Corwin's presentation at the 1982 conference, Corwin sent BASPCAN some 'tapes,' and asked Brendan McCarthy to evaluate whether they were 'suitable for copying' but the outcome of McCarthy's review is not to be found in the archives. BASPCAN Exec Committee minutes, 16 Jul 1981.

[146] *ISC Newsletter*, Dec 1983.

[147] *ISC Newsletter*, Sept/Oct 1982.

[148] *ISC Newsletter*, Sept/Oct 1982.

[149] *ISC Newsletter*, Dec 1981.

own offspring, conditioned as they are by their upbringing.' In the programme, Bentovim 'kindly pointed out that survivors commonly become homosexuals, prostitutes and drug addicts' and in adulthood 'go around making victims of themselves.'[150] Campaign members had been interviewed but their footage was not used in the programme. Osborn bemoaned the lack of information about brother-sister incest on the show even though 'this was precisely what we'd talked about with her, from a personal as well as a Campaign point of view, and there she was even denying our whole existence.' They phoned into the programme and wrote to Capital Radio but got only 'the usual guff' in response.[151]

They created a rota to make sure that someone was always available to write to the publications to protest against misrepresentations. The work to challenge stereotypes was exhausting and took time away from the proactive steps the Campaign wanted to take such as teaming up with others to fundraise to set up a girls' refuge. A conference about this was held in Birmingham on 21 June 1982 with seventy women from across Britain. The aims were 'to stop the abuse' and 'to create space for girls who at present have no options.'[152] By winter 1983, there were active refuge planning groups in Dundee, Glasgow, Leeds, London, Manchester and Stirling.[153] By the mid-1980s, there were virtually no services specifically providing accommodation for homeless young women. Hill and Wendy Hammon of Bradford Rape Crisis Centre set up a multiracial collective and established a safe house called One in Four for young women fleeing sexual violence in Bradford.[154]

The Incest Survivors' Campaign made some efforts in their early days to reach out to medical professionals, although they were sceptical about whether or how they would respond. In February 1981, they noted that their links to doctors were not 'too strong' and they were unsure 'how impervious the whole medical profession is to our feminist cause.' But they emphasised that if 'any nurses or doctors are reading this, we would be glad to meet you.' Aware that there was a group meeting regularly at CIBA, the Campaign asked whether they could get involved. Although they were 'brushed … off' by an unnamed group member and told that

[150] *ISC Newsletter*, Apr 1983.
[151] *ISC Newsletter*, Apr 1983.
[152] *ISC Newsletter*, Sept/Oct 1982.
[153] *ISC Newsletter*, Winter 1983.
[154] London Met/ The UK Women's Liberation Movement UK/ Violence Against Women, Sat 31 Jan 2009 Hillside Leeds, 'Sexual Violence' panel.

'the Committee only wanted to talk to 'Experts,' the survivors were keen to 'overcome that obstacle' by 'sounding out' other members.[155] They may have succeeded in making contact. There was a small section at the end of the CIBA book entitled 'Self-Help Groups and Alternative Networks,' which referred to a 'strong self-help component' working well in the US (citing Giarretto but omitting Parents United). The Great Ormond Street groups were also mentioned. It was a very brief segment that did not mention survivors, ending with a contact list that included Incest Survivors' Campaign, OPUS and Rape Crisis Centre branches, the Incest Crisis Line, Taboo, Safeline in Bradford and SAVES in Hull. Its brevity encapsulated the decentring of survivors from the medical and psychiatric narrative about child sexual abuse.[156] By including only a truncated list and little description of the work of the other 'faction,' the spirit, ethos and expertise of those with lived experience were diminished in value.

## Conclusion

Perhaps a good place to end this chapter is with Smith and Warner whose personal experiences galvanised them to work in the field of child sexual abuse. When Smith's Aunt Lily was raped and murdered, she was 77 years old, an 'odd' old lady with kyphosis, a spinal condition which used to be commonly called a 'dowager's hump.' Smith experienced what happened to her aunt as a powerful confirmation that sexual violence had nothing to do with behaviour, physical attractiveness, flirtation or collusion. Both Smith and Warner saw clearly that violent acts were merely one end of a spectrum of violence that was part of every girl and woman's experience.[157] And yet, when UK activist survivors of the period spoke out, that experience was discounted; they were silenced and belittled, they were revictimized. Many of the 'Experts' of the 1980s at best blamed girls and women as complicit for the abuse; at worst, held them at least partially responsible.

The various factions struggled to develop a shared understanding and language to describe child sexual abuse, its aetiology, its impact and how best to respond to it. If it was a battle between factions, the medical and psychiatric perspective seemed to win the first phase. Politicians and officials at the national level paid attention to them, they were on the platform at conferences and quoted often in the media whilst survivor voices were

[155] *ISC Report*, 7 Feb 1982.

[156] CIBA Foundation, *Child Sexual Abuse within the Family*, 114.

[157] Liz Kelly, 'Continuum of Sexual Violence,' in *Women, Violence and Social Control*, ed. J. Hanmer and M. Maynard (London: Macmillan Press Ltd, 1987).

literally silenced. They were influential in shaping policy messages and statutory guidance to the children's workforce. Theirs were the ideas that were apparently despatched to practitioners in GPs' surgeries, health centres, child guidance clinics, social work departments and to other members of the children's workforce.

Some psychiatrists continued to promote family therapy methods in relation to child sexual abuse treatment. Warner recalled a video of a therapy session played by Bentovim at a conference in the early 1990s. It showed a daughter (who had been abused by her father) waiting with her mother in a room. The father

> walked straight in, sat really close to this girl … and leaned into her and the girl's … squashed down and that… So the girl and mother were terrified. They're leaning down, screwed up. Dad's leaning into them, all powerful. One, I wouldn't have had him in the room to begin with but, two, having seen what he did, before he even sat down, you would have made him leave because nothing had changed.[158]

Warner reflected that at the time the feminist position was 'once an abuser, always an abuser.' The perspective was 'they should not be part of family life, so we were—yeah, a hundred per cent, no negotiation.' Decades later, she was more hopeful that there might be some situations in which a perpetrator could change, but that could not emerge through family therapy in an environment where the perpetrator could wield that sort of untrammelled power. The Great Ormond Street model, in her view, failed to grasp the way that not just the particular children, but 'all family members [were] groomed and managed within that abusive system.'[159]

In November 1989, the Feminist Coalition against Sexual Abuse announced a conference entitled 'Challenging the professional takeover.' It was called to give women, particularly survivors of child sexual abuse,

> the chance to talk to each other from our own experience; to look at how professionals are taking over and making decisions about our lives without taking account of what we as survivors or carers want, nor how being female, black, working class, disabled or lesbian affect both our experience of abuse and how professionals treat us.[160]

[158] Interview with Warner.
[159] Interview with Warner.
[160] Incest and Child Sexual Assault newsletter, 21 Nov 1989.

From as early as 1984, Louise Armstrong had seen the birth of an 'incest industry' in the US, 'a staggering array of clinicians and counsellors and therapists and researchers and authorities and experts.'[161] In Britain, Liz Kelly called out the 'people whose careers (and notice how many of the most "successful" are men) have been built on the investigation, treatment and "prevention" of child sexual assault.' Some, Kelly noted, were 'passionately committed to supporting women and children,' but most lacked the 'coherent political position' that would enable them to recognise the obstacles to achieving real change.[162] Many years later Smith remembered how the manner in which medics and psychiatrists 'colonised' the field was galling. She regretted that while their reputations grew, there was a distinct lack of recognition for the 'hundreds and hundreds, thousands of unpaid hours of work' done at the London Rape Crisis Centre. Without that, the organisation did not have the financial stability to do the work and 'to allow people, women and girls, the choice to decide how to manage the situation that they found themselves in.'[163]

Some members of the medical elite moved on from sexual abuse in the family to other interests. This was partly due to scandals such as Cleveland which I will explore in Chap. 5. But it was also simply that they felt that the specialists had done their bit. Glaser returned to Great Ormond Street in the mid-1990s, taking up Bentovim's post shortly after he left to go into private practice. She had delivered a child sexual abuse assessment and treatment service in Lewisham for ten years and been heavily involved in driving forward the knowledge base internationally. She felt that by that time, there were 'answers to quite a lot of the questions,' but that

> [u]nfortunately, the understanding doesn't always lead to change. The main frustration is actually getting people to change once you have an idea about what it's about … we'd learned so much about it but at this point, there was a need for people to do things differently.[164]

As a specialist hospital, Great Ormond Street was set up to develop and treat interventions for rare or complex conditions. Glaser felt that it was

[161] Louise Armstrong, *Rocking the Cradle of Sexual Politics: What Happened When Women Said Incest* (London: Women's Press, 1996), 77–78.

[162] Liz Kelly, 'Bitter Ironies: the professionalisation of child sexual abuse,' *Trouble & Strife* 16 (Summer 1989): 15.

[163] Interview with Smith.

[164] Interview with Glaser.

obvious by then that child sexual abuse 'was *not* rare' and that much of the work in developing assessment and treatment protocols had been done. In terms of 'offering an intervention service and a consultation service,' she believed that this should no longer be delivered at Great Ormond Street but should instead be made available in local community settings. The way that leading medics and psychiatrists moved on from child sexual abuse having gained prestige and authority can be viewed cynically. But Glaser had assisted more than a thousand sexually abused children and their families in Lewisham over a decade, she continued to help children by deploying her knowledge of sexual abuse in court cases, and under her leadership many children in a range of abusive situations were treated at Great Ormond Street. It was undoubtedly the case that if change were to happen in terms of identifying child sexual abuse in the family earlier and responding better, practitioners in primary care settings would need more knowledge and better skills to make that happen. But to what extent would they be trained and supported to respond to children locally? In Chaps. 5 and 6, I return to those frontline practitioners to find out.

CHAPTER 5

# 'Turn to the colour plates.' Training Before and After Cleveland

## Introduction

One point of agreement between feminists, survivor activists, medics and psychiatrists in the 1980s was about the need for community-based practitioners to recognise and respond swiftly and compassionately to sexually abused children and non-abusing parents. This chapter looks at the extent to which paediatricians, GPs and health visitors were equipped to do that. It chronologically traces changes in training and work-place support to doctors and nurses who cared for children and families in local clinics, doctors' surgeries, health centres and schools. This is important since very little is known about the recent history of medical and nursing education relating to child sexual abuse, either in terms of formal taught programmes or in relation to supervised practice. From the late 1970s, government, professional organisations and commentators encouraged practitioners to respond to child sexual abuse, but historical sources demonstrate that information about this form of maltreatment and exactly how the different disciplines should respond was not incorporated into professional education swiftly or consistently.

Health visitors' training was lengthy; they had to first qualify as hospital nurses, then train in midwifery or obstetrics and finally undertake the specific one-year health visiting course. The intention was to teach them the basics of hospital nursing, provide them with an understanding of pregnancy and childbirth, and give them an education in the key components



R. Beecher, *Community Health Practitioners and Child Sexual Abuse in the Family, 1970s–2010s*, Genders and Sexualities in History, https://doi.org/10.1007/978-3-031-80052-8_5

of public health work, but it left them poorly equipped in terms of the knowledge and skills needed to deliver an effective response to child sexual abuse. Meanwhile, what doctors learned about the phenomenon depended more on the attitudes of the individual consultants they encountered during their training than on the formal curriculum. There was also a difference between the two professions in terms of their potential roles in relation to child sexual abuse, with much greater clarity for doctors about what they were expected to do than was the case for health visitors. For although there were debates between different types of medical specialisms (police surgeons, paediatricians and GPs), their responsibilities in terms of child sexual abuse were fairly clear. They were to observe the signs of injury, gather information about the patient's history in order to diagnose, and treat pathology.[1] The health visitor's exact remit was less clearly defined.

## Part 1: Starting Out - Nurses' Training and Motivation

In the decades in which Jennifer Xavier, Jane Bramwell and Diana Quigley* trained (1960s and 1970s), most hospital-based nursing schools delivered three-year courses; the first two years comprised academic lectures and practical experience, the third year was supervised practice.[2] After written and practical examinations, they became State Registered Nurses (SRNs).[3] State Enrolled Nurses (SENs) had only two years training and were paid less; structural racism meant that nurses from overseas were often encouraged to become state-enrolled rather than state-registered.[4] There was little to no child abuse content within nurse education until the late 1980s and almost none on sexual abuse. Neither did the lectures nor the 'on the job' supervision equip nurses with the knowledge and skills that would help them to spot the signs of abuse and respond effectively.

[1] These signs or indicators could be physical or psychological. This chapter will focus mainly on the physical signs.

[2] 'Nursing schools in the 1960s,' People's history of the NHS, https://peopleshistorynhs.org/galleries/nursing-schools-in-the-1960s/. Accessed 23 Jan 2024.

[3] Adrian O'Dowd, 'A history of nursing in Britain: the 1960s,' *Nursing Times*, 11 Oct 2021.

[4] Royal College of Nursing, 'Hidden in plain sight: celebrating nursing diversity,' https://www.rcn.org.uk/library-exhibitions/Diversity-Exhibition. Accessed 24 Sep 2024.

Some nurses, like Xavier, remembered the work on the wards as routine and mundane: winding bandages, making porridge and poached eggs, arranging patients' flowers and testing blood samples.[5] Others, such as Bramwell, recalled that she and her colleagues on the children's leukaemia ward at Great Ormond Street Hospital (GOSH) 'were doing a most extraordinarily responsible job and taking on huge tasks, you know, life and death tasks.'[6] What both women had in common was that they were under the age of majority and had been passed from their parents' care to the guardianship of the hospital Matron.[7] They lived in a nurses' home and felt overprotected. Many nurses thought like Bramwell did, that they were 'still children in [Matron's] eyes.'[8]

They were also infantilised within the hospital setting where they were taught to be seen and not heard. The expectation was that a student nurse should not question more experienced colleagues. Quigley remembered her nurse training in the late 1970s as dominated by rote learning. If she asked a question, the typical response was 'because we've always done it this way' or 'because that's what the doctor wants you to do.' It was a world in which the nurses were easily identifiable by their old-fashioned uniforms, their white, starched aprons and stiff hats. The consultants (who were mostly men) 'tended to wear suits, no white coat' and they did not wear name badges because they expected 'everybody to know who they were.' The doctors rarely used the nurses' names, '[they] were just "nurse"... Or "you there."'[9]

The expectation that nurses should stifle any budding professional curiosity extended to patients. Quigley recalled that when people were admitted who were self-harming, 'whether it was physical or whether it was an overdose of medication ... you treated what they presented with.' If they had cut their arm, the nurse was to clean and dress the wound, not to ask why they might have hurt themselves. Other professionals such as social workers or psychiatrists could ask questions but nurses had to provide patient care with very little contextual knowledge, and were not encouraged to put forward their own ideas. Neither should they attempt to build

[5] Oral history interview with Jennifer Xavier by author, 2 Aug 2019.

[6] Oral history interview with Jane Bramwell by author, 4 Jul 2019.

[7] In 1969, the age of majority was reduced from 21 to 18. Family Law Reform Act 1969, Section 1, https://www.legislation.gov.uk/ukpga/1969/46. Accessed 24 Sep 2024.

[8] Interview with Bramwell.

[9] Oral history interview with Diana Quigley* by author, 23 Jan 2020.

rapport with patients. They were taught to address them formally as 'Mr' or 'Mrs' and there was a 'bit of frowning upon anything which suggested a relationship with a patient.'[10] It was seen as unprofessional.

Senior nurses took on a protective role in relation to those in training. Xavier nursed on the children's ward at St Mary's, Paddington, in London for a year after she qualified. She remembered seeing 'a large baby in a cot all day long and he was blind, and I was told he'd been battered and that was the result.' She was told nothing more.[11] In another hospital, an infant admitted with a head injury was the subject of 'hushed conversations' between senior doctors, the ward sister and the hospital social worker. Quigley was a staff nurse; she recalled that 'everything was immediately closed down.' Nurses were left in the awkward position of looking after a child's injuries or the 'physical health needs' that were the result of parental abuse, but not 'necessarily in that loop that this is what we're worried about.' Quigley thought that the senior nurse deliberately chose to keep the trainees away from discussions about maltreatment, 'almost like… that people think you might become tainted in some way because of the shame.' It was all 'kept very, very hush, hush.'[12]

Jane Hutcheson recalled a similar silencing when she was assigned to a paediatric ward. She was looking after a young girl aged eight who had been repeatedly admitted with stomach pain for which the doctors could find no cause.[13] Hutcheson noticed the girl's interactions with a little boy in the adjacent bed and thought, 'that's overtly sexual behaviour.' She recalled that one day the girl gave the boy a note and that too 'was very overtly sexual.' Concerned, Hutcheson gave the note to the ward sister. She thought at the time that 'the chances were that child was being abused,' but the senior nurse never spoke to her about it, and she did not know whether it was ever investigated or discussed with the parents. There was neither criticism nor validation of her actions. It was as if she had never said anything at all.[14]

[10] Interview with Quigley.

[11] Interview with Jennifer Xavier.

[12] Interview with Quigley.

[13] Oral history interview with Jane Hutcheson by author, 7 Jan 2019. This is an indicator that would later appear on many lists of possible signs of child sexual abuse.

[14] Bentovim described this tendency to stifle certain 'junior staff' as a coping strategy. Arnon Bentovim, 'Treatment: A medical perspective,' in Jan Carter, ed. *The Maltreated Child* (London: Priory Press, 1974).

Conversations about what had happened to these children were not permitted. Nevertheless, these nurses had witnessed the injured child and noted the hushed conversations from which they were excluded. By contrast, nurses who left the hospital wards and trained as health visitors often heard nothing at all about child abuse in the years that followed. Detecting child abuse was not, in any case, what had motivated them to become health visitors.

For some, health visiting was a sort of 'preparation for having a family and being married.' The hours of work were appealing; it was a nine-to-five job, without the punishing night shifts of hospital nursing. Then there was the status and the pay, which was at a significantly higher rate than that of a staff nurse.[15] The opportunity to work in preventative healthcare was important too. Hutcheson loved working on a general ward but, time after time, she saw middle-aged men 'coming in with heart disease and dying.' She thought 'maybe I could do something that, you know, prevents that or starts a bit earlier.'[16] Many health visitors wanted to work with 'the needs of ... people who weren't necessarily ill.'[17]

Some individuals left hospital nursing because they wanted to move away from its physicality: they did not want to see the effects of illness and injury on patients' bodies, tend to wounds or monitor symptoms. Most had not foreseen the physical and emotional impact of what they would witness as hospital nurses when they started as eighteen-year-olds. Abramovich had thought nursing was about 'putting bandages on people and taking their temperatures.' She was horrified by the procedures, by the 'thought of putting a catheter into somebody's bladder .... And ... you know all the incontinence to start with, [she] found really tough.' Her memories of that time were all about the sensations she felt on the wards; the sound of her shoes sticking to the floor, the smell of urine, the sight of soft food falling out of a patient's mouth as another student nurse spoon-fed her.[18]

These young nurses and midwives also had to cope with serious illness and death. Bramwell was on a leukaemia ward, and she found 'the stress of the atmosphere, and the children who were not going to make it, terribly

[15] Interview with Quigley.
[16] Interview with Hutcheson.
[17] Interviews with Charles, Scowen, Quigley and Bramwell.
[18] Interview with Abramovich.

traumatic.'[19] Similarly, when Chloe Duncan* trained as a midwife at the Jessop Hospital for Women in Sheffield, she was twenty-two and 'quite raw.' She remembered a baby dying as his mother gave birth, she said he was 'a little boy, I remember quite clearly.' It was still indelibly imprinted on her mind decades later. She was just 'expected to take it in [her] stride.' The only comfort she got was from her peers when they gathered together in their rooms after work to 'share our experiences and support each other.'[20] Similarly, Abramovich delivered a baby that 'wasn't breathing and the mother was bleeding really, really heavily and [Abramovich] pulled the emergency cord and it just seemed forever until somebody came.' She was frightened and felt unsupported by the senior midwives.[21]

Facing up to child abuse meant dealing with injury and distress inflicted deliberately by a parent on a baby or child. It required paying attention to the body and to the symptoms and signs of harm. Some health visitors found this difficult. Duncan* remained in health visiting for decades but she remembered that even much later on, when more was known about sexual abuse and local social workers provided training to her and her health visitor colleagues, she did not like to think about it. 'Why,' she wondered, 'should people want to do that sort of thing?'[22] Abramovich expressed similar feelings; child sexual abuse filled her with 'horror and disgust,' and she could not 'perceive how anybody would have the desire to do anything like that, how they could inflict anything like that on a child. Maybe,' she said, 'it's an area I don't really want to go to that much.'[23]

They certainly did not have to 'go to' it much on their health visiting training. Although this was very different to their training as hospital nurses, it was not noticeably better in relation to child welfare. However, it did provide a more holistic perspective on health. As student nurses, they had been taught basic anatomy and physiology and 'what [they] weren't ever taught about at the time was what health looks like.'[24] Health visiting training by contrast included consideration of the social determinants of health, child and human development, social policy and principles of practice. In comparison to the rote training of general nursing, it offered 'proper studying, proper debate, encouragement to read, some practice.'[25] Hutcheson

[19] Interview with Bramwell.

[20] Oral history interview with Chloe Duncan* by author, 19 Feb 2020.

[21] Interview with Abramovich.

[22] Interviews with Duncan and Abramovich.

[23] Interview with Abramovich.

[24] Interview with Quigley.

[25] Interview with Quigley.

recalled learning about health promotion, screening, child development, immunisations 'and all those kind of practical things.'[26] Part of the job would be screening for developmental delay or problems in the family environment, but their main focus would be on supporting children's normal progression and supporting parents in relation to childcare—feeding, play, or walking and talking. As well as their college classes, health visitors had supervised practice, usually one day a week and then towards the end of the course, they would do a ten- or twelve-week placement overseen by an experienced practice teacher.

Post-qualification, some health visitors wondered whether the advanced training had been necessary in order to tend to poor or 'problem' families. Xavier recalled that when she 'got on to the community' in South Leeds 'which was a sort of [sighs], how can I put it? It was a housing estate, anyway,' she wondered 'why one needed all this training, just to ... tell people where to go for mattresses at the Salvation Army and provide free baby milk and stuff.'[27] She felt that anyone could have done the job of providing practical support, encouraging mothers to keep the home clean and to discipline their children appropriately. Health visitors were also taught that many of these households contained 'problem families.'[28] Xavier recalled an example of a couple who went off to the horse races and left the children at home alone.[29] In Newcastle, Donna Salter,* who qualified as a health visitor in 1969, remembered they referred to these as families where there was 'cause for concern.' These were the types, she recalled, whose 'children went hungry and took food out of bins.'[30]

Some training courses did not refer at all to 'problem families,' 'battered babies,' 'child maltreatment' or 'child abuse.' In the late 1960s, when Duncan* trained in Sheffield and Manchester, she was not taught anything about it.[31] Twenty years later, Anne Hackett* trained as a nurse under the old-style three-year apprenticeship model in a general infirmary in the northeast of England. She could not remember any information about child abuse and thought that 'if it was there, it was minute. It might

[26] Interview with Hutcheson.

[27] These classed attitudes to 'problem families' are described in John Welshman, 'In Search of the 'Problem Family': Public Health and Social Work in England and Wales 1940–70,' *Social History of Medicine* 9, no 3 (1996).

[28] Michael Lambert, '"Problem Families" and the Post-War Welfare State in the North West of England, 1943–74; Vol One' (Lancaster University, 2017).

[29] Interview with Xavier.

[30] Interview with Donna Salter* by author, 15 Mar 2019.

[31] Interview with Duncan.

have come under general safety, patient safety, but I can't remember anything.'[32] Training in London around the same time, Abramovich had a similar experience. She recalled that it 'wasn't a very big thing' in her training, 'not like it is now.'[33]

Patricia Scowen's health visiting course in Chiswick in 1967 was unusual in that she was told about 'battered babies': the infants would have a look of 'frozen watchfulness' and she should watch out for 'bruising or unexplained incidents … the parents would tell you … the child had banged its head or fallen off the changing mat.' She was told to report any unexplained injuries to the Heads of Health Visiting and then on to the local authority's Children's Officer. She remembered that 'incest' was also mentioned in passing on her course—that it 'happened … in some … rural communities….' This [myth] about incest being more commonly found in isolated places was not explained, leaving Scowen with a vague sense that 'perhaps it had been discovered or found out about in … the Forest of Dean … East Anglia.' Her class were also told that incest might happen when a man's sexual appetite could not be 'satisfied' by his wife because she had 'become almost prematurely old and had had several children—was worn out basically.' In that circumstance, Scowen was informed, 'the father might turn to the eldest daughter for sexual needs.' She recalled that there was no sense that they should look out for 'incest,' only 'battered babies.'[34] Most colleges delivered a brief session on child abuse at most. Sheffield City Polytechnic invited in a paediatrician, medical officer, area nurse and a social worker to deliver a two-hour lecture.[35] At Gloucester College of Arts and Technology in 1982, Quigley 'had an afternoon' on the subject delivered by a visiting social work manager. She recalled that the speaker was preoccupied by organisational changes in social services and how social workers were affected by them. She learned nothing about how to identify abuse.[36]

[32] Oral history interview with Anne Hackett* by author, 11 Jul 2019.

[33] Interview with Abramovich.

[34] Scowen's training preceded the 1970 Local Authority (LA) Social Services Act which replaced children's, welfare and mental health departments in each LA area with one social services department. Oral history interview with Patricia Scowen by author, 19 Sep 2019.

[35] Other colleges had similar content. See, for example, North East Surrey College of Technology and University of Southampton syllabi. 1975–77. TNA DW4/3; DW4/6; DW4/10.

[36] Interview with Quigley.

In 1982, there was some recognition at the national level that health visiting training was inadequate in relation to child maltreatment. A report commissioned by the Council for the Education and Training of Health Visitors tacitly acknowledged that qualifying courses should be updated, noting that the curriculum did not equip health visitors to meet the government requirement that practitioners have the 'special knowledge, skills and experience to be able to recognise when [abuse] is taking place or is likely to take place.' The author felt that perhaps some relevant information was conveyed on current courses by, for example, the psychiatrist who might cover 'abuse, physical and sexual, as a manifestation of mental illness or personality disorders.' However, specific sessions about predictors or the 'physiological signs of violence and sexual abuse; and the clues which may be found in the child's social interaction with others' might be needed.[37] Despite these recommendations, the proposal went nowhere, and courses remained largely devoid of content on child abuse. In 1987, Shirley Richardson, nursing officer responsible for in-service training at Middlesbrough Hospital, could not recall having received any formal training in relation to physical or sexual abuse.[38] Health visitors often called for their long professional training to be recognised, but it was training that was completely inadequate to the task of child protection.

## Part 2: Compassionate Consultants

In some ways, doctors' training gave them a better grounding in terms of detecting and responding to child sexual abuse, even though the taught curriculum at medical schools would not incorporate the topic until at least the end of the 1980s. Medical education usually consisted of two years' pre-clinical training following by three clinical years. After they qualified, all doctors had at least one supervised year as a 'houseman' (later updated to 'house officer' as more women took up training), before they could be registered as a medical practitioner.[39] The quality of the

[37] Sharman analysed messages for health visitors from the Lucy Gates Inquiry as well as previous reports. Ruth Sharman, *Child Abuse: A Discussion Paper* (London: Council for the Education and Training of Health Visitors, 1983); Department of Health and Social Security, *Child Abuse: A Study of Inquiry Reports 1973–1981* (London: HMSO, 1982), 2, 4–5.

[38] Inquiry into Child Abuse in Cleveland, TNA, BN68/18 Day 16 hearing – Shirley Richardson (Middlesbrough General Hospital), 4.9.1987, 26–27.

[39] The House Officer was the term used for the first stage of training in medicine. Laura Jefferson, Karen Bloor, and Alan Maynard, "Women in Medicine: Historical Perspectives and Recent Trends," *British Medical Bulletin* 114, no 1 (2015).

supervision was variable,[40] but where the relationship with the supervising consultant worked well, it had an overall positive effect on early career doctors, giving them more confidence in themselves as doctors.[41] As we will see below, this extended to the skills and knowledge related to child abuse.

A good example of this was Judith Trowell's experience when she worked as a paediatric registrar at Hemel Hempstead hospital in Hertfordshire. She had not had any formal training in child abuse, but she had 'a very good consultant' called Israel Kessel and it had come up in her 'sessions with him and on the ward rounds.' Kessel, she recalled, was extremely supportive in relation to a case that had 'a profound effect' on her. When a child was admitted with a severe head injury, it transpired that rather than permit her ex-husband to have contact with her daughter, the mother had deliberately attacked the toddler with the stiletto heel of her shoe. Initially, Trowell viewed the mother's behaviour as 'horrendous' and 'sort of unbelievable.' Her incredulity was compounded by the fact that the woman appeared to be 'entirely rational and reasonable,' and it was only later that Trowell realised that she was 'very disturbed.' It was her first 'traumatic experience' of child abuse, but she appreciated that afterwards, Kessel 'talked it all through' with her and accompanied her to the various follow-up conferences. She learned how to respond appropriately under the leadership of an interested and compassionate consultant.[42]

In Leeds, Chris Hobbs and Jane Wynne had a similar role model in Michael Buchanan, whose interest in child abuse was evident not only in the way he recorded details about non-accidental injuries in the notebooks that he carried about with him, but also in the empathy he showed children on the wards.[43] Deborah Hodes remembered that when she was a senior house officer at the Queen Elizabeth Hospital in Hackney in London in 1979, her supervising consultant, paediatrician Tony Jackson, explained the case of a child who had multiple bruises, 'a very sad, pathetic

[40] I. C. McManus, Diana N. J. Lockwood, and J. K. Cruickshank, 'The Preregistration Year: Chaos by Consensus,' *The Lancet* 309, no 8008 (1977).

[41] Consultants were the most senior NHS doctors who were fully qualified in a specialist area. Elisabeth Paice et al, 'The Relationship between Pre-Registration House Officers and Their Consultants,' *Medical Education* 36, no 1 (2002).

[42] Interview with Trowell.

[43] C. J. Hobbs and J. M. Wynne, "Management of Sexual Abuse," *Archives of Disease in Childhood* 62, no 11 (1987).

two-year-old' to her and the other doctors accompanying him on the ward round. His sympathy and understanding impressed her.[44] Speaking to researchers in the late 1970s, Jack Brown* recalled that paediatric consultant Christine Cooper had 'introduced' him to child abuse when he worked as her senior paediatric registrar in Newcastle. When he in turn became a consultant at a general hospital in Yorkshire, he took the lead in 'social problems, handicaps and NAI [non accidental injury].'[45] Similarly, Marietta Higgs recalled that she found working with Cooper in Newcastle 'very inspiring.' Under Cooper's leadership, she 'recognised the important part that paediatricians need[ed] to play' in the field of child abuse.[46]

Even if the consultant was not specifically interested in child maltreatment, they could provide trainees with opportunities to develop relevant knowledge and skills. Danya Glaser would ultimately become a child psychiatrist and specialise in child protection, but she had many different medical jobs during her training and early career in the late 1960s and early 1970s, a period in which she skilfully balanced the competing demands of work and childcare. She held various house officer posts in medicine, surgery and paediatrics, she filled in as a locum GP and she was a school doctor for a period. Under the influence of Tom Oppé, a consultant at St Mary's, Paddington, she became interested in developmental paediatrics, and he recruited her for multiple concurrent posts. These included running a clinic for premature babies at Paddington Green Children's Hospital, a paediatric outpatients' clinic at the Royal Free Hospital and an educational project for community paediatricians. She recalled that in all of this work, there 'was no child abuse in that at all, I can tell you, at all, at all, at all.'[47] What she was learning, however, was wholly relevant to understanding what was 'normal' or 'abnormal' in babies and young children; how to communicate with parents and other professionals; and the importance of gathering and analysing data.

Like Glaser, Stephen Amiel had no teaching on child abuse during his clinical training at University College London Hospital in the early 1970s. He did not remember 'anything about battered babies as such. And

[44] Oral history interview with Deborah Hodes by author, 31 May 2019.

[45] TM interview with Dr Jack Brown,* paediatrician, Yorkshire, 19 Oct 1979. Professor Robert Dingwall, ESRC QUALIDATA Study: 'The Protection of Children', Wellcome Collection, GC225.

[46] Inquiry into Child Abuse in Cleveland, TNA, BN 68/66 Day 54 hearing - Dr Marietta Higgs (Middlesbrough General Hospital), 16.11.1987, 7.

[47] Oral history interview with Danya Glaser by author, 20 July 2020.

certainly not a—not a whiff of child sexual abuse … for a number of years after that.' However, he had been interested in social problems from an early age. His parents were part of the Jewish diaspora, leaving Poland (which was part of Tsarist Russia at the time) to come to London as refugees. They brought their son up in a left-wing, socially conscious milieu. Amiel was admitted to hospital with suspected appendicitis as a small child. He remembered 'lying in bed watching this huddle of people in white coats, talking about cases and just desperately wanting to know what they were talking about.' He 'wanted a piece of that,' because he had an 'intense curiosity / nosiness' and an 'overdeveloped sense of social justice.' In his year as a house officer, he spent six months working to a consultant professor of geriatric medicine who had previously been a GP. Amiel thought he was 'completely inspirational' in the way he treated patients and his staff, having those 'two … key things' that were important in a doctor, which were 'empathy on the one hand and curiosity on the other.'[48]

Of course, not every doctor had a compassionate and supportive supervising consultant. Some had negative memories of consultants' attitudes to abused children. Charlotte Donaldson* heard nothing about child abuse during her training in Manchester or when working as a registrar in Kent in the early 1980s and when she moved to a leading London teaching hospital, she was shocked by the attitude of some consultants. They 'managed to not go down and see [children who had been abused] on ward rounds and things like that. They were not seen as important.' Donaldson had been sexually abused as a child herself and she felt her own experience made her more aware of this poor treatment. She decided to educate herself on the topic by reading recent scholarship such as Roland Summit's theory of the accommodation syndrome and Dante Cicchetti's ideas about developmental psychopathology.[49]

Where good quality supervision was provided and there was a positive relationship with the supervising consultant, junior doctors expanded their skills in a range of areas that were relevant to child abuse: an understanding of normative child development, communication skills, an awareness of the importance of data and evidence, curiosity and compassionate

[48] Amiel recalled hearing the phrase 'every story starts in the middle' in a radio play and it influencing his practice and teaching. Oral history interview with Stephen Amiel by author, 3 March and 6 Oct 2022.

[49] Interview with Charlotte Donaldson* by author, 9 Apr 2021.

care. Although child abuse was not a specialism in its own right, doctors could choose a specialty (such as paediatrics, general practice, emergency or forensic medicine) that would enable them to develop experience in identifying, assessing or treating child abuse. Doctors who were not interested in the topic could ignore it entirely.

## Part 3: Health Visitors as Catalysts

Whether the abuse was physical, related to neglect, poisoning or sexual abuse, the doctor's role was fairly clear. At the core of medical practice was the need to directly confront the signs and symptoms of illness or injury, ask questions, gather a history, physically examine patients and make a differential diagnosis. What might be causing this medical problem and what further investigations were required in order to arrive at an answer? Knowing what to look for was essential. Where there were suspicions of child abuse, they would follow the same process.

The situation was less straightforward for the health visitor. In 1982, their Training Council had suggested that the health visitor was 'most appropriately placed to make an assessment of childcare and an early identification of child abuse.' She might 'act as a catalyst by collecting information from all possible sources, collating the data collected, and presenting an informed case with a strategy for action.'[50] However, what information was she to collect, what was she assessing and how could she present 'an informed case' to others in a way that would establish her credibility and ensure that action would be taken?

Health visitors did recall attempt to 'act as catalysts,' but it was rarely uncomplicated. Scowen, for example, described a time when she was worried about a family. She felt that 'something was wrong somehow' in the relationships between the different family members and she observed that one of the girls 'was withdrawn and she wasn't developing quite as one would expect.' She told the superintendent health visitor that she was worried about sexual abuse and the family was asked to attend the local child guidance clinic. Once the referral was made, Scowen was 'absolutely shut out' and no feedback was shared with her. At the family home, she was confronted by angry parents; they told her that they 'didn't like' the clinic because 'a lot of questions were asked about their sexual life and their

[50] Sharman, *Child Abuse: A Discussion Paper*, 3.

private life, and they were shocked by this and hostile.' She had no information to help her to manage those interactions. Had her intervention made any difference? There were no mechanisms for her to give an outlet to her own feelings and her sense of her own professional standing was undoubtedly diminished by the process. After this bruising encounter, she did not 'notice' worrying signs of child sexual abuse in any subsequent case.

Scowen's supervisor had, at least, paid attention to her worries, whereas other health visitors felt their concerns were dismissed. Bramwell recalled having 'grave concerns' about a particular family. The younger girls were often only partially clothed, the older girls' poor school attendance was unexplained, and they were all somewhat 'watchful and a bit guarded' and she 'didn't feel it sat right with [her], but [she] wasn't quite sure.' She felt that it was her duty to go to the senior GP but he acted as if her concern did not deserve any serious consideration, saying that 'he knew them well and that there was nothing to worry about.' She was aware that there was no 'actual evidence' or disclosure, but she felt that 'there was something as they say "not quite right"... it was more a feeling and wanting some more senior advice to say, "well where do we go with this and could this be a concern."' But Bramwell 'didn't feel that [she] was listened to at that stage.'

Hackett* similarly sought advice from a doctor. She was suspicious of a father who, she thought, was possibly abusing his baby. The mother was vulnerable because she had an intellectual disability. Hackett examined the father's medical records and 'could see he had a whole raft of child abuse himself .... Every form: sexually, physically, every form, had a horrific childhood.' She felt there was a risk of physical, sexual and emotional abuse of both the child and the mother in that situation, but she found it 'very difficult to get underneath' what was happening. Hackett noticed that the child 'always had an erect penis.' As this happened very frequently, she mentioned it to the doctor. He said,

> it's probably just that he's going to have a wee or that he's maybe a bit overexcited or something like that, and that was the end of it. But I was thinking, 'is he being sexually abused?' But it's almost too—too horrific to think about, do you know?[51]

The doctor had dismissed her concern about sexual abuse. This compounded her own difficulty in accepting the possibility that a father could sexually abuse his very young baby. In fact, she was unsure about whether

[51] Interview with Hackett.*

small babies could be victimised in that way, stating, 'babies—did they get sexually abused at that—in that era? Not really.'[52] When a crisis of a different sort occurred in the family, she was relieved that the facts were more easily verifiable and that when the case went to court, it was accepted that the child was unsafe and needed protection.[53]

Whether the practitioner actively suspected sexual abuse or had a 'feeling' that something was wrong, finding out later that a child had been abused provoked guilt. Xavier was concerned about a schoolchild whom she often saw waiting outside the nurse's room and, she recalled, 'if she wasn't there, if I didn't see her, the mother would usually be round at the clinic saying she'd lost her [contraceptive] pills.' On a visit to the family home, the 'rather young and immature father' insisted on taking her upstairs to show her the bedroom for reasons she could not fathom. The child seeking attention, the mother constantly asking for extra oral contraceptives and the father eager to show her the bedroom were pieces of a puzzle that worried her, but that never coalesced into concrete concerns that she could express. Later, she met the school nurse who told her that there had been a court case because the child had been sexually abused. She thought 'should I have known? Was I too stupid or could I have stopped something, or could I have done it better?' There was no forum for her to share her concerns and no one to offer professional advice.[54]

Neither were health visitors' professional opinions always taken seriously in multi-disciplinary settings and, accordingly, they could lack confidence in asserting their views, particularly at case conferences.[55] Hutcheson recalled attending one such meeting about a pre-school child who had a sexually transmitted disease. The professionals were arguing about 'how accurate the test could be, you know, it got into all of that and then there was something about the dog ....' She remembered thinking, 'there's something about this that isn't right .... I can't articulate what it is.' In conversation with the child protection advisor a few days later, she realised

[52] This speaks to philosophical ideas of what can be named and understood about child abuse, and to the extent to which empirical data about the sexual abuse of babies and infants was known about which is discussed below. Ian Hacking, 'The Making and Moulding of Child Sexual Abuse,' *Critical Inquiry* 17 (1991); Carol Smart, 'A History of Ambivalence and Conflict in the Discursive Construction of the "Child Victim" of Sexual Abuse,' *Social & Legal Studies* 8, no 3 (1999); Christopher J. Hobbs and Jane Wynne, 'Buggery in Childhood: A Common Syndrome of Child Abuse,' *The Lancet* 328, no 8510 (1986).

[53] Interview with Hackett.*

[54] Interview with Xavier.

[55] Sharman, *Child Abuse: A Discussion Paper*, 4.

that 'there was a lot of anger in the room ... lots of trying to placate and ...no-one was really focusing on what does this mean for the child.' She remembered thinking 'do we know if this child's at risk or not?' When she left the case conference, she thought 'actually I don't, I don't really.' Everyone around the table had focused on the adults in the family and in that fraught space Hutcheson was not able to assert herself and articulate her concern for the child.[56]

'Accurate factual reporting,' the ability to analyse information, interpret it and 'state a professional opinion' were essential skills for a health visitor, according to their Training Council.[57] What did 'factual' look like in relation to a hidden form of abuse where there were usually no witnesses, there was rarely a direct disclosure from a child or other family member and there was seldom any physical evidence? Health visitors struggled to voice their concerns in ways that would be accepted by other disciplines as legitimate professional opinions. A feeling that 'something was not quite right' could be dismissed as subjective, a hunch, and thus open to bias. Of course, intuition could be rooted in a health visitor's professional expertise and grow out of their skills in relationship-building, their knowledge of child development and child health, their understanding of family dynamics, as well as what a healthy parent/child relationship looked like. But this was not articulated. Nor did anyone within or outside the profession specify exactly what might be expected of a health visitor in terms of the knowledge and skills they would need in order to prevent or interrupt sexual abuse in the family.

## Part 4: Drawing in All the Disciplines

In a speech given in London in 1978, US paediatrician C. Henry Kempe advocated extending the 'closed system of child protection' beyond social workers to 'physicians, nurses, police, the judiciary ....'[58] Inquiries into child fatalities also emphasised that effective working relationships between the professions were of great importance in keeping children safe.[59] And in

[56] Interview with Hutcheson.

[57] Sharman, *Child Abuse: A Discussion Paper*, 4–6.

[58] C. Henry Kempe, 'Recent Developments in the Field of Child Abuse,' *Child Abuse & Neglect* 2, no 4 (1978): 262.

[59] Department of Health and Social Security, *Child Abuse: A Study of Inquiry Reports 1973–1981.*

these years, when medicine and nursing education did not address child abuse, health practitioners seeking to educate themselves on the subject had to look to multi-disciplinary training.

The Open University (OU) and Newcastle Polytechnic worked together to develop the first comprehensive multidisciplinary course on child abuse published in Britain in 1978. The project's advisers were leading voices in the emerging field of child protection and medics exerted the greatest influence. There were four paediatricians including consultant Cooper from Newcastle; Margaret Lynch of the Park Hospital for Children in Oxford; Catherine Peckham of Charing Cross Hospital Medical School; and Alfred White Franklin, convenor of the influential Tunbridge Wells Study Group.[60] These were joined by an accident and emergency doctor, a psychiatrist, psychologists, a nurse and six university or charity affiliated researchers.[61]

This course aimed to attract 'medicine, nursing, therapy, psychology, child care, social or welfare work, teaching, social administration, police work, the law or some related discipline.'[62] It would require a significant time commitment from students, with each of its twenty-six units expected to take about two hours of study time.[63] Those who signed up received a red and a blue book, each about the same size as a paperback novel. The red *Reader and Sourcebook* contained a range of articles and book excerpts.[64] It is the first four pages, however, sandwiched between the

[60] This was the first medically led group to consider non-accidental injury in Britain in the early 1970s; White Franklin was also the founder member of the British Association for the Prevention and Study of Child Abuse and Neglect (BASPCAN). John Pickett, 'The BASPCAN Founders,' *Child Abuse Review* 1, no 1 (1992).

[61] Malcolm Hall, Preston represented accident and emergency medicine. Marie-Thérèse Gilbert, nursing. Winifred Cavenagh was the lawyer. Israel Kolvin, University of Newcastle and the Nuffield Psychology and Psychiatry Unit was the psychiatrist; William Reavley, the clinical psychologist, Maurice Chazan the educational psychologist. The researchers were social worker Olive Stevenson and Christine Desborough at Keele; Jacquie Roberts at the Park Hospital; Anna Kerr at the NSPCC; Carolyn Okell Jones at the National Children's Bureau; Megan Jobling at the Institute for Research into Mental and Multiple Handicap.

[62] Perhaps this alluded to social workers, as child abuse was certainly not incorporated into nursing or medical education at this time.

[63] Carver, ed., *Child Abuse: A Study Text*, xviii.

[64] Constance M. Lee, ed., *Child Abuse: A Reader and Sourcebook*; Vida Carver, ed., *Child Abuse: A Study Text*; Colin Harris and Constance M. Lee, 'Child Abuse: Finding Further Information,' (Milton Keynes and New York: The Open University Press, 1978).

table of contents and the introduction, that stuns the contemporary reader. These contained seven colour photographs of children who had been physically injured, each accompanied by a descriptive caption. The images included the mark of a strap on a young child's face, a festering rash on the arm of a baby said to be severely neglected and to have multiple fractures, babies with fingertip bruises on their faces, a child with cigarette burns to her lips and the chubby feet of a toddler scalded by being lowered into hot water. One photograph was a close up of teeth marks on a child's buttocks, the caption noting that the two-year-old boy also had part of one testicle removed by a very severe bite. These were (and are) deeply unsettling photographs. They were taken at close quarters and some of the infants stared into the camera, with expressions that the captions described as 'frozen awareness,' the look Scowan had been taught about on her health visitor training, seen in children who had suffered cruelty over a long period.[65]

The *Study Text* instructed students to 'turn to the colour plates,' look at the photographs and captions closely and not to take notes or read anything else. After examining the photographs, they were to complete a questionnaire about their personal feelings. These included horror, anxiety, physical nausea, sorrow, incredulity, pity for the child, feelings of uselessness, shame and guilt. There was a feeling that some forms of abuse were worse than others. There was pity for, and anger at, the abusers and some people ticked that they felt disturbed that they might be personally capable of hurting a child. Some felt a need to help, others an inability to look at the photographs at all. Some ticked detachment or clinical objectivity. The purpose of the graphic photographs was to provoke these intense reactions.[66] Without feeling, the authors claimed, 'we would be little more than human vegetables, and we would certainly lack understanding of other, more warm-blooded human beings.' However, there was a risk that when 'gripped by' emotion, 'cool judgement and wise action' might come under threat, creating what psychologists called

[65] Lee, ed., *Child Abuse: A Reader and Sourcebook*, plates 3 and 4 (pages unnumbered).

[66] The fourth category, 'a need for more information,' was ticked by many respondents and seemed to stem from respondents' desire to distinguish between impulsive and premeditated acts of cruelty. The chapter authors went to some lengths to encourage students to empathise with abusive adults who had deliberately hurt their children in a way that later training materials seemed to avoid.

'selective perception,' affecting what was seen and believed about the situation to hand.[67] Emotion was required to motivate people and to help make sense of others' behaviour, but it must be contained.

There are no records of who might have purchased the course.[68] We do not know whether the materials reached their intended audiences in the different disciplines, whether people paid for the course themselves or were subsidised by their employers, or whether they studied alone or in groups. Unsurprisingly, given the year of publication, there were only a handful of references to sexual abuse. It was mentioned in passing by White Franklin alongside 'fear, nagging, quarrelling, and [being] kept in isolation' and listed as one of the features of an 'abusive environment' by Cooper.[69]

The OU training course was one route to learning more about child abuse. It prepared students intellectually and emotionally to respond, but it required a significant time commitment on the student's part. Many less time-consuming alternatives became available from the mid-1980s in the shape of short workshops and courses. These were most commonly provided by not-for-profit organisations run by feminists and survivors, by social services departments, and by Area Review Committees (later Area Child Protection Committees) which began to take on a greater leadership role in multi-disciplinary training.

Some courses were superficial in terms of the knowledge imparted to participants. Kidscape fell into that category. Founded by an American educational psychologist Michele Elliott, its main aim was to promote primary prevention programmes for children and for professionals who could assist children to protect themselves from sexual abuse. Although Elliott claimed that Kidscape had trained over 20,000 teachers, social workers, education welfare officers, health visitors, police, nurses and others by 1989, the majority of those were probably teachers. There was a *Kidscape Kit* (1986) for teaching children aged five to eleven about body ownership, touching, secrets, intuition, saying no and getting support. Training included awareness-raising days at schools, as well as teachers'

[67] Carver, ed., Child Abuse: A Study Text, 12.

[68] Author correspondence with OU archive, 12 Oct 2021. There were other short courses running at universities, e.g. a one day per week, 20-week course on Child Protection run by King's College Law Faculty and LSE Department of Social Sciences was advertised to take place in Oct 1989. See Incest & Child Sexual Assault newsletter, 11, 21 May 1989.

[69] 'Normal' and 'abnormal' parent-child relations within the context of the course, Carver, ed., *Child Abuse: A Study Text,* pp. 33–45.

and parents' workshops.[70] Practitioners such as Christine Judson of Riverside Child Health Project in Newcastle raised concerns about putting so much responsibility onto children to protect themselves. Nevertheless, she thought school doctors should be aware of child sexual abuse and be present at parents' meetings to answer questions. If training the children encouraged disclosures, they might also need to assist in assessing the children or referring them on to 'a suitably experienced colleague.'[71] Kidscape also produced a Training Guide for adults (1989) to be used for a single or three-day course; this covered feelings, disclosure, multi-disciplinary working, helping children to express themselves, child protection materials for use with children, statistics and next steps. Sexual abuse was a complicated and fraught topic and yet the time allocated to tasks was brief and the treatment of the topics was simplistic.[72]

The Child Sexual Abuse Prevention and Education project (CSAPEP) delivered a very different kind of training. Established in 1984 with a grant from the Greater London Council the project's primary beneficiaries were children, but it also offered training to practitioners. Reflecting later on the work, founder Emily Driver acknowledged 'the difficulties faced by workers battling against the massive institutional powers of their agencies … forcing some into silence and others into collusion.' The lack of professional training and the absence of reflective spaces combined with large caseloads often prevented practitioners from bringing 'their own insights and understandings to the work, [and] actually militated against self-expression and therefore against useful communication with both clients and colleagues.'[73] It was surprising to Driver that professionals expected children to 'disclose all their feelings to adults when adults have not yet even dared to break their own silence in the workplace.'[74] The suppression of the voices of those with lived experience was widespread: a

[70] *Kidscape Primary Kit.* London: Kidscape (1986)

[71] *Community Paediatric Group Newsletter* in association with British Paediatric Association, Autumn 1989, 6. For a critique of primary prevention programmes directed at adult women, see Lesley Macmillan and Deborah White, 'The Missing and Imagined Perpetrator in Rape Prevention Efforts,' *Women's History Review* 32, no 7 (2023).

[72] Michele Elliott, *Dealing with Child Abuse : The Kidscape Training Guide* (London: Kidscape, 1989).

[73] Emily Driver, 'Through the Looking Glass: Children and the Professionals Who Treat Them,' in *Child Sexual Abuse: Feminist Perspectives*, ed. Emily Driver and Audrey Drioisen (Basingstoke: Macmillan, 1989), 107–108, 129.

[74] 'Through the Looking Glass: Children and the Professionals Who Treat Them,' 107–108, 129.

social worker explained that she and other female colleagues who were survivors of child sexual abuse 'don't share that fact of our abuse with our managers' because they 'say it blinkers us—that we'll feel, automatically, that the man is guilty.' She argued that her own abuse gave her insight into working with children, 'because they'll tell you maybe an inch of what's on their mind, and if they feel you believe them, they'll keep telling you more.'[75]

Many other organisations put on short training courses on sexual abuse in this period and in those pre-internet days, activists like Rasjidah St John played a vital role by collating the information and distributing it to interested individuals in the NHS, local authorities and charities in her monthly Incest and Sexual Assault newsletters. The British Association for the Study and Prevention of Child Abuse and Neglect (BASPCAN) was also important in delivering conferences and study days nationwide. Paediatricians and child psychiatrists had been heavily involved in forming the organisation and it continued to draw doctors and health visitors to its events.[76]

Local organisations in different areas also ran training. To give just a few examples, City and Hackney Association for Mental Health ran a free introductory workshop on preventing child sexual abuse at Hackney Hospital in London in October 1985.[77] The Child Abuse Studies Unit at the Polytechnic of North London hosted conferences, lectures and workshops, often open only to women participants. These included the 'Child Sexual Abuse: Towards A Feminist Professional Practice' conference in April 1987 and a talk on 'Working with sexually abused boys' on 27 Apr 1989. The Family Rights Group provided short workshops on topics such as 'Work with mothers of sexually abused children' while the Women's Therapy Centre ran (on multiple occasions) a training course for 'women working with incest survivors.'[78] Lambeth Women and Children's Project planned a training day for Black women 'working with and living with the effects of child sexual assault' to take place in February 1990.[79] In

[75] Melba Wilson, *Crossing the Boundary: Black Women Survive Incest* (London: Virago, 1993).

[76] BASPCAN events were advertised frequently in the Incest and Sexual Assault newsletter throughout the 1980s, archive of Rasjidah St John.

[77] CHAMH flyer and programme, archive of Rasjidah St John.

[78] Incest and Sexual Assault newsletter, 12, 21 Jun 1989; 15, 21 Sep 1989.

[79] Incest and Sexual Assault newsletter, 17, 21 Nov 1989.

Shrewsbury, the Sexual Abuse Child Consultancy Service (SACCS) regularly advertised workshops with invited speakers including, for example, a one-day session led by psychiatrist Tilman Furniss from the Tavistock Clinic on 'The adolescent sex offender—abused and abuser' on 24 October 1989. The Standing Committee on Sexually Abused Children (SCOSAC) provided workshops in different venues nationwide, including residential training courses.[80] Rape Crisis and community services for survivors of child sexual abuse like Taboo in Manchester and CHOICES, the Cambridge Incest Survivors Refuge also delivered training, often for a low or even no fee.[81] Many social services departments across the country offered training and developmental activities to the agencies in their areas that worked with children.[82]

Health practitioners, then, could engage with a diverse array of training if they had a particular interest in child sexual abuse. Even if they were keen, however, there was no guarantee that they would get agreement for time away from their everyday duties to attend the training as it was not part of any agreed plan of professional development or formally supported by employers. It could only have a marginal effect on practice.

## Part 5: Training the Specialists

At the frontline of community healthcare, there was no consistent training for GPs or health visitors up to the late 1980s. Paediatricians, however, were developing more specialist training with an emphasis on the technical skills needed to respond to child sexual abuse. Leeds paediatricians Hobbs and Wynne were highly influential figures in this process. The pair met in Leeds in the early 1970s and then went their separate ways to develop their careers before reuniting approximately ten years later when they were appointed to two new lectureships in community paediatrics in the city. When Buchanan asked for volunteers to form a multi-disciplinary child abuse team, Hobbs and Wynne signed up along with clinical psychologist

[80] Incest and Sexual Assault newsletter, 13, 21 Jul 1989.

[81] Helen Jones and Kate Cook, *Rape Crisis: Responding to Sexual Violence* (Dorset, UK: Russell House Publishing Ltd, 2008), 19–26; Norwich Consultants on Sexual Violence, 'Claiming Our Status as Experts: Community Organizing,' *Feminist Review*, 28 no 1 (1988); Jenny Kitzinger, 'Defending Innocence: Ideologies of Childhood,' *Feminist Review*, 28, no 1 (1988).

[82] Interview with Beth Fuller;* oral history interviews with Gerrilyn Smith and Sam Warner by author.

Helga Hanks and social worker Jill McMurray. They met weekly, seeing children on ward rounds and discussing cases. Around 1982, Buchanan invited American psychiatrist David Corwin to give a lecture on the 'new area' of child sexual abuse to his team,[83] along with colleagues from the NSPCC, child psychiatry and social services. As local awareness grew, so did the number of sexual abuse cases referred, with a steep climb from ten cases in 1983, to 106 in 1985 and 237 in 1986.[84]

Buchanan's notebooks were replaced with detailed records of the team's assessments and findings. In the mid-1980s, Hobbs and Wynne submitted an article to *The Lancet*, based on data they had gathered on a cohort of eighteen girls and seventeen boys over an eight-month period. Under the arresting title, 'Buggery in childhood: a common symptom of child abuse,' they described some of the signs of 'penile penetration' of the vagina but noted that it was uncommon in the very young. Their main and most controversial finding was that 'buggery' in infants, toddlers and young children was a 'serious, common, and under-reported type of child abuse.' The physical evidence they documented related to 'fissures, dilation and reflex dilation, loss of sphincter, shortening and eversion of the anal canal, external venous congestion and generalised reddening and thickening of perianal tissues.'[85] The exact definition of these signs is not important here, but the article would cause consternation amongst medics and have serious implications for children, families and practitioners.

Hobbs's colour photographs were an essential component of the article, captioned 'anal appearances in anal abuse.'[86] Although colour plates had been published in the medical journals since the early twentieth century,[87] they were used infrequently due to prohibitive printing costs. *The Lancet's* editor, Ian Munro, predicted that the article's main contention (that very young babies and children were anally raped) and the use of the images would be controversial, but following a meeting with the

[83] See Chap. 4.

[84] Hobbs and Wynne, 'Buggery in Childhood: A Common Syndrome of Child Abuse.'; C. J. Hobbs and J. M. Wynne, 'Sexual Abuse of English Boys and Girls: The Importance of Anal Examination,' *Child Abuse & Neglect* 13, no 2 (1989).

[85] Hobbs and Wynne, 'Buggery in Childhood: A Common Syndrome of Child Abuse.'

[86] 'Buggery in Childhood: A Common Syndrome of Child Abuse.'

[87] See colour plates of men and women with leprosy 'Explanation of Special Colour Plate,' *British Medical Journal* 1, no 2349 (1906).

two paediatricians, he decided to proceed with publication. Reactions were swift and vociferous with many angry letters sent to Munro, not only from paediatricians but also from doctors in surgery, medicine, forensics and other specialties.[88] Wynne and Hobbs had emphasised that consideration of the child's history and their behaviour (for example, 'particularly explicit behaviour manifest in the child's play') was essential and that differential diagnosis should be considered, as well as highlighting the need for further research on the physical signs. Lastly, they pointed out that seventeen of the 35 children had said that someone had done something to their bottoms, commenting, for example, that 'a snake bit my bottom,' or 'he put a knife in my bottom.' In five other cases, a sibling had given the abuse history.[89] The authors concluded that 'a clear history given by the child of interference with his bottom' was of the 'greatest importance.'

Despite their caution, they were criticised for presuming that the physical signs they documented were pathological. Letter writers put forward other possible explanations for anal dilatation, fissures and other signs.[90] More than one correspondent described the dangers of destroying families 'on circumstantial evidence that prove[d] to be misleading.'[91] Elizabeth Tylden described a seven-year-old who 'burst into tears' telling her that she was frightened of 'lady doctors.' Tylden explained that the child had been

> referred to the social services for masturbation and disturbed behaviour at school. She had violently resisted inspection of her 'bottom' by a woman doctor and was threatened with examination under anaesthetic. Instead she had been subjected to a session with 'dirty dolls.'[92]

[88] Elizabeth Tylden, letter to the editor, *The Lancet*, 31 October 1987: 1017; John A. Davis, 21 November 1987: 1217; H. B. Keen, 31 October 1987: 1018; George Russell, 12 December 1987: 1397; R. Sunderland, 31 October 1987: 1018; B. L. Priestley, 12 December 1987: 1396; J. K. H. Wales and L. S. Taitz, 12 December 1987: 1396–1397; C. M. Ridley, 31 October 1987: 1017–1018.

[89] Hobbs and Wynne, 'Buggery in Childhood: A Common Syndrome of Child Abuse.'

[90] H. B. Keen, letter to the editor, *The Lancet*, 31 October 1987: 1018; George Russell, 12 December 1987: 1397; R. Sunderland, 31 October 1987: 1018; B. L. Priestley, 12 December 1987: 1396; J. K. H. Wales and L. S. Taitz, 12 December 1987: 1396–1397; C. M. Ridley, 31 October 1987: 1017–1018.

[91] John A. Davis, letter to the editor, *The Lancet*, 21 November 1987: 1217; Elizabeth Tylden, letter to the editor, *The Lancet*, 31 October 1987: 1017.

[92] Tylden, letter to the editor.

Tylden claimed that she was not criticising Hobbs and Wynne's paper or an article by child psychiatrist Harry Zeitlin in the same issue; both of which, in her view, demonstrated that doctors must stick to the principle that 'correct diagnoses are arrived at as a result of weighing up the large number of clinical factors presented to the doctor.' Her disapproval was directed at those [unnamed] who saw sexual abuse at the root of any number of symptoms: 'molestation,' she commented, 'preferably incestuous, is the fashionable diagnosis.'[93] Hobbs and Wynne had explained their use of anatomically correct dolls to 'help the child talk more precisely about the nature of the abuse,' but stressed that their use could 'precipitate emotional disturbances which the examiner must feel confident to handle.'[94] Tylden felt examiners were poorly qualified; she was particularly disturbed by the 'merciless grilling' of children in badly executed disclosure interviews using anatomically correct dolls while 'voyeurs behind one-way glass create a Kafka like setting for the perversion of innocence.'[95]

Doctors looked to the prestigious medical journals to continue their education and keep up to date with developments. Within their pages, paediatricians and police surgeons disagreed about how to interpret the signs of sexual abuse on children's bodies. Some of these debates were territorial. Police surgeons had seen themselves as the experts in this area. They had the technical skills to examine children's bodies and document their findings to enable their use in court. But their photographs had also been used to teach doctors about child abuse. The colour plates reproduced in the OU/Newcastle training course reader were credited to *The Police Surgeon* journal.[96] In 1983, the *Police Surgeon Supplement* advertised 'An Atlas of Non-Accidental Injuries in Children' which provided 87 'mostly colour' illustrations from past issues of the journal. It was promoted as an essential resource for other police surgeons and police officers, GPs, those working in casualty, social workers, probation workers, health visitors and NSPCC officers.[97]

[93] Tylden, letter to the editor.

[94] Hobbs and Wynne, 'Buggery in Childhood: A Common Syndrome of Child Abuse,' 796.

[95] Tylden, letter to the editor.

[96] Lee, ed., *Child Abuse: A Reader and Sourcebook*, 313.

[97] The contributors were consultant M H Hall from the Accident and Emergency department at Preston Royal Infirmary, John Furness forensic odontologist, Liverpool and James Hilton, force surgeon at Norfolk Constabulary. 'An Atlas of Non-Accidental Injuries in Children,' Advertisement in *Police Surgeon Supplement,* 14 (May 1983): 4.

While Buchanan had captured data about child abuse with a pen and a notebook, Hobbs gathered visual images used a handheld camera, and later via a colposcope machine which incorporated built-in magnifying lenses, an intense light source and a 35 mm camera. Originally used in Germany in the 1930s to try to detect early signs of cervical cancer, the colposcope was not used much in Britain until the late 1970s when gynaecologists increasingly deployed it to support the diagnosis of women with abnormal cervical smears and prevent unnecessary invasive medical procedures.[98] With this technology at his disposal, Hobbs could capture close-up colour photographs of children's genital and perianal anatomy to be used for diagnosis and sometimes to be produced as evidence in court. The data could also be analysed for research and teaching purposes. Through compiling collections of photographs, Hobbs hoped to provide clarity on the physical signs of sexual abuse in much the same way as radiographers and paediatricians had previously used x-ray images 'to make the invisible visible … and bring new attention to the child's physical injuries.'[99]

Paediatricians, therefore, were encroaching on police surgeons' area of authority. Some were also openly critical of police surgeons' treatment of children. Paediatrician N. J. Wild claimed that there was 'growing evidence that the collection of evidence by police and police surgeons may be damaging and that abused children often do not subsequently receive advice or treatment.'[100] This opinion was denounced by two women police surgeons, Phyllis Turvill and Raine Roberts, in subsequent letters to the *British Medical Journal (BMJ)*. Roberts pointed out that her profession was aware of the need for improvements and, furthermore, doctors required forensic, as well as paediatric, skills in order to provide accurate reports to the court if they were needed. Roberts also warned that the use of the anatomically correct dolls, while being a 'very helpful tool in skilled hands, [was] open to grave errors of interpretation.' Interviews should be videorecorded, in her opinion, so that interpretation was not left to just the 'subjective opinion of one observer.'[101] It was ironic that while Roberts

[98] 'Colposcopy,' *British Medical Journal (Clinical Research Edition)* 282, no 6260 (1981): 250–251.

[99] Jennifer Crane, *Child Protection in England, 1960–2000: Expertise, Experience, and Emotion* (Cham, Switzerland: Palgrave Macmillan, 2018), 29.

[100] See Chap. 3 in relation to Nesta Wells had argued back in 1961 that such treatment was outside the police surgeon's remit. N. J. Wild, 'Sexual Abuse of Children in Leeds,' *BMJ (Clinical Research Edition)* 292, no 6528 (1986): 1115.

[101] P. Turvill and Raine Roberts, letters to the editor, *BMJ*, 7 Jun 1986: 1527.

called for greater transparency through video documentation, the tone of the letters sent following the publication of the Hobbs and Wynne article suggested that other doctors found the increased visibility of child sexual abuse—whether achieved through photographic evidence of anal injuries or video recordings of children telling adults what had been done to them—deeply disturbing.

## Part 6: Cleveland and After

That Hobbs and Wynne's research on the physical signs generated dissent was not in itself particularly problematic. After all, differences of opinion were at the heart of the peer review process. The system was based on colleagues scrutinising each other's research findings for methodological problems, biases or flawed arguments. Research in the area of the physical signs of sexual abuse was in its infancy, there was not yet a great deal of accountability. Neither were there any 'normative standards for the appearance of the hymen, peri-hymenal tissues, or perianal tissues.'[102] Hobbs and Wynne had described some of the limitations of their study themselves, but their caveats went unnoticed. Ultimately, it would be doctors in Cleveland rather than in Leeds who would be subjected to the most vociferous public criticism about the validity of the physical signs.

Marietta Higgs and Geoffrey Wyatt were the Cleveland paediatricians under scrutiny. In 1987, they came under fierce attack from politicians and the press for precipitating the removal of children they had diagnosed as sexually abused from their parents' care and admitting them to hospital under Place of Safety Orders.[103] This created what would later be described as 'a phenomenal rise' in admissions of children suspected of being sexually abused to Middlesbrough Hospital, from two children in 1986 to 104 between March and July of 1987.[104] Much of the press attention honed in on a specific physical finding of 'reflex anal dilation.' This was a 'sign' that

[102] Patricia A. W. Brennan, 'The Medical and Ethical Aspects of Photography in the Sexual Assault Examination: Why Does It Offend?,' *Journal of Clinical Forensic Medicine* 13, no 4 (2006): 199.

[103] Prior to Children Act 1989, under Section 28 of Children and Young Persons Act 1969, 'Place of Safety' order allowed the Local Authority to detain a child without considering the parents involvement for up to 28 days with no duty to promote contact between the child and their parents.

[104] Inquiry into Child Abuse in Cleveland, TNA, BN68/02 Day 1 hearing - Matthew Thorpe QC, 11.08.1987, 3–4.

had previously been associated with homosexuality between adult men. More than a century earlier, it had been at the centre of an infamous court case, R v. Boulton and Park, relating to two men who had been 'accused of conspiring to commit, and of committing, unnatural acts.' The 1871 proceedings were a site of medical controversy, with seven medical practitioners called to give evidence. Police surgeon James Thomas Paul testified that the accused men had 'an extreme dilation of the anus,' that the 'muscles were relaxed' and that the anus 'readily opened.'[105] After Wynne and Hobbs identified it as one of the possible indicators that a child had been anally abused, the Cleveland doctors incorporated the test into their practice. As the number of children admitted to hospital rose, two individuals (politician Stuart Bell and vicar Michael Wright) brought the situation in Cleveland to the attention of the national media.[106] They styled themselves as advocates for the parents (who were painted as the 'real' victims in this situation).[107] On 9 July 1987, the government announced an Inquiry.[108]

To combat the accusation that she and Wyatt had relied solely on anal dilation as the basis for a diagnosis of sexual abuse, Higgs attempted to emphasise early on in her evidence to the Inquiry that she was acting on the latest discoveries in the field. She described a conference hosted by the Leeds Sexual Abuse Team that she had attended the previous year. It was there, listening to Wynne give a presentation and seeing the photographs, that she 'realised for the first time the numbers of children that could be involved in this problem' and the 'importance of the medical examination.'[109] She claimed that one of the first things she had learned from the Leeds team was not to rely on physical signs alone, but to also think about the history and listen to what the child had to say.

[105] Ivan Dalley Crozier, 'The Medical Construction of Homosexuality and Its Relation to the Law in Nineteenth-Century England,' *Medical History* 45, no 1 (2001): 68–69.

[106] Mica Nava, 'Cleveland and the Press: Outrage and Anxiety in the Reporting of Child Sexual Abuse,' *Feminist Review*, no 28 (1988); Jenny Kitzinger, 'Media Templates: Controversial Allegations and Analogies,' in *Framing Abuse: Media Influence and Public Understanding of Sexual Violence against Children* (London: Pluto Press, 2004); Beatrix Campbell, *Secrets and Silence: Uncovering the Legacy of the Cleveland Child Sexual Abuse Case* (Bristol: Bristol University Press and Policy Press, 2023).

[107] 'Crisis that has doctors on attack,' *Daily Mail*, 25 Jun 1987;'I could weep for some of these children, *Daily Express*, 26 Jun 1987; 'The first child is set free, *Daily Mail*, 26 Jun 1987.

[108] 'Child abuse Cleveland,' HC Deb 09 July 1987 vol 119 cc528–38.

[109] Inquiry into Child Abuse in Cleveland, TNA, BN 68/66 Day 54 hearing - Dr Marietta Higgs (Middlesbrough General Hospital), 16.11.1987, 20.

She also emphasised that she had learned from Wynne that once other professionals became aware that there were doctors in their local area who could diagnose child sexual abuse, the numbers would rise swiftly. Higgs had made this connection in an earlier interview given to *The Observer*, stating that 'once social workers know there is someone at the hospital who is concerned about child abuse, they send up all the children they have been worried about for some time,' adding that she thought that the anger directed at her was 'a direct analogy of what happens to children when they disclose that they have been abused or when abuse is detected.' This, she believed, justified removing children 'to a safe environment' at that point 'to protect them from pressure.'[110]

Many of the practices for which Higgs and Wyatt were being criticised (admission to hospital, carrying out a full body examination, the reflex anal dilation test) had been used in Leeds and in some other areas as well, and yet the scandal arose in Cleveland. One key difference between the two areas was, as counsel to the Inquiry Matthew Thorpe QC explained, that 'all sorts of conflicts' between doctors themselves and between doctors and other 'relevant agencies' had arisen in Cleveland.[111] This was in contrast to Leeds where Buchanan had from the outset involved other agencies in discussions about child abuse and how to combat it. The Sexual Abuse Team had built on that, running large multi-agency, multidisciplinary training sessions every year for people across the city and generally promoting relationships across the agencies.

The details of how the professions fell out in Cleveland (the paediatricians and social workers positioned in one corner, the police and police surgeons in the other) are not important here.[112] Ultimately, the abused children and the two paediatricians were the losers. The government and the mainstream press amplified the news that 98 of the total 125 children who had been removed on place of safety orders had been returned home by July 1988 and that proceedings in 27 wardship cases had been dismissed.[113] The fact that the Second Opinion Panel had judged that the diagnoses of sexual abuse were correct in at least 80 per cent of the cases was not circulated publicly.[114] And although the Inquiry report was

[110] 'Child abuse doctor slams her critics,' *The Observer*, 28 Jun 1987

[111] BN 68/02 Day 1 hearing - Matthew Thorpe QC, 11.08.1987, 3–4.

[112] Sue Richardson and Heather Bacon, *Child Sexual Abuse: Whose Problem? Reflections from Cleveland* (Birmingham: Venture Press, 1991).

[113] Summary of the Cleveland Inquiry,' *BMJ* 298 (16 July 1988): 190–191.

[114] R. B. Saunders, memo to John Major, Chief Secretary to the Treasury, 5 July 1988 (TNA HPSS T632/139. Cleveland Enquiry into Child Abuse Documents).

complex, most newspaper cited its summary which contained little negative commentary about the police, police surgeons or the MP but did include criticisms of Higgs, Wyatt and the social work consultant Sue Richardson.[115]

The Cleveland Inquiry had an important influence on national policy. The White Paper that would become the Children Act (1989) was amended to strengthen parents' rights and the balance of power in terms of childcare decisions shifted away from medicine and towards social work and the judiciary.[116] However, what is important here is that the consequences of the Inquiry were different for specialist doctors (police surgeons and paediatricians) and frontline community-based practitioners (health visitors and GPs).

Research after Cleveland concentrated heavily on the physical signs of sexual abuse and the development of a shared language to describe doctors' findings. The notion that one could somehow diagnose child sexual abuse on the basis of a 'single, conclusive diagnostic sign' was dismissed as 'invalid.' It was somewhat redundant to say so, as none of the research papers had claimed that there was a single sign, but perhaps it reflected a lingering desire across the child protection field for conclusive proof in sexual abuse cases, a 'smoking gun.' Paediatrician Frank Bamford and police surgeon Roberts ruled that out, explaining that the only way to prove sexual abuse by clinical examination was to find 'semen or blood of a group different from that child' in the 'vagina or rectum, or in the perineum in a prepubertal child,' but these were 'wholly exceptional in paediatric practice.' The presence of lubricants or hair was also important as was genital infection with *Neisseria gonorrhoeae*.[117]

When *Child Abuse and Neglect* published a special issue on the 'medical aspects' of child abuse, six out the ten papers were on sexual abuse. Hobbs and Wynne were included, with an expanded version of the paper they had published in *The Lancet* three years earlier. They now had a bigger cohort

[115] Nigel Parton, *Governing the Family: Child Care, Child Protection and the State* (Hampshire: Palgrave, 1991), 114.

[116] Adrian Bingham, "'It Would Be Better for the Newspapers to Call a Spade a Spade': The British Press and Child Sexual Abuse, C. 1918–90," *History Workshop Journal* 88 (2019): 104; Parton, *Governing the Family: Child Care, Child Protection and the State*, 115.

[117] Frank Bamford and Raine Roberts, 'Child Sexual Abuse - II,' in *ABC of Child Abuse*, ed. Roy Meadow (London: BMA Publications, 1989), 31. In the international journal, Krugman made a similar statement that apart from the exceptions of acquired gonorrhoea or syphilis, or the presence of sperm or semen, there were no 'pathognomic findings for sexual abuse.' Richard D. Krugman, 'Editorial: The More We Learn, the Less We Know "with Reasonable Medical Certainty"?,' *Child Abuse & Neglect* 13, no 2 (1989): 165–166.

of 337 probable or confirmed cases.[118] John McCann and his colleagues in Fresno, California, published a study of perianal findings in non-abused prepubertal children. They had designed a recruitment and screening process that aimed to reduce the likelihood of sexually abused children being included in their study. Two hundred and sixty-seven children were examined for the sorts of changes in the soft tissue of the perianal region that Hobbs, Wynne and other scholars had observed. Although researchers accepted that forced anal intercourse could cause lacerations, abrasions and hematomas, there was up until that time, no normative data available about findings in relation to what they described as 'less violent and ongoing anal abuse.' What the researchers discovered was that some of the 'signs' of anal abuse were found so often in the non-abused cohort of children that they 'appeared to be variants' of normal, while others were found very infrequently.[119] The article could be read as a repudiation of Hobbs and Wynne's findings.

Richard Krugman, editor of the special issue, disclosed that some US peer reviewers of the Hobbs and Wynne article had refused to accept their findings, since the numbers of children the British doctors identified with physical signs were so much higher than those in their own practices.[120] He dismissed these objections. In his opinion, the higher levels of awareness of sexual abuse in the US meant that children were seen by physicians 'before many physical findings exist.' He believed that Hobbs, Wynne and others were seeing the 'battered children' of sexual abuse.[121] In other words, they were examining the children whose injuries had been ignored or denied until they were more severe, or as Higgs had suggested at the

[118] Hobbs and Wynne, 'Sexual Abuse of English Boys and Girls: The Importance of Anal Examination.'

[119] John McCann et al, 'Perianal Findings in Prepubertal Children Selected for Nonabuse: A Descriptive Study,' *Child Abuse & Neglect* 13, no 2 (1989): 189.

[120] The admission that some US peer reviewers were sceptical of the high rates of CSA found by Hobbs and Wynne was later wielded against them. See for example Robert Sunderland's negative review of their *Physical Signs of Child Abuse: A Colour Atlas* in which he referred to US criticism and implied that the authors had not given the 'fraught area' the 'careful reflection, repeated reassessments of objectivity together with full assessment of all aspects of the children's history' that was warranted. R. Sunderland, 'Physical Signs of Child Abuse,' *Archives of Disease in Childhood* 75, no 4 (1996); Christopher J. Hobbs, Jane M. Wynne, and J. E. S. Fortin, *Child Abuse (Bailliere's Clinical Paediatrics)* (London; Philadelphia: Bailliere Tindall, 1993).

[121] Krugman, 'Editorial: The More We Learn, the Less We Know "with Reasonable Medical Certainty"?,' 165.

Cleveland Inquiry, once social workers knew there were doctors that cared about sexual abuse and were prepared to 'see the signs,' they referred the children that they had been worried about for some time.

The year after Cleveland, the Royal College of Physicians established a working party to adjudicate on disagreements about the significance of anogenital signs. They set out to agree a common terminology, describe the range of normative findings, produce evidence on the signs and their significance, as well as to provide advice on conducting examinations. The results were published in 1991.[122] By the time a second issue of the booklet appeared in 1997, many more studies were cited demonstrating a growing literature, and the controversy surrounding reflex anal dilation appeared to have 'settled,' with changes in the recommendations of what counted as threshold for suspicion. Specialisation was the trend with an increasing proportion of assessment and management said to be carried out by 'experienced and well-trained individuals.'[123]

Photographs continued to be central in educating health practitioners on the signs of child abuse. Both the Hobbs and Wynne and the McCann articles in the 1989 medical special issue of *Child Abuse and Neglect* were accompanied by colour plates of the children's anuses. A number of textbooks and atlases of child abuse were published. Early editions still gestured towards their usefulness to the wider children's workforce in community settings, whereas later editions specified that their main audience was the emerging paediatric specialist in child abuse. For example, the first edition of Meadow's *ABC of Child Abuse* (1989) featured a quotation by Henry Kempe in large red typeface stating: 'child abuse is the difference between a hand on the bottom and a fist in the face.' Inside, the book made extensive use of graphic colour plates of all types of abuse. The back cover advertised it as a book that provided 'clear guidance on how to recognise child abuse' and 'should be read by everyone concerned with the care of children.'[124] The 2007 edition of the Meadows book, by then renamed as the *ABC of Child Protection*, had a much blander cover, illustrated by a non-descript image of a paper-chain family. The book's target audience was defined much more clearly, noting that that it was 'a text for

[122] 'Physical Signs of Sexual Abuse in Children: A Report of the Royal College of Physicians,' (The Royal College of Physicians, 1991).

[123] Mark Hunter, 'Physical Signs of Sexual Abuse in Children,' *Archives of Disease in Childhood* 78, no 3 (1998).

[124] Roy Meadow, ed. *ABC of Child Abuse* (London: BMA Publications, 1989).

doctors' written to the level of knowledge 'to which a paediatrician should aspire,' but also useful for 'nurses and other staff of the health service who deal with children and who may be the first to notice abuse or be informed of it and all those concerned with child protection in other services to understand how medical diagnosis is made and the strengths and weaknesses of medical opinions and reports.'[125] The intended audience for these textbooks was becoming clearer as was a clear delineation between specialists and generalists.

In the second edition of the Royal College of Physicians' *Physical Signs* booklet (1997), colour photographs had replaced line drawings. Paediatricians on both sides of the Atlantic also produced anatomical atlases to assist those carrying out medical assessments where sexual abuse was suspected. In the US, Astrid Heger and S Jean Herriot Emans published a well-regarded textbook and photographic atlas which aimed to help practitioners learn 'what the variants of normal are to the genitalia and anus of children.'[126] Not everyone was keen on these graphic images. When the Leeds team produced a clinical handbook and a colour atlas of the physical signs,[127] paediatrician Robert Sunderland's review of the latter was scathing. His main criticism was of the authors' failure to describe 'the normal' or to consider differential diagnoses. Interestingly, however, he associated line drawings with objectivity. For example, he noted that a book by Edward Arnold used 'line drawings rather than photographs in a balanced comprehensive text,' and a textbook called *Clinical Forensic Medicine* included 'clear uncontentious text with line illustrations' in its chapters on child abuse.[128] He seemed to find the photographs highly contentious, associating them with subjectivity and overstatement. Given the tradition of photography in medical atlases more generally, Sunderland's objections hint at a wish by some paediatricians to reduce the visibility or make more obscure the physical signs of sexual assaults on babies and children.

[125] S. R. Meadow, Jacqueline Y. Q. Mok, and Donna Rosenberg, ABC of Child Protection 4th edition (Chichester: John Wiley & Sons, 2009).

[126] Astrid Heger, S. Jean Emans, and Carole Jenny, *Evaluation of the Sexually Abused Child : A Medical Textbook and Photographic Atlas* (New York: Oxford University Press, 1992), x-xi.

[127] Christopher J. Hobbs, Helga Hanks, and Jane M. Wynne, *Child Abuse and Neglect: A Clinician's Handbook* (Edinburgh, New York: Churchill Livingstone, 1993); Hobbs, Wynne, and Fortin, *Child Abuse (Bailliere's Clinical Paediatrics S.)*.

[128] Sunderland, 'Physical Signs of Child Abuse.'

Cleveland generated immense pressure on Hobbs and Wynne. A group of 75 Leeds parents campaigned against them and called for a second opinion on their cases; there was extensive coverage in the local and national press. The scrutiny was intense, and Wynne stated that she was considering giving up child abuse work altogether and concentrating on her other specialism of disabled children.[129] At the same time, the Leeds team was in great demand to train paediatricians from across the UK and further afield. Back in 1987, they had issued a public appeal through the *Yorkshire Post* for donations to help them raise the £20,000 needed to purchase colposcopes for St James's Hospital and the Leeds General Infirmary. They framed their public appeal by claiming that 'because it is more accurate than the human eye it will mean we will be able to ... rule out child sexual abuse at a much earlier stage than we would otherwise be able to do.'[130] By investing in the colposcopes, they made it possible to introduce better peer review and transform teaching.[131]

The five-day course for paediatricians that they developed ran at least five times per year for usually up to a dozen doctors. Paediatrician Deborah Hodes remembered that in 1990, she thought to herself that as she was planning to 'do safeguarding,' she would 'see children being sexually abused as in Cleveland' and she had 'better not make a mistake and ... better know what [she was] doing.' She booked herself on to the Leeds training which she found to be 'very, very good.' Hobbs introduced the visiting doctors to the patient and asked permission for them to observe the examination. The course attendees would sit behind a one-way screen and watch Hobbs (or Wynne) and Hanks interview the child. Then Hodes recalled, 'he had the colposcope and examined the child, in the room where you were sitting, which was this tiny little room with some chairs, you had a screen with the picture that he was seeing on the child.' Hodes thought observing the colposcopic examination had facilitated excellent

[129] 'New child abuse inquiry urged,' 11 *The Guardian*, Apr 1988.

[130] Angela Friend, 'Plea in child sex abuse war,' *Yorkshire Post*, 1987.

[131] Health authorities have never been prevented from accepting charitable legacies or donations. In 1953, a court held that it was 'legitimate to permit charitable support of the NHS, on the basis that the state would never be able to meet all conceivable health needs.' Helen Abnett, James Bowles, and John Mohan, 'The Role of Charitable Funding in the Provision of Public Services: The Case of the English and Welsh National Health Service,' *Policy & Politics* 51, no 2 (2023); Hunter, 'Physical Signs of Sexual Abuse in Children.'

learning for the doctors and was kinder for the child who did not have to have a junior doctor 'breathing over her shoulder'.[132]

Despite Cleveland, paediatricians gained confidence and authority as specialists in the arena of sexual abuse. That authority was constrained for sure by the increasing bureaucratic control that social services and the police held over the processes of investigation. Police and social services were now more cautious in using the medical evidence. That was beyond the paediatrician's control. Their authority was restricted to the medical assessment; not just the physical anogenital signs but what Wynne, Hobbs and Hanks described as the whole 'jigsaw' of evidence to be considered by medical practitioners working in a multidisciplinary context.[133] Paediatricians' expertise would be further recognised once the 'designated' and 'named' doctor roles were introduced in the 1990s. Health authorities had to identify a senior paediatrician to act as the designated lead on 'all aspects of the health service contribution to safeguarding.' Within each NHS Trust there was a named doctor to take a professional lead within the Trust itself on all child protection matters.[134]

## Part 7: Back at the Frontline

Where did this increasing specialisation leave GPs and health visitors? What effect did Cleveland, combined with the legislation and guidance that followed, have on the training and support provided to them? Firstly, there is no evidence to suggest that it had a strong negative impact on GPs or health visitors on the ground. Prior to the Cleveland Inquiry, most community-based practitioners simply had not had the training or support to equip them to routinely recognise and respond to sexual abuse in the family.[135] Far from being hyperaware of sexual abuse or overreacting to potential signs, it would be more accurate to say that as professional groups they had been made aware of its existence and that there was an

[132] Oral history interview with Deborah Hodes by author, 31 May 2019.

[133] Hobbs, Hanks, and Wynne, *Child Abuse and Neglect: A Clinician's Handbook*.

[134] 'Working Together to Safeguard Children,' (London: The Stationery Office, 1999), 17–18.

[135] Ruth Beecher, 'Children, Sexual Abuse and the Emotions of the Community Health Practitioner in England and Wales, 1970–2000,' *Journal of the History of Medicine and Allied Sciences* 78, no 4 (2023).

expectation that they should do something about it. Cleveland represented an opportunity to improve their response to sexual abuse rather than to discourage them. The episode clarified what were specialist and what were generalist roles for doctors and provided some new government funding for training.

Around the same time that John Moore, the Secretary of State for Health and Social Security, decided to set up the Cleveland Inquiry, he asked the Standing Medical Advisory Committee and the Standing Nursing and Midwifery Advisory Committee to each meet and draw up guidance for their profession. The former was asked to formulate guidelines for the medical profession on the diagnosis of sexual abuse; the latter to 'consider and report on child abuse, including sexual abuse, and the implications for the [nursing] profession of the sharp increase in the number of cases.' Guidance booklets for both professions were published in 1988.[136]

*Diagnosis of Child Sexual Abuse: Guidance for Doctors* was specifically about sexual abuse and forthright about the fact that it had been produced as a result of concerns about diagnosis in the Cleveland cases. It acknowledged that many cases occurred 'within the family circle,' emphasised that the 'medical aspects were only one element in the diagnostic process' and stressed that close cooperation across agencies and disciplines was essential. It was predicated on the fact that any doctor might encounter sexual abuse in the course of their working day. In the event of a disclosure from a child or an allegation from another person, the booklet provided very clear information on how to act; the range of physical signs was described, along with the sorts of emotional concerns that might give rise to serious, moderate or mild suspicion. Ultimately, the role of the doctor was to make an accurate diagnosis by taking a 'careful history' and undertaking 'relevant clinical examinations.' This should be followed by 'an assessment of what investigations might be needed and how to use referral for specialist opinion.' It was, as the guidance stated, the same for sexual abuse as for 'every other condition in medicine.'[137] This sharply (and helpfully) delineated the boundaries around the GP's territory and its relationship to the particular role of the specialist. The GP must be familiar with the warning signs, but they should always have the support of a specialist opinion in relation to medical assessment.

[136] *Child Protection: Guidance for Senior Nurses, Health Visitors and Midwives*, (London: HMSO, 1988), 5, 1988.

[137] 'Diagnosis of Child Sexual Abuse: Guidance for Doctors,' (London: HMSO, 1988), 2,5.

The medical guidance was addressed to each and every doctor, but the Standing Committee for nursing only addressed supervisors/ seniors in its guidance. The booklet did not spell out how *every* nurse or health visitor should respond to a physical sign or a disclosure, or what exactly they were expected to do. It seems they were unable to find answer to these questions. They showed no leadership and offered no help to the rank and file of their profession in how to respond. Instead they focused on the systems of oversight that senior nurses should establish and maintain over the rank and file in each locality to ensure compliance with local policies and guidelines. The committee's chair Suzanne Mowat emphasised the negative findings of various child death inquiries, which

> demonstrated certain recurring characteristics in the management arrangements for all practitioners, but particularly for health visitors and school nurses. These characteristics include uncertainty about incident reporting; confusion about case conference outcomes and review decisions; and inadequate monitoring of incidents and concerns.[138]

The solution to this problem was clear to the committee. The senior nurses responsible must rectify matters through liaison with other disciplines, caseloads reviews, systems for formal notifications of case conferences and monitoring of non-attendance, maintaining lists of missing families, managing systems for handover from midwife to health visitor to school nurse, managing workloads, having an overview of record-keeping systems.[139] The list went on. Rather than supporting professional autonomy, expertise and reflective practice in order to respond better to these often very complex cases, the Standing Committee confined the health visitor and school nurse within a rigid bureaucratic framework. Moving forward, everything should be checked, counted and documented.

As Hutcheson put it, the Cleveland report and new guidance following the Children Act (1989) were presented to them as important documents and events that they must learn from. 'But,' she continued, 'the analysis and understanding of what that meant was quite limited, it was more kind of—[they] recommended we do this, therefore we'll set up a system.' The focus was on process; what series of actions was to be taken, which procedures were to be followed. The professional insecurity of the profession

[138] *Child Protection: Guidance for Senior Nurses*, 5.
[139] *Ibid.*

made them grateful for the emphasis on process. Hutcheson recalled that it was valued because it gave them 'a very clear role [and] a sort of importance in the system and the process.' Each 'child protection' family had a named health visitor and 'outside of the social work arena, we were the kind of next most important thing was kind of the message.'[140] This was helpful in terms of straightforward cases, particularly where the abuse was already verified. But how helpful could it be in developing the potential for early identification of sexual abuse?

Cleveland was not mentioned at all in the nurses' guidance and the topic of sexual abuse was avoided almost entirely. Mowat noted that abuse, particularly sexual abuse, 'stirs up feelings which can be deeply troubling and may be difficult for the professional to accept and that they 'may unconsciously use various defence mechanisms in order to cope.'[141] But nothing more was said about it. Sexual abuse was not tackled again until a few pages before the document's conclusion where five short paragraphs were provided, which focused on training for senior nurses to enable them to recognise how sexual abuse differed from other forms of abuse and the 'emotional impact of dealing with these cases.' This should enable them to provide advice and counselling for their staff, keeping in mind that some staff might find it 'a difficult subject to discuss.' The senior nurse should also keep up to date with current publications, ensure that she and practitioners attend multidisciplinary training and familiarise herself with local guidance and procedures.[142]

The doctors' guidance had identifed the health visitor as one of the community practitioners that 'in many cases a child would present to .... and be found to have a story or symptoms or signs which cause child sexual abuse to be suspected.' And yet, the final clause of the brief sexual abuse section in the nursing guidance demonstrated the deep ambivalence held within the professional committee about whether nurses should expect to encounter sexual abuse. The section of the *Guidance for Doctors* that described 'grounds for suspicion' might, it noted, 'provide a useful checklist' for nurses, midwives and health visitors.[143] This section worked through disclosure, information or allegations from others, differential diagnosis, behavioural or emotional grounds for concern and family circumstances and described when mild, moderate or serious suspicion

[140] Interview with Hutcheson.

[141] *Child Protection: Guidance for Senior Nurses*, 5.

[142] *Child Protection: Guidance for Senior Nurses*, 27.

[143] *Child Protection: Guidance for Senior Nurses*, 27.

should be aroused.[144] The implication was that it was completely up to the individual nurse to decide whether such information was relevant.

The qualifying curriculum for health visiting did begin to address child abuse, albeit awkwardly. It 'came up in lectures' on Hutcheson's training in Manchester in the 1990s but 'it was treated as a kind of separate thing.' Her group were shown a television programme about child abuse. She reflected that

> the lights went down and—I don't know—It was almost like something we had to do and it was important but it was almost too difficult for us to do somehow in any meaningful way.[145]

Quigley could not recall an increase in in-service training or support in the period after Cleveland. There were no forums for team reflection or case discussion. At infrequent team meetings, they talked about holiday rotas, mileage forms and 'new forms of artificial milk'. She felt that 'it literally was about the bureaucracy of the organisation and not about professional practice.' Quigley recalled that there were no opportunities to bring a group of practitioners together to say, 'what's really concerning you?' or 'what are the issues of the moment?' She remembered that she 'might run something past someone' while making coffee but she had no formalised one-to-one supervision of practice in training: 'Or after. Or as a qualified health visitor. Ever.'[146]

When the roles of designated and named nurses and doctors were introduced in the 1990s, this did gradually improve training provision. Grace Norland* was one of a new generation of nurses (post Project 2000). She had a BA in nursing and health visiting (1997) and she subsequently undertook another BA to achieve RN Child status.[147] She had child protection training on both her degree courses although it was very 'basic,' they only 'learned the different categories of abuse.' But in her first health visiting job in a small team of two other health visitors and two health-trained nursery nurses, they worked the five hundred families' cases together. They also had

[144] 'Diagnosis of Child Sexual Abuse: Guidance for Doctors,' 7–10.

[145] Interview with Hutcheson.

[146] Interview with Quigley.

[147] Project 2000 saw the demise of the nurse apprentice delivering hands-on practical care to patients on the hospital ward, replaced by degree-level nursing courses designed to produce what the Royal College of Nursing described in 2024 as 'highly skilled professionals,' carrying out a safety-critical job 'Transforming to meet the future of nursing,' Royal College of Nursing, accessed 8 Feb 2024, https://www.rcn.org.uk/About-us/What-the-RCN-does/Transforming-to-meet-the-future-of-nursing. Interview with Grace Norland by author, 18 Jan 2019.

access to monthly supervision with the area's designated nurse for child protection cases or cases where they had 'cause for concern.'

In 2000, eight-year-old Victoria Climbié was murdered. She had been brought to London (via Paris) from the Ivory Coast by her great-aunt Marie-Therese Kouao, who had promised her parents that she would have a 'better life' in England. Instead, she was grotesquely tortured by Kouao and her boyfriend Carl John Manning over a nine-month period and finally killed by them. It was the publicity about Climbié's suffering and the 'gross failure of the system' that should have protected her that led to an Inquiry,[148] and ultimately to the first Intercollegiate Guidelines for Training in Safeguarding, published in 2006. These provided clarity on the level of competence required for each type of practitioner in health to recognise child maltreatment and take appropriate action.[149] GPs and health visitors were classified at level three, the highest level for non-specialists, the two levels above were for specialist 'named' (level four) and 'designated' (level five) doctor and nurse roles.

In that same year, Michelle Cutland went to Leeds as a registrar on a two-year training post and stayed on until she had completed her clinical training in paediatrics. Hobbs retired shortly after she arrived, but she was mentored by a 'very smart, dedicated, passionate woman' called Mandy Thomas who had joined the Leeds team in the early 1990s and was well known in the field. Cutland found the child protection work 'interesting, stimulating, different,' whereas her peers often did not want to take on those cases. She thought that they did not like 'the greyness… the feeling of—the fear of getting it wrong, the fear of getting it right.' Even in the mid-2000s, she thought that 'it didn't feel like a solid field with a good evidence base underneath it at that stage.' She learned a lot at Leeds; they 'took all the sexual abuse medical appointments for the patch.' There were at least three clinics a week with two or three children for medical assessment at each, from 'teenagers down to littlies.' There was a 'good mix of disclosures and suspicions without disclosure,' and they had a colposcope and a play therapist to see each child with you, 'so it was a good set up.' Peer review was prioritised and she recalled that

[148] 'The Victoria Climbié Inquiry: Summary Report of an Inquiry by Lord Laming,' (London: HMSO, 2003).

[149] 'Safeguarding children and young people: roles and competences for health care staff. Intercollegiate Guidance,' (2006).

> once a month, two and a half hours every month, was like closed off on everyone's job plan. And we'd all come and we'd all look at each other's images and we'd all read each other's reports and then we'd discuss it and, you know, see if we agreed or disagreed and what were the challenges and what did we learn, that kind of thing. So that was quite a good model.[150]

The features of a good learning environment for child sexual abuse had been established in Leeds twenty-five years earlier and were still working well. These included a multi-disciplinary approach, supportive colleagues, protected time for reflection and support, non-defensive practice and a commitment to learning. In Leeds there was continuity, it was a model of best practice. This model was used to good effect in other areas in relation to medical assessments, but there is no sense of it being adopted widely or wholeheartedly in relation to early intervention in child sexual abuse in general practice or health visiting.

## Conclusion

By the mid-2000s, specialists were in place within nursing and medicine. Consultant paediatricians and health visitors functioned as strategic leaders and as technical experts when it came to safeguarding, child abuse and child sexual abuse. Some were in acute trusts, but most were community-based. Hodes approved of this because she believed that 'children have a right to see a specialist when something like this happens to them.' She gave an analogy of a GP hearing a heart murmur and referring to a 'cardiologist to see if there's a heart defect.' They do not do the tests themselves 'even if [they have] learned about it and been trained because [it is] quite difficult.' She thought that, similarly, children should be referred to a specialist because sexual abuse should be treated 'in the same way that we think of any medical condition.'

Child abuse is now included in medical and nursing education. There are clear expectations about the content and frequency of in-service training for GPs, school nurses and health visitors. There are many additional training courses available on specific topics such as harmful sexual behaviour, sexual exploitation and, in recent years, online abuse. When attending generic safeguarding training, participants are no longer shown the sort of graphic photographs that Hobbs used to display at conferences, designed to shock them into accepting that child sexual abuse in the family

[150] Oral history interview with Michelle Cutland by author, 28 Sep 2020.

is a reality that they might expect to encounter in their daily working lives. The expectation is that there is no need to use such disturbing images because practitioners know that responding to abuse is part of their job. The consistently low rate of identifications of sexual abuse by health practitioners suggests the opposite but this inconvenient fact is ignored. Furthermore, even though there is a continuing expectation that GPs, health visitors and other disciplines should recognise the 'warning signs,' often there is no medical input at all on safeguarding training. Hodes regretted that because, she said, if the paediatrician takes part, they can get

> an idea of the physical signs and it's not to show them gory pictures, it's to say, 'if you see a bruise along the thigh which isn't explained, worry,' 'if you see strangle marks on the neck, worry.' Just those sorts of things and I think it's more effective coming from a doctor.[151]

It seems that the preferred mode of training in the 2020s is bureaucratic and abstract. Perhaps the doctor's presence would bring children's bodies into the room, make them visible and call all practitioners to account. As this chapter has demonstrated, that has not happened.

[151] Interview with Hodes.

CHAPTER 6

# 'Seeing it Everywhere' or Oblivious to It. Clinical Child Psychology and Child Sexual Abuse in the Family

## Introduction

> I told the story of my childhood and adolescence to a group of mental health workers who asked me 'So for all of those years, did you not try to tell anyone what was going on for you?' I starved myself, I stole, I vomited, I cut myself, I banged my head, I wore black, I overdosed, I beat myself up, I wrote unhappy poetry, I listened to Leonard Cohen. How much more loudly could I have spoken?
>
> Clare Shaw, *poet and mental health trainer*, 2023[1]

Some researchers have argued that about half of all women who use psychiatric services have experienced sexual abuse in childhood.[2] Clinical psychologist Lucy Johnstone has suggested that this raises 'rather embarrassing questions' about how 'all this trauma in the early lives of women psychiatric patients' can go 'undetected by professionals for so long.' 'So-called

[1] Clare Shaw, 'I do not believe in silence,' accessed at https://poetryschool.com/essays/i-do-not-believe-in-silence, 11 Nov 2023.

[2] Women who survive childhood sexual abuse are at a higher risk of mental health and substance abuse problems and this cannot be explained by background factors in the family. Kenneth S. Kendler et al, 'Childhood Sexual Abuse and Adult Psychiatric and Substance Use Disorders in Women: An Epidemiological and Cotwin Control Analysis,' *Archives of General Psychiatry* 57, no 10 (2000); Jennie Williams and Gilli Watson, 'Mental Health Services That Empower Women: The Challenge to Clinical Psychology,' *Clinical Psychology Forum* 1, no 1 (1997).



R. Beecher, *Community Health Practitioners and Child Sexual Abuse in the Family, 1970s–2010s*, Genders and Sexualities in History, https://doi.org/10.1007/978-3-031-80052-8_6

"symptoms" of their "mental illnesses"' (low mood, despair, self-destructiveness, dislike of their bodies, fearfulness and so on) seemed to Johnstone to be 'entirely understandable reactions to the traumas that have been inflicted upon them.' Beliefs that were labelled 'delusional,' in her view, could also reflect experiences of sexual abuse in a 'disguised form' and the apparent traits of borderline personality disorder were hard to distinguish from what is known about the impact of abuse.[3]

Johnstone raised these 'embarrassing questions' in *Users and Abusers of Psychiatry* (1989). At that time, a handful of her clinical psychology peers were pushing the profession to detect sexual abuse in children. Gerrilyn Smith, for example, gave talks about child sexual abuse to the British Psychological Society's annual conference, the North West Thames Division of Clinical Psychology and the Institute of Family Therapy, as well as publishing articles directed at her peers in books and journals.[4] In Ved P. Varma's *The Secret Life of Vulnerable Children*, she explained that children gave 'caring adults clues to the existence of an unspeakable problem,' but were ignored. The way adults overlooked the often 'gross and obvious indicators' of sexual abuse, combined with the potential of that abuse to generate a trauma response, meant children were left with 'little choice but a psychic retreat into self,' a 'depressed numbness or manic madness,' which was 'often infinitely preferable to the reality they are forced to live with, and to keep secret.'[5] Smith's aim was to persuade her peers to play a greater role in protecting children from sexual abuse: to be curious about what lay behind the outward signs of their mental distress and to believe them if they disclosed; to understand the serious consequences for them stemming not only from the sexual abuse itself, but from how they were treated in its aftermath; and lastly, to help children make sense of what had been done to them.

Identification of child sexual abuse comes usually in two ways: through signals and signs (or 'symptoms') or via a child or a protective adult telling their secret ('disclosure'). Where clinical practitioners are concerned, the

[3] Lucy Johnstone, *Users and Abusers of Psychiatry: A Critical Look at Psychiatric Practice*, 2nd ed. (London: Routledge London, 2000), 115–116.

[4] Gerrilyn Smith, '"The Traumatic Response Cycle." Paper Presented to the North West Thames Division of Clinical Psychology,' (Unpublished, 1988); '"Collusive Women: Power and Sexual Abuse in the Family." Paper Presented at the Institute of Family Therapy,' (London: Unpublished, 1989); 'Essay Book Review,' *Journal of Family Therapy* 14 (1992).

[5] 'Child Sexual Abuse,' in *The Secret Life of Vulnerable Children*, ed. Ved P. Varma (London: Routledge London, 1992), 154.

'symptoms' of mental distress are usually already evident; the next step might be to build enough trust for the child to disclose or so that they can ask the young person 'what happened to you?' In order to offer psychological support to a child, a clinician must exhibit 'warmth, attunement, and sensitivity to their feelings,' be 'understanding and accepting of their experience' and able to help the child to feel 'safe and supported.' Young people want mental health practitioners to convey a sense of professional competence, to demonstrate not only 'good intentions' but also the professional skills that can actually help them.[6] These are the important aspects of the therapeutic relationship as defined by young people; they sound remarkably similar to the qualities that might encourage a child or non-abusing parent to disclose sexual abuse. A practitioner working in child or adolescent mental health would also have the material conditions to create a place of safety: a room in a clinic, health centre or school where they could see a child privately, often over multiple sessions that gave them time to get to know the child.

Some clinical psychologists and counsellors have committed to working with sexually abused children and I will discuss some of those experiences below. In comparison to other community-based health practitioners, however, child sexual abuse has had a low profile within clinical child psychology. The phenomenon is strongly associated with the profession, but it is thought about in relation to very particular aspects of their work, (e.g. the techniques of disclosure interviews, the reliability of children and adults' memories or whether children lie about abuse), rather than in terms of the potential positive role of the clinical psychologist in the early detection and prevention of child sexual abuse in the family.

Curiously, since the 1970s, child and adolescent mental health services have been *both* heavily involved in responding to child sexual abuse and, paradoxically, oblivious to it. This chapter explores how this strange incongruity came about. Although psychological services to children have been delivered by a range of disciplines, here I focus mainly on clinical psychologists, exploring their motivation to join the profession and work with children, their professional training and their experiences once qualified. This was a profession coalescing in the context of competing disciplinary perspectives, and I examine how that context affected psychologists'

[6] Eva Wilmots et al, 'The Therapeutic Relationship in Cognitive Behaviour Therapy with Depressed Adolescents: A Qualitative Study of Good-Outcome Cases,' *Psychology and Psychotherapy: Theory, Research and Practice* 93, no 2 (2020).

reactions to the proposition that protecting children from child sexual abuse should be a core function of the discipline. The chapter centres the experiences of six individuals who qualified as clinical psychologists at various points between the late 1970s and 2015. Each went on to develop considerable expertise in responding to disturbed, abused and traumatised children and young people, some of whom had been sexually abused by someone close to them. These individuals all became part of what was a nascent profession: clinical *child* psychology.

## Part 1: Motivation

Individuals were motivated by a range of factors to join the budding profession of clinical child psychology. They were not medically trained but the close association to medicine and science meant a higher status and better pay than most other reparative or welfare work with children. Whether drawn to join the profession for personal or political reasons; because of a desire for excitement, autonomy or by the opportunities for innovation that could flourish in a relatively new discipline, new recruits would find themselves operating on shifting ground. Structural changes in the landscape of child and adolescent mental health services brought a sense of flux in terms of role ambiguity and interprofessional competition. This was the context in which practitioners were called upon to respond to child sexual abuse.

Stephen Frosh was not sure which direction to take in his terms of his career when he finished an undergraduate developmental psychology degree at Sussex in the late 1970s. He was interested in exploring the theory and history of psychoanalysis and hence, one option was to study for a PhD. Alternatively, he could gain some clinical experience by working directly with those in psychological distress via 'abnormal psychology,' as it was then known. He decided to take a year out to see if he was suited to work with children. Although he was only twenty-two and had no previous practical experience, he was offered a job as a 'house parent' at a school for 'maladjusted' children aged seven to twelve in Exeter. There he came into contact with a mixture of children, ranging from the 'very, very behaviourally difficult' children to the passive and withdrawn. There were children who had been expelled from school for challenging behaviour and then, in stark contrast, there was 'a bunch of … mostly girls,' who were labelled 'delicate' and 'manipulative;' they had asthma which was thought to be 'psychologically manufactured.' Frosh found the work quite hard at the beginning and he was very lonely, but he did 'get very involved with it.' It convinced him that clinical psychology training was the right choice for him. At the school, he had only been able to provide basic care to and containment of the children, clinical psychology training would equip him to move beyond that, by giving him the knowledge to assess and treat children and adolescents. And it would also provide him with more authority in the professional context, 'to put it bluntly, more power.'[7]

Like Frosh, Gerrilyn Smith wanted her career to provide her with power, recognition and fair remuneration. Influenced by the rape and murder of her aunt and 'all fired up' by feminist writings about rape and sexual assault,[8] she knew that she wanted to work in the field. As she approached the end of her undergraduate degree in English literature and psychology at Carleton University in Canada, a professor advised her to train in the low-paid traditionally 'female' role of nursery nurse.[9] She rejected his advice and explored alternative careers for herself. Wavering between social work or clinical psychology, she realised the stark gendered differences between the two professions. Social work was 'eighty per cent women, twenty per cent men and paid ... say twenty-five thousand;' clinical psychology was exactly the opposite in terms of gender and pay: 'twenty per cent women, eighty per cent men and paid fifty thousand.' She couldn't 'see the difference' between the two professions, so she flew to London in 1976, began volunteering at London Rape Crisis Centre and enrolled on clinical psychology training at the Institute of Psychiatry.[10]

Sam Warner also came out of sexual violence services. She had worked for the sexual abuse survivors' organisation Taboo in Manchester for a number of years in the late 1980s, which was rewarding but had not brought her any 'power, money or status.' Because she had a first degree in psychology, she thought that her 'quickest route into getting all three ... was to go and train as a clinical psychologist.' She had been brought up by

[7] Oral history interview with Stephen Frosh by author, 22 Jan 2020.

[8] See Chap. 4, part four.

[9] Although the Royal Commission on the Status of Women in Canada had made many recommendations to combat 'sex role stereotypes' and had commented on the inadequacy of career counselling in 1970, their efforts to promote women's equality were slow to take hold. Rebecca Priegert Coulter, 'Gender Equity and Schooling: Linking Research and Policy,' *Canadian Journal of Education / Revue canadienne de l'éducation* 21, no 4 (1996).

[10] Oral history interview with Gerrilyn Smith by author, 2 May and 25 Jun 2021.

three strong women: 'my mum, my nan and my auntie Bet' and had a core belief in feminism, alongside 'a concern with inequality and doing something about it.' Her mum's family were travellers who had lived in a horse-drawn carriage in the 1930s and, Warner supposed, 'always had a sense of not being in … acceptable society, nevertheless there was an awful lot of acceptance within that community.' That affected her own political perspective. She admired her mother's determination and independence; she had defied convention by having 'an illegitimate baby [Warner] in the 1960s and keep[ing] her.' Lastly, her convent school education brought her under the leadership of another group of women 'in charge,' as well as 'a sense of belonging but also a sense of needing to learn and perhaps through that a desire to change the world.'[11]

Whereas Frosh, Smith and Warner were searching for status and politically motivated, Peter Fuggle was looking for exciting and challenging work. He had been a teacher in private schools and worked in adventure playgrounds. His decision to become a clinical psychologist 'was the sort of second order of choice really, the first order of choice was children.' It was not that he felt sentimental about them but rather to the contrary, he was drawn to them because he felt that 'the work would be dangerous, risky, unpredictable; you never know what will happen with children.'[12]

Natasha Rahman* was looking for something different; she wanted to understand the dynamics of families and communities. She had initially rejected the idea of studying psychology and applied to study law.[13] She felt that was what her parents wanted her to do. They had arrived in the UK from Bangladesh in the 1970s and were part of a London-based Bangladeshi immigrant community that, she felt, did not really understand the point of psychology. Ultimately, Rahman 'had a total change of heart' and she enrolled in a psychology course at Royal Holloway in 1997. Her motivation to study psychology came from being an observant and curious child who noticed what was happening in her family and their community. She felt that she had 'always been the one in the family that [was] particularly emotionally connected to everything.' Her father had been part of the Freedom movement in Bangladesh and although he retained close ties to the struggles of his home country, he had made an active choice to move to England. Her mother had to leave her large

[11] Oral history interview with Sam Warner by author, 28 Jun 2021.

[12] Oral history interview with Peter Fuggle by author, 6 Jun 2019.

[13] Pseudonyms marked with * on first use.

sibling group behind and felt isolated and depressed at times. Both of her parents were heavily involved in supporting Bangladeshi families who had recently arrived in London. Her mother visited local bed and breakfast accommodation to recruit children for the Bengali school she ran at the weekends. Her parents were in touch with

> many, many families who had all sorts of stories as to how they came over, why they came over, their circumstances once they arrived and, yeah, things that they were struggling with potentially, or thriving and living a great life.

Psychology, Rahman thought, would give her the tools to understand them better.[14]

Kim Underhill's* decision to study psychology at Durham in the mid-1990s was based on 'a leap of faith.' As a working-class girl from an armed forces family, the subject and the place were unfamiliar to her. She worked 'four or five jobs' during her gap year to gather the money to support herself through university. Her mother had bipolar disorder, 'there'd been violence in the household,' her parents' marriage had broken down and she found it 'quite a challenging environment to grow up in.' A teacher at her school in London had taken her 'under her wing,' helped her to think about careers and suggested psychology. She reflected later that the teacher was a gay woman from a Muslim background who perhaps 'understood what it was like—although we weren't from similar backgrounds—understood what it was like to be looking for something different.' Her teacher persuaded her that psychology was about people and relationships which could enable her to help individuals 'like her mum' or 'children like you.' Underhill felt she could not tell her parents she was going to enrol in a subject like drama or English, on the contrary, the subject she chose had to have 'some rigour to it' in order to 'justify' her choice to go to university rather than straight into a job. And like Frosh, Smith and Warner before her, 'there was this thing in me that I felt like I had to have some status when I'd graduated.'[15]

These six individuals, who trained at various different points between the late 1970s and 2015, held some features in common. They initially chose the profession for a range of reasons including a commitment to feminism or social justice; a desire for recognition and fair remuneration;

[14] Oral history interview with Natasha Rahman* by author, 16 Sep 2022.
[15] Oral history interview with Kim Underhill* by author, 26 Sep 2022.

and an interest in how children and families functioned, sometimes linked to feelings about their own family, racialisation or class. Some of the six who trained in the 1980s spoke explicitly about their own political positions and saw themselves as activists. Rahman and Underhill, who trained a little later, articulated a clear personal political position centred around their identities as an Asian woman and a working-class woman respectively in relation to race, community, class and clinical psychology.

Although some of the mental health practitioners may have been survivors of sexual abuse, none divulged that in the course of their interviews with me. As consultant clinical psychologist Khadija Rouf has highlighted, survivors who are open about their childhood experiences in the professional environment of psychology have been subjected to prejudice, an 'unhealthy and invasive level of scrutiny,' as well as assumptions about their past and how it might affect their capability for different sorts of clinical work. She commented that it was 'a strange kind of binary, where a profession built on understanding the human psyche, cannot cope with a person who happens to be both a survivor and a clinician.'[16] The next section explores professional training from the late 1970s and explores how it equipped practitioners to be vigilant and curious about abuse.

## Part 2: Professional Training

Clinical *child* psychology was a nascent profession in the 1970s and there was no specific training available; potential practitioners enrolled on generic clinical psychology courses. The Institute of Psychiatry (IoP), linked to the Maudsley Hospital in south London, was highly influential in training psychologists as 'scientific practitioners' but the approach did not appeal to every potential psychologist. Getting accepted on to a course anywhere in Britain was challenging; there were few spaces. Those who succeeded in obtaining places tended to be white, middle-class and, in the majority, female. Although the curriculum would change over the ensuing decades, there was little input on child sexual abuse. Neither were great efforts made to take the issue on as a core professional responsibility. Individual trainees and early career psychologists who developed an interest in sexual abuse often felt that they were perceived as slightly fanatical in terms of 'seeing it everywhere.'

[16] See also Chap. 5. Khadj Rouf, 'Who Looks and Sounds Like a Psychologist' *The Psychologist*, 10 Sep 2020.

Prior to 1987, a psychologist had to hold an honours degree in psychology or 'equivalent' and to be at least twenty-five years old in order to work in the NHS. In addition, they were required to have either completed an approved clinical psychology training course plus one year's supervision (University route); served for three years under supervision to their employer's satisfaction (Independent Probationer route); or have completed two years' training, with the employer deciding whether a third supervised year was needed (In-service route).[17] One could not train specifically as a clinical *child* psychologist and, in fact, when Michael Berger was appointed as a lecturer at the IoP in 1965,[18] most of his colleagues worked across the age ranges. Until William Yule arrived four years later, Berger was the only clinical psychologist at the Institute who worked solely with children.[19] Across Britain, those who trained in the late 1970s and became clinical *child* psychologists were joining a nascent profession. The training was deliberately generic and comprehensive; students were expected to complete practice placements across the age range and with different client groups. It was possible to navigate around those expectations. For example, Fuggle recalled that his training 'was a little bit skewed;' he managed to do solely child-focused placements and 'did surprisingly little work with adults.'[20]

Smith and Frosh enrolled in clinical psychology training at the IoP in the late 1970s. Established in 1924 as the Maudsley Hospital Medical School, by 1938 the Institute had a reputation as the top site in Europe for research and teaching in psychiatry.[21] After the Second World War, Monty Shapiro joined the Institute and, when Hans Eysenck was appointed as head of psychology, he asked Shapiro to run the clinical psychology training course. The discipline had previous focused narrowly on psychological testing; Shapiro and Eysenck took it in a new direction, developing

[17] Tony Lavender and Graham Turpin, 'The Development and Training of the Clinical Psychology Workforce,' in *Clinical Psychology in Britain: Historical Perspectives*, ed. John Hall, David Pilgrim, and Graham Turpin (Leicester: The British Psychological Society, 2015), 93–110.

[18] It was a dual academic and clinical role; he was also staff psychologist to the adolescent units of the Bethlem Royal Hospital and the children's department at the Maudsley. https://pure.royalholloway.ac.uk/en/persons/michael-berger. Accessed 5 Jan 2024.

[19] Professor William Yule 1940–2023. https://www.kcl.ac.uk/people/william-yule. Accessed 5 Jan 2024.

[20] Interview with Fuggle.

[21] Bonnie Evans, Shahina Rahman, and Edgar Jones, 'Managing the "Unmanageable:" Interwar Child Psychiatry at the Maudsley Hospital, London,' *History of Psychiatry* 19, no 76 (2008).

psychological treatments based on 'scientific principles.'[22] When Smith and Frosh arrived, the department remained under the leadership of Eysenck who was 'famously antagonistic' to psychoanalysis,[23] and was wedded to behavioural approaches.[24] He believed that 'by virtue of their training and experience psychologists are (or should be) experts in the fields of conditioning and learning theory, laboratory procedures, and research design,' and should focus on those areas rather than to deliver therapeutic interventions.[25] By now, Jack Rachman was leading the training. Described as someone with an 'endless stream of new ideas for research, innovative clinical interventions or a combination' and a clinical style that his patients experienced as like a 'concerned friend,' he was an important influence on emerging developments in learning theory and cognitive behavioural therapy (CBT).[26]

Not everyone was attracted to the theoretical bent at the IoP. Smith was deeply uncomfortable with the intense concentration on the 'empirical research, evidence based, behavioural, pharmacological,' and as soon as she started the course, she thought, 'oh my gosh, what have I done?'[27] Frosh was dismayed by the 'distanced technical approach' by his 'teachers at the Maudsley.' He felt that 'there was such a mismatch' between the 'sense of the … emotionality of children's lives' and the engagement he had experienced with them at the school for 'maladjusted' children, in contrast to the emphasis on 'what they called the scientific practitioner model' at the IoP.[28] That approach could be largely attributed to Michael Rutter, who was the first professor of child psychiatry in Britain. His tenure at the IoP was seen as instrumental in moving the profession away from its dependence on clinical 'opinion' and 'unproven psychoanalytic

[22] Stephen Morley, 'Obituary Monte Shapiro,' *The Guardian,* 2 May 2000. https://www.theguardian.com/news/2000/may/02/guardianobituaries1. Accessed 24 Sep 2024.

[23] Interview with Frosh. Eysenck concluded that psychotherapy was not effective in the treatment of mental disorders. Hans J. Eysenck, 'The Effects of Psychotherapy: An Evaluation. 1952.' *Journal of Consulting Psychology* 60, no 5 (1992).

[24] '"Eysenck and the development of CBT:" Jack Rachman's Hans Eysenck Memorial Lecture,' at the 2003 Annual Conference in Bournemouth, 18 Nov 2003. https://www.bps.org.uk/psychologist/eysenck-and-development-cbt. Accessed 20 Nov 2023.

[25] Hans J. Eysenck, 'Learning Theory and Behaviour Therapy,' *Journal of Mental Science* 105, no 438 (1959): 73.

[26] David Clark, Paul Salkovskis and Roz Shafran, 'Jack Rachman 1934–2021,' 10 Sep 2021. https://www.bps.org.uk/psychologist/jack-rachman-1934–2021. Accessed 24 Sep 2024.

[27] Interview with Smith.

[28] Interview with Frosh.

theory.' By using 'objective research methods from areas such as epidemiology, developmental psychology and genetics,'[29] Rutter was said to have transformed child psychiatry 'from an incoherent set of theories and practices into a rigorous and humane discipline.'[30] The idea, as Frosh interpreted it, was that you 'knew the science from psychology and then you practised it by applying it.' He appreciated 'the way in which Michael Rutter could take the literature and say "oh, this child's an example of [a specific disorder]."' That, he thought, was 'very helpful to somebody's learning,' but the idea that it could be applied in such a direct way was, in his view, 'completely wrong.'[31]

Perhaps as a consequence of the 'scientific practitioner' approach and the antipathy to psychoanalysis, there was a void within the training when it came to the effects of the work on the practitioner. Trainees were not required to be in therapy themselves and Frosh felt that there was no recognition that they would 'somehow need to work on [themselves] as opposed to [solely] learning something factual.' The course did not equip them for the messy realities of treating children and young people in the community or for delivering therapeutic interventions with abused and traumatised children. Frosh remembered that during his training, a trainee committed suicide and the topic was 'just shut down.' The emotional impact of this on the other students was not addressed and 'no space was given to us to think about the effect of this at all on us or what it might mean.' He characterised this as a 'sense of disconnection between the ... significance and difficulty of the work and ... how we were being trained and ... avoidance I think of the difficult issues.'[32]

The behavioural approach always ran alongside other tendencies at the IoP and the Maudsley, however, and there were some opportunities for those who were interested in psychoanalysis or family therapy. For example, Smith found 'areas where [she] could grow,' particularly in relation to family therapy and psychoanalytical approaches to the family with psychiatrists Robin Skynner and Christopher Dare.[33] Skynner, in particular, was a driving force in group and family therapy and was one of the founding

[29] Peter McGuffin, 'Sir Michael Rutter Obituary' *The Guardian,* 8 Nov 2021.

[30] An earlier version of this obituary referred to Rutter as transforming child psychiatry 'from a dismal and incoherent state.' Uta Frith and Francesca Happé, 'Mike Rutter 1933–2021: Obituary,' *Nature* 9 Nov 2021.

[31] Interview with Frosh.

[32] Interview with Frosh.

[33] Interview with Smith.

members of the Institute of Group Analysis and the Institute of Family Therapy.[34]

From the 1970s, the behavioural and increasingly cognitive behavioural therapies that would gradually come to dominate clinical psychology training flowed out to other settings as Maudsley-trained personnel took up positions elsewhere.[35] By the end of the decade, there were thirteen clinical psychology training courses running in England, seven of which were in London or southern England.[36] The remaining courses in England were at Liverpool, Newcastle, Leeds, Birmingham and Oxford, as well as In-service option at Lancashire. Four courses ran in Scotland and one In-service option was offered in South Wales.[37] The IoP had a disproportionate influence on programmes elsewhere and that may partly explain why clinical training that embraced a psychoanalytical approach became increasingly hard to find during the last two decades of the twentieth century. Ingrid Jacobs* did succeed in finding such a course in Leeds in 1978, where they 'already knew Winnicott and Bowlby and others who were working with children.'[38] In the early 1990s, Warner found it difficult to find clinical training that would support her interest in the long-term impact of childhood trauma. Many universities were offering courses that

[34] Skynner joined the IoP in 1970 and having previously been a consultant at Woodberry Down Child Guidance Unit and the Queen Elizabeth Hospital for Children. John Schlapobersky, 'Obituary Robin Skynner,' *The Guardian*, 28 Sep 2000. Schlapobersky, 'Obituary Robin Skynner,' *The Guardian*, 28 Sep 2000. Accessed 24 Sep 2024.

[35] Sarah Marks, 'Psychologists as Therapists: The Development of Behavioural Traditions in Clinical Psychology,' in *Clinical Psychology in Britain: Historical Perspectives*, ed. John Hall, David Pilgrim, and Graham Turpin (Leicester: The British Psychological Society, 2015), 196–202.

[36] The IoP, North East London Polytechnic, University of Surrey, University of Exeter, along with In-service training at South East Thames, North West Thames and Wessex. Lavender and Turpin, 'The Development and Training of the Clinical Psychology Workforce,' 100–101.

[37] 'The Development and Training of the Clinical Psychology Workforce,' 100–101.

[38] Interview with Ingrid Jacobs.* Donald Winnicott was a paediatrician who trained as a psychoanalyst in the late 1920s. He had a great deal of clinical experience, including many years as a paediatric consultant at Paddington Green child guidance clinic. This led him to realise that 'if you show me a baby you certainly show me also someone caring for a baby, or at least a pram with someone's eyes and ears glued to it;' in other words, that mothers played a 'crucial role' in caring for their babies in their early years. Jan Abram, 'Donald Woods Winnicott (1896–1971): A Brief Introduction,' *The International Journal of Psychoanalysis* 89, no 6 (2008); Bowlby similarly emphasised the importance of infant/mother attachment or 'continuous mothering' in early childhood. John Bowlby, *Attachment and Loss: Vol I Attachment* (London: Penguin, 1971); Sula Wolff, *Children under Stress*, Second edition ed. (Suffolk: Pelican Books, 1969).

'were very restricted around cognitive behavioural approaches.' She settled on the programme at the University of Liverpool which, she felt, had an eclectic approach that emphasised psychodynamic therapy.[39]

The British Psychological Society (BPS) had discussed potentially introducing a three-year PhD and this seemed to make sense once a Charter and Register was adopted in 1987 because that required three years' postgraduate training. Following the splitting of purchaser/provider functions within the NHS, changes in the management structure in the regions drove the In-service schemes out of the NHS and into universities or other organisations. However, there was opposition to the establishment of the PhD within the NHS and the profession itself, due in large part to concern about the shortage of clinical psychologists. Increasing the length of the training would increase costs and divert funds away from creating additional training places. Dissent notwithstanding, by 1995, all providers were offering doctorates as well as additional input for previously qualified staff to achieve the PhD.[40]

The number of clinical psychology training places available in the UK crept above two hundred at the beginning of the 1990s; it had doubled by 2000 and at the end of that decade it hovered at nearly six hundred.[41] Despite the increase in the number of places available, getting a place felt increasingly competitive to those wishing to train. To succeed in getting a place, potential trainees had to be able to navigate the system and to have sufficient financial resources to support themselves through a three-year programme (with the additional expense of therapy which was now recommended). Structural racism meant that only a tiny minority of those accepted to courses were people of colour and it could be an uncomfortable experience for them.[42]

As a child of immigrants, Rahman knew nothing about the possibility of progressing to clinical training, but a friend on her undergraduate degree was the daughter of a doctor and hence, she felt, was more 'clued in' to navigating the system; she found them both a volunteering opportunity assisting a doctoral student with her research on post-traumatic

[39] Liverpool's programme began in 1962. Interview with Warner.

[40] Lavender and Turpin, 'The Development and Training of the Clinical Psychology Workforce,' 102–103, 105.

[41] 'Appendix 4: Selected Workforce Data,' in *Clinical Psychology in Britain: Historical Perspectives*, ed. John Hall, David Pilgrim, and Graham Turpin (Leicester: The British Psychological Society, 2015), 390.

[42] Nick Wood and Nimisha Patel, 'Special Issue: Racism During Training in Clinical Psychology,' *Clinical Psychology Forum* 323 (2019).

stress disorder. This led to other opportunities; the doctoral student, knowing that Rahman was 'politically and socially aware and motivated,' helped her to get her first assistant psychologist job working with survivors of torture. In 2002, the year after the 9/11 terrorist attacks in the United States, Rahman was put in touch with a psychologist doing a study on children's responses to watching the attacks on TV and whether they developed symptoms of PTSD. She found 'different parts of [her] world colliding' because, she reflected,

> if you think about the social context at that point, there's very much a backlash against the Muslim Community and all the narratives around … terrorism and looking closely at the Muslim population. And it's at that time actually that I'd started to wear a headscarf …[43]

Rahman recalled 'trying to make sense of who I was within … psychological services which [were] predominantly — yeah I'll say it, predominantly white.' She remembered the importance of certain 'incredible women' who supported her career development: the doctoral student and later a supervisor who helped her to get a place on doctoral training. Coming from the British Bangladeshi community, she reflected, 'even now it's really hard to enter these professions if you don't have the contacts, the connections, the people who … have experience … I didn't know what a clinical psychologist was or looked like, you know, growing up.' These two female mentors helped her to work out what she wanted to do in her career and how to progress.

Rahman was keen to attend the clinical training programme led by Mary Boyle at the University of East London because of its focus on the wider social context to psychological difficulties and mental wellbeing. Boyle (together with Lucy Johnstone and others) would go on to develop the 'Power Threat Meaning Framework.' It challenged models of understanding mental health based on medical and psychiatric diagnosis and was rooted in the idea that inequalities of power were major causes of 'mental health problems,' including power imbalances because of racialisation and gender, between adults and children and between the state and individuals.[44] Despite that ethos, as a visibly Muslim woman and 'one of a

[43] Interview with Rahman.

[44] The framework was funded by the British Psychological Society's Division of Clinical Psychology and launched in 2018. Mary Boyle and Lucy Johnstone, *A Straight Talking Introduction to the Power Threat Meaning Framework: An Alternative to Psychiatric Diagnosis*, Straight Talking Introductions (Monmouth, UK: PCCS Books, 2020).

handful of non-white trainees,' Rahman felt isolated during her training. The day she heard that she had been accepted onto the course was the seventh of July 2005, when 'the tube attacks in London … happen[ed] just down the road from where I was.' Even though she saw little of her family and friends during the three very intensive years of the training and her peers on the course became her support network, she felt that there was 'all of this stuff going on for me in the background which [was] difficult to talk about.' Racism was acknowledged in her courses and they talked about 'whiteness in clinical psychology.' But at the same time, her family and community were the targets of 'some harsh and attacking conversations,' yet she did not feel that she had enough of a 'safe core network of people … or allies' to enable her to 'bring in some of what was going on for [her] outside.'[45]

Experiences of training were gendered as well as racialised. Across Britain, the vast majority of applicants to courses were women.[46] Once on the training, women often had to balance course work and placements alongside pregnancy and raising young children. Underhill worked for ten years and had a family before she started training in her thirties. Most of her peers were in the same age group and, like her, relying on a partner to support them financially. The IoP became the Institute of Psychiatry, Psychology and Neuroscience in 2014,[47] and Underhill learned about 'MRI machines and taking brain slices.' She recalled that the gender balance on her course was different from others; about fifty per cent of the students were men and she wondered if this was perhaps because of the explicit inclusion of neuroscience. She also noticed that the course makeup was more diverse ethnically than often found on clinical psychology programmes, although the people of colour on her course were mostly international students rather than coming from minoritised communities in the UK. Underhill found the course to be carefully balanced in terms of incorporating different approaches and the tutors used studies that

[45] Interview with Rahman. See also Anuradha Sayal-Bennett, 'Equal Opportunities - Empty Rhetoric?,' *Feminism and Psychology* 1, no 1 (1991).

[46] In fact, the gender breakdown of trainees in the UK was exactly the opposite to what Smith remembered finding when she researched helping professions in Canada. In the UK, women were the majority group on clinical psychology training. See Linda Morison, Christina Trigeorgis and Mary John, 'Are mental health services inherently feminised?' https://www.bps.org.uk/psychologist/are-mental-health-services-inherently-feminised. 27 Jun 2014. Accessed 24 Sep 2024.

[47] 'From IoP to IoPPN,' https://web.archive.org/web/20150222140955/https://www.kcl.ac.uk/ioppn/about/from-iop-to-ioppn.aspx. Accessed 30 Oct 2023.

demonstrated the efficacy of both neuroscientific and therapeutic approaches, sometimes in combination. They were taught about neuroanatomy; 'we were talking about basal ganglia [and] executive function maladaptions;' they learned how different medications worked and the implications for clients. This was alongside a good grounding in what different interventions looked like, particularly cognitive behaviour therapy, talking therapies, psychodynamic and interpersonal approaches.[48]

There was little input on child sexual abuse within the taught elements of clinical psychology training through to the early 2000s. Neither Smith nor Frosh could recall any specific mention of child maltreatment of any sort on their training at the IoP, nor did it feature at the University of Leeds in those years. Fuggle made no mention of child abuse training at the North West Thames Regional Training Scheme where he trained in the 1980s.[49] At the University of Liverpool, a tutor came in from the regional psychology service to deliver a lecture on the topic for Warner's course. She recalled that they were merely told about 'the limits of what you should and shouldn't do' and her impression was that child sexual abuse was not taught well on any of the clinical psychology training at the time.[50] The majority of clinical psychology trainees' two (and later three) years in training was spent in practice placements and that is where some would learn about child protection and child sexual abuse.

## Part 3: 'A Psychological Phenomenon'

In the 1980s, messages about detecting child sexual abuse in the family and how to respond were regularly directed at GPs, health visitors, school nurses and the like.[51] It is peculiar that even although many clinical psychologists worked in community settings, they were not persistently assailed by these sorts of exhortations to be vigilant about the potential signs or how to respond if they were suspicious that an adult close to the child might be molesting them. As will become evident below, neither did child sexual abuse become more visible within the taught element of clinical psychology training programmes. Once trainees were out in the field in supervised practice placements, those who developed an interest in child

[48] Interview with Underhill.

[49] This was based in a hospital in Hertfordshire until the late 1980s when it merged with the North East Thames scheme run by UCL. Interviews with Fuggle and Frosh.

[50] Interview with Warner.

[51] See Chap. 3.

sexual abuse often felt that their more experienced colleagues did not approve. Although those who trained after 2000 or so felt that there was more input in the workplace on child protection, plenty of barriers remained in terms of recognition of sexual abuse.

At the British Psychological Society, a working party had been established on child sexual abuse. A March 1990 report produced by the group noted that 'the majority of the professionals involved [with cases] will have had no realistic exposure to the issue in their original training,' and that many would 'have to come to terms with the fact that they must have, in the past, missed cases that they might now recognise as involving sexual abuse.'[52] The authors made strenuous efforts to encourage psychologists to accept that child sexual abuse was a psychological phenomenon and thus within their purview. They pointed out that physical signs were found 'relatively infrequently.' Many more cases were identified through disclosures, behavioural disturbance or other non-medical indicators. In other ways too, this was a psychological matter. 'Abuses of trust and power' were 'always present,' the child's feelings of guilt, the perpetrator's inappropriate sexual arousal and the boundaries that were transgressed—each had a psychological component. The report also highlighted that when medical and legal investigations had positive and negative 'psychological sequelae,'[53] the psychologist could support victims to cope with their impact.

Despite these efforts to persuade psychologists that they had a role to play in child sexual abuse, professional training curricula were not updated swiftly. Psychologists who qualified in the 1990s did not recall much about the topic. Sam Simpson* trained at the IoP in the early 1990s, he remembered one lecture on child protection in the two-year programme and felt that the syllabus was heavily weighted towards adults.[54] Sarah Kitson* and Davina Young* recollected that child protection did feature in some form on their clinical programme at the University of Surrey in the latter part of the decade,[55] but neither could say much about it. Kitson remembered there were vignettes of different types of abuse. Young recalled that her group was given specific chapters of books or articles to read about aspects of abuse, and that she was also recommended to read something specific in relation to a

[52] 'British Psychological Society Report: Psychologists and Child Sexual Abuse,' *The Psychologist* 1990, 344.

[53] 'Psychologists and Child Sexual Abuse,' 345.

[54] Interview with Sam Simpson* by author, 14 Mar 2019.

[55] The Surrey programme was set up in 1971. Lavender and Turpin, 'The Development and Training of the Clinical Psychology Workforce.'

child who had been sexually abused that she had come into contact with on a placement. The training had left little impression on these clinicians, and their responses to my questions about it were slightly guarded, the implication was that the training was adequate and to imply otherwise was somehow to impugn the course organisers or their own professional integrity.

Some clinical child psychologist trainees began to encounter the presenting signs of child sexual abuse during their practice placements and in their first post-qualifying jobs in the early 1980s. They often found that their developing interest in sexual abuse was ignored or deemed unsavoury. Jacobs* recalled that when she was a newly qualified psychologist in a hospital child psychiatry department, colleagues used to say, 'this is a new child referred and they are soiling,' or 'this child is very badly behaved.' She and her colleagues were beginning to wonder 'why are there all these children with horrendous behaviour problems?' But when she asked questions about sexual abuse, she felt isolated because 'nobody else' spoke about it.[56] She began to work in partnership with the hospital's paediatricians to provide clinical sessions, and her head of department commented that they 'didn't think I would get involved with something seedy like this.' When colleagues came to talk to her about cases and she queried whether the child's distress could be caused by sexual abuse, they would say 'you see it everywhere.' She found it frustrating that other 'people were starting to see it,' but, at the same time, they criticised her for what they felt was her hyper-vigilance. Their response, to her mind, went beyond a personal criticism of her practice and had wider consequences because it 'fed into this thing, that sexual abuse was in the mind of the therapists and the clinicians, that it didn't really happen.'[57]

Smith had a similar experience. After a year on Michael Rutter's Family Research Project at the IoP,[58] she took up a full-time psychologist post at a child guidance clinic in Medway in south-east England. There she found that colleagues did not want to know about sexual abuse. She attended enuresis and encopresis clinics where she sometimes asked whether children might be 'peeing their bed to keep someone out of it' or 'maybe

[56] Interview with Ingrid Jacobs* by author, 25 Sep 2019.

[57] Interview with Jacobs.

[58] This was a follow-up study with adults who had been in care as children. Smith said some of the interviewees had 'clearly been taken into care because they'd been sexually abused in their families,' but this 'couldn't be talked about.' David Quinton, Michael Rutter, and Christine Liddle, 'Institutional Rearing, Parenting Difficulties and Marital Support,' *Psychological Medicine* 14, no 1 (1984).

they're pooping themselves because someone's poking something up their bum.' Her colleagues' response was, 'oh Gerrilyn, you're so disgusting.' A psychiatric social worker who worked in the Sexual Abuse Team at Great Ormond Street recalled that their colleagues in the Department of Psychological Medicine were not 'hostile' to the team, but they did not want to know anything about the topic. And echoing Jacobs* ('something seedy') and Smith ('you're so disgusting'), the GOSH practitioner felt that there was an 'implication that you've all got dirty minds.'[59]

Other psychologists felt that some of their peers in mental health services in the 1980s and 1990s were too quick to suspect sexual abuse. Fuggle recalled that it was quite common for his colleagues to speculate about sexual abuse when they treated 'kids with soiling.' Given that there was some research linking encopresis to sexual abuse,[60] and that it appeared on many checklists as *one* of the possible physical indicators, this was unsurprising. But some of the studies suggesting that soiling was linked to sexual abuse had methodological weaknesses. For example, research by Jan Morrow, Catherine Yeager and Dorothy Otnow Lewis claimed a high level of encopresis in a sample of twenty-three boys who were placed in a residential unit in Connecticut, US, because of emotional and behavioural problems, but they had failed to compare their sample to general clinic populations.[61] Rushing to assume sexual abuse, Fuggle thought, was 'deeply flawed' and contrary to the research evidence.[62]

This sense that certain people 'saw' child sexual abuse 'everywhere' was a persistent trope. Beth Fuller* considered that perhaps there was some truth in it at times. If you worked in a team with a high number of cases

[59] Interview with Beth Fuller* by author, 26 Sep 2019.

[60] J. E. Oliver and A. H. Buchanan, 'Generations of Maltreated Children and Multi-Agency Care in One Kindred,' *British Journal of Psychiatry* 135, no 4 (1979); G. S. Clayden, 'Anal Appearances and Child Sexual Abuse,' *The Lancet* 8533 (1987).

[61] Jan Morrow, Catherine A. Yeager, and Dorothy Otnow Lewis, 'Encopresis and Sexual Abuse in a Sample of Boys in Residential Treatment ' *Child Abuse & Neglect* 21, no 1 (1997); 'Letter to the Editor,' *Child Abuse & Neglect* 22, no 5 (1998).

[62] See, for example, Israel Kolvin's Special report to the Cleveland Inquiry which put enuresis and encopresis in the 'low or possible association with CSA.' I. Kolvin et al, 'Child Sexual Abuse: Principles of Good Practice,' *British Journal of Hospital Medicine* (1988); Mellon et al suggested that sexually abused children and psychiatrically referred children where sexual abuse had been ruled out had similar rates of soiling. Michael W. Mellon, Stephen P. Whiteside, and William N. Friedrich, 'The Relevance of Fecal Soiling as an Indicator of Child Sexual Abuse: A Preliminary Analysis,' *Journal of Developmental and Behavioral Pediatrics* 27, no 1 (2006).

of sexual abuse, 'your level of suspicion, especially of men' initially rose. It might subsequently decrease as one became more able to 'process the whole thing' but there 'certainly can be a period when it rises.'[63] Sam Simpson* felt that by the time he trained in the early 1990s, clinicians were suitably cautious about child sexual abuse, having been overly eager in the 1960s and 1970s to the extent that they 'used to see it everywhere.'[64] These dates were wholly inaccurate as sexual abuse was hardly mentioned in child mental health circles until the late 1970s and, in fact, the major criticisms of practitioners for being too keen to identify child sexual abuse were in the late 1980s and early 1990s, amplified by media reporting about child sexual abuse diagnoses in Cleveland in 1987 and reporting on the removal of children in Orkney in 1991 because of suspicions of ritual sexual abuse.[65] These 'scandals' occurred at the time that Simpson had trained, and the fact that he shifted these supposedly 'hypervigilant' practitioners into the more distant past reinforces the sense that it was not within his consciousness or that of those delivering the course he attended.

Back in the 1970s when Frosh had worked at the school for 'maladjusted' children, he had encountered girls whom he later realised had been abused; they were 'very explicitly sexualising,' which, 'as a completely naïve … young man coming in to work with them in those days before anybody had really talked about it,' he found hard to deal with. He remembered having no idea 'what was normal and what wasn't really in a group of … pretty disturbed children.' There was no training and despite being part of a caring staff team that regularly discussed the children, nobody talked about the sexualised behaviour.[66] In contrast, by the time Rahman and Underhill began to work in CAMHS in the early 2000s, there were short in-service training courses in child protection and forums where staff teams could reflect on child abuse even before they enrolled on the training to get their clinical qualifications.

In 2003, while working as a Bengali-speaking assistant psychologist based in an early years centre in east London, Rahman recalled that they had a half-day's mandatory training which taught her 'the definitions, the processes and procedures. This is what you need to do in the situation. This is what it is. This is how you identify it.' Although it was just an

[63] Interview with Fuller.*

[64] Interview with Simpson.*

[65] 'The Report of the Inquiry into the Removal of Children from Orkney in February 1991,' (London: HMSO, 1992).

[66] Interview with Frosh.

introduction, strictly procedural and fairly basic, once in the job she had regular opportunities for reflection. There was individual and group supervision where they discussed the kind of 'conflict and abuse' that young people were experiencing and a broad perspective in relation to 'mental health and how that links to ... child safeguarding, child protection and child abuse.' She was personally very familiar with the local community and aware of live issues, and she noticed that particularly with 'young Asian girls ... there was a lot of self-harming.' She felt well-supported to do her work; she assisted in running a therapy group in Bengali for women who had experienced family violence and were now living with their children in a refuge. It helped that there were other Bangladeshi practitioners in the service who, she thought, 'were very strong in being able to name sexual abuse.' Even so, managing relationships with clients from the same culture as herself could be challenging. The shared culture helped with her own understanding and to build trust with families, but she worried about 'potentially hav[ing] to report something that could have a life changing impact on all involved.'[67]

Underhill was also required to attend a short training course at the outset of one of her early jobs working directly with young people as an assistant psychologist in a youth offending institution. It was a one-day NSPCC training course on sexual abuse, which covered the ways in which young people might try to communicate that something was wrong, how they could help the child to feel safe and how to conduct a conversation that would not be discredited if the case went to court. Although a major thrust of the training was procedural (e.g. it involved learning how to report effectively and take the information 'straight away to the right person'), Underhill remember it as 'child-centred' and 'pretty good.' She also had group supervision and, less frequently, one-to-one meetings. The work itself was 'emotionally draining' and, looking back, she felt there were limitations to the supervisory spaces; personal resilience was so highly valued that it probably made practitioners less able to reflect on their own feelings. She felt that it might have affected 'how much [they] were willing to admit that [they] ever struggled.'[68]

In this setting, she worked mostly with Black or mixed race boys who had been pulled into the criminal justice system, often because of drugs offences, petty theft and gang activity. They acted 'really tough and really

[67] Interview with Rahman.
[68] Interview with Underhill.

bombastic,' but, she thought, they were 'really quite infantile and quite lost,' and she felt 'almost like this mother object to them.' Even though she saw the boys for a short time each day, they did not speak to her about the 'really messy parts of themselves.' She felt that racialisation and class might have been a barrier; she was working class and had been through a lot in her own family but she 'looked like a white middle-class young woman.' Reflecting back years later, she thought it was likely that some of the boys had been sexually abused. Even though a lot of their mothers 'were doing an incredible job' in difficult circumstances, many of the young men had come from homes where 'there were men coming and going,' creating 'opportunities for these young men to have been abused and assaulted and even just made to feel really uncomfortable.' She remembered the culture of the 1990s within gangs was that 'any homosexuality was very, very shameful. And I think that probably dissuaded young men from thinking about it or talking about [sexual abuse].' That culture continued within the youth offending institution where, she felt, there was 'some shame around sexuality, particularly between men,' which manifested itself in frequent homophobic slurs and jokes.

Abuse might be described in a young man's case history which the psychologists reviewed when they started work with them, but once the work was underway the focus was entirely future-oriented. The question 'what is it that made you do this in the first place?' was not asked. Instead, they worked to encourage the boys to think about reaching 'a more positive place in the future.' It was about how the boys could be constructive members of society, how they could be rehabilitated and change their behaviour patterns. The mode of intervention was cognitive behaviour therapy (CBT); they delivered sessions and assessed their efficacy, although, Underhill wondered 'how can you test that in an environment where they're not in the community?' There was not much therapy provided to the boys and there was no physical space in which they might feel comfortable enough to discuss historical abuse. She felt that no one said to the young men that they had been 'treated very badly,' that 'something's happened to [them] that never should have happened…' and helped them to think about how that might link to them 'seeking out security in a gang.' There was no acknowledgement that 'what had happened to a young person up to this point where they offended is really, really important.'[69]

[69] Interview with Underhill.

Underhill was attuned to the possibility of sexual abuse in the boys' past lives, but she recalled the organisational attitude to possible disclosure as being quite procedural. Safeguarding was 'something that you—you reviewed at the start of a project and like, these are your reporting lines if anyone discloses anything to you.' There were no messages from her supervisor or from professional leadership encouraging practitioners to help the boys explore past experiences, as noted above, it was rather the opposite, the emphasis was on the future. Although each of the mental health practitioners' experiences were different, what they held in common in relation to sexual abuse was that they did not receive strong signals from the leaders of their profession that early intervention in child sexual abuse or encouraging disclosures should be a core function of their role. Consequently, their responses to it varied enormously. There is no simple schematic that can explain why some clinical child psychologists were open to the possibility of such abuse and others were not. However, what those who 'saw' sexual abuse in the family shared was a sense of professional curiosity about children's past lives, a thoughtful attitude to their own positionality in relation to those they supported, an empathy for children that surpassed other adults' disapproval (for whatever reason) of discussing the possibility of child sexual abuse, and a feeling of being supported in a space where such a frequently shunned topic could be broached. The latter, of course, exactly mirrored what children had to weigh up in deciding to disclose that they had been, or were still being, raped or sexually assaulted by a family member.

## Part 4: From Child Guidance to CAMHS

Between the 1970s and the 2010s, the shape of services for children and young people affected by psychological distress or displaying 'challenging' behaviour changed significantly. Debates about the structure of services and the nature of the work also consumed professional time and energy. At the beginning of the period, on-the-job training and early career job opportunities for those wanting to qualify as clinical psychologists and work with children tended to take place in child guidance clinics, in hospital psychiatric services or via area psychology teams. Jacobs began her career in a hospital psychiatric department; Smith and Frosh had placements in child guidance clinics; Fuggle worked in a local authority run psychology service. Each type of service had evolved in a distinct manner and in response to specific drivers; they had their own distinctive ethos, professional and interprofessional structures, and working protocols. This changed slowly until, by the early twenty-first century, Rahman and Underhill worked in the completely different landscape of integrated child and adolescent mental health (CAMHS) services. In the next section of the chapter, I will examine in more detail the changing shape of provision and what that meant in relation to early intervention in child sexual abuse, beginning with child guidance.

In the early twentieth century, progressive reform impulses in the United States drove the 'mental hygiene' movement which placed great emphasis on the early detection and amelioration of 'maladjustment' in early childhood. The child guidance clinic was seen as the place to do that. The idea was to influence school systems so that preventative work could be undertaken and children 'saved' from sliding into delinquency.[70] The Commonwealth Fund of New York promoted the expansion of the child guidance model to London; they funded a Child Guidance Council in 1927 and the London Child Guidance Clinic in 1929. British philanthropists also funded some clinics. In 1932, the Institute for the Scientific Treatment of Delinquency was set up to 'initiate and promote scientific research into the causes and prevention of crime' and to 'establish observation centres and clinics for the diagnosis and treatment of delinquents' of all ages.[71] The fear was that, if left 'untreated,' a maladjusted child could detrimentally affect the stability of their family, community and ultimately, society as a whole.[72] The child was labelled a 'nuisance' if they would not learn or 'conform' at school; if their 'tantrums, aggression, enuresis or encopresis' were disrupting their family; or if they were drifting into truancy, violence and petty crime. Very few were considered to have severe psychiatric disorders.[73] The enterprise of child guidance was constructed

[70] Sol Cohen, 'The Mental Hygiene Movement, the Commonwealth Fund, and Education, 1921–1933: Every School a Clinic,' in *Counterpoints: Challenging Orthodoxies: Toward a New Cultural History of Education* (New York: Peter Lang, 1999).

[71] Janet Weston, 'Sexual Crimes, Medical Cures: The Development of a Therapeutic Approach toward Sexual Offenders in English Prisons, C. 1900–1950,' *Canadian Journal of History* 49, no 3 (2014): 400.

[72] John Stewart, "The Dangerous Age of Childhood': Child Guidance in Britain C.1918–1955,' https://www.historyandpolicy.org/policy-papers/papers/the-dangerous-age-of-childhood-child-guidance-in-britain-c.1918–1955. Accessed 24 Sep 2024.

[73] June D. Mills, 'Child Guidance Clinics (A Review of their Development, Present Structure and Future Trends),' *The Journal of the Royal Institute of Public Health and Hygiene* 31, no 2 (1968): 41.

on a moralistic foundation and it was assumed that children and families, 'and not the circumstances of their lives,' were primarily responsible for the 'maladjustment.'[74] It followed, therefore, that with the right intervention, rehabilitation was possible. This assumption drove the Board of Education to provide funding to local authorities to set up child guidance clinics; the Education Act, 1944 drew the clinics under the auspices of school medical services and the local education authorities. By 1955, there were about 300 clinics in England and Wales.[75]

Within the clinic, the staffing team usually consisted of a lead psychiatrist, a psychiatric social worker and an educational psychologist; they assessed, tested and treated the child and parent (usually the mother) to root out the cause of the 'maladjustment.' The clinics were often situated in economically deprived neighbourhoods and had to deal with increasing community tensions. Frosh, for example, had a six-month placement at the Camberwell Child Guidance Clinic on the North Peckham Estate, a huge complex comprised of more than 1400 homes in sixty-five blocks on a forty-acre site. He remembered it as a 'really scary' place and 'one of the roughest bits of London at the time.'[76] When construction commenced in the late 1960s, the *Southwark Civic News* described the estate as a place where residents would be able to 'walk freely along this two and half miles of deck away from the dirt, noise and danger of London traffic.'[77] However, changes in housing allocation policy to ensure that vulnerable groups were given priority access to housing meant that council accommodation was more and more seen as a place of last resort. Rising unemployment and the shifting of people with mental health problems from institutions to living in the community with little support created a 'combustible mix' to which race 'could

[74] Michael Berger, 'Towards a History of Clinical Child Psychology,' in *Clinical Psychology in Britain: Historical Perspectives*, ed. John Hall, David Pilgrim, and Graham Turpin (Leicester: The British Psychological Society, 2015).

[75] Christopher J. Wardle, 'Twentieth-Century Influences on the Development in Britain of Services for Child and Adolescent Psychiatry,' *British Journal of Psychiatry* 159, no 1 (1991): 56.

[76] It became notorious after the murder of ten-year-old Damilola Taylor in 2000. Nick Allen, 'Nothing has changed since Damilola died,' *The Guardian* 25 Apr 2002.

[77] 'Life at Deck Level,' *Southwark Civic News*, July 1968 quoted by John Boughton on the Municipal Dreams website. https://municipaldreams.wordpress.com/2016/10/11/the-five-estates-peckham-part-one/

add an ugly element.'[78] Racist rhetoric increased. Long-standing white, working-class residents on the nearby Brandon Estate in Southwark interviewed in the early 1980s commented on the new arrivals: 'Every one of them are all problem families … and all blacks, or nearly all of them.'[79]

This rhetoric was reflected in a more genteel way in the clinics. Smith worked in child guidance in Medway Towns from about 1979 to 1984. It was a white working-class area where a fifth of the population were 'breadline poor,' with resource levels that were 'so low that people [were] excluded from participating in the norms of society.'[80] Even though the stressors on families were evident, she recalled that the 'problems' that generated the referrals were presented in very 'psychiatric ways' that ignored environmental factors including, for example, family violence. The individuals were pathologised, and 'the etiological factors which is the relational violence going on in the background [was] totally blinkered, not picked up at all.'[81]

There were increasing tensions between different types of professionals and skirmishes in relation to what disciplinary stance or treatment approaches would predominate in assessing and treating children. At Alder Hey in central Liverpool, Warner was one of six or seven child psychologists in a regional team in the 1990s; they were completely 'separate' from the Child Mental Health service which operated 'very much on medical lines.'[82] Fuggle's first post-qualifying job was in Croydon's Psychology Service. All of his colleagues worked with adults, he was the only clinical *child* psychologist. He worked completely separately from the local child guidance clinic who 'weren't particularly enthusiastic about having a clinical psychologist.'[83] There was overlap between the newly arrived clinical child psychologists and educational psychologists who had traditionally focused on psychometric testing, clinical work in the child guidance

[78] John Boughton, *Municipal Dreams: The Rise and Fall of Council Housing* (London: Verso, 2018), 143–144, 212.

[79] Tony Parker, *The People of Providence: A Housing Estate and Some of Its Inhabitants* (London: Hutchinson, 1983), 26.

[80] Source data files kindly provided by Danny Dorling and Ben Wheeler. Daniel Dorling, *Poverty, Wealth and Place in Britain, 1968 to 2005* (Bristol: Policy Press, 2007), 9.

[81] Interview with Smith.

[82] Interview with Warner.

[83] Interview with Fuggle.

centres and supporting schools to deal with 'maladjusted' children.[84] The 1974 Trethowan consultation had heard from witnesses who proposed that child and educational psychology should be combined into a new discipline, but this was not taken forward.[85]

Equally, as clinical child psychologists moved into delivering therapeutic interventions, they encroached on medical and psychiatric territory. They were far cheaper to employ than child psychiatrists and this created an element of competition between the two disciplines. Lastly, it was assumed that clinical child psychologists were oriented towards behavioural approaches, which drew the ire of psychoanalysts. When Fuggle took up a post in Islington in 1987, he experienced 'pretty intense hostility' from the psychotherapy community towards the 'sort of new discipline' of clinical child psychology. He recalled that 'we were not welcome, not at all actually.' 'Generally,' Fuggle recalled, 'we were a bright, perhaps somewhat enthusiastic new profession. And we caused a lot of trouble really because of that.'[86]

Child guidance was increasingly criticised by all sides in the wake of a growing interest in family therapy on the one hand, and behavioural approaches on the other. Although behavioural therapy had not initially been successful in treating disturbed children, psychologists such as Rachmann believed that rather than trying to 'extinguish' children's 'bad habits,' building up 'adaptive behaviour' would lead to better outcomes.[87] Unfortunately, some of those advocating behavioural and social learning techniques based on the work of American psychologists BF Skinner and later Albert Bandura, 'denigrated other approaches, talking of "Romantic psychiatry" and "medical" or "disease" models, and curiously applying the latter epithet against psychoanalysis.'[88] As Fuggle remarked, in the rivalries between different types of treatment such as psychotherapy, family therapy and behavioural therapy, 'there was no real interest in integration of these ideas; it was about which was best.'[89]

[84] Geoff Lindsay, 'Educational Psychology in England and Wales,' *Journal of School Psychology* 23, no 4 (1985): 309.

[85] Berger, 'Towards a History of Clinical Child Psychology,' 223–225.

[86] Interview with Fuggle.

[87] S. J. Rachman, 'Learning Theory and Child Psychology: Therapeutic Possibilities,' *Journal of Child Psychology and Psychiatry* 3 (1962): 149–163.

[88] Wardle, 'Twentieth-Century Influences on the Development in Britain of Services for Child and Adolescent Psychiatry,' 59.

[89] Interview with Fuggle.

Nevertheless, the sense of flux offered opportunities and certain freedoms to clinical child psychologists. They were often the first of their kind to work in a service. In 1982, Frosh started a part-time job as a clinical psychologist in a new outpatient clinic at what was then called the Lewisham Park Day Hospital. Led by child psychiatrist Kirk Weir, it consisted of two psychiatric nurses, a social worker, a registrar or senior registrar and Frosh. They took on all sorts of cases and delivered individual, couples and family therapy. Frosh remembered that he 'just packed the days,' seeing five or six families in each clinic to get as much experience as possible. And although there 'was no great guidance because everybody in that team was quite young and quite new,' it was 'very stretching.' He recalled that 'there was a good feeling about it, you felt—I felt like we were discovering something.'[90]

Fuggle had a similar experience in Croydon's psychology service (and in a later role in Colchester). Even though he was newly qualified, he was appointed to develop work with children across the whole borough. He was the first child psychologist in the service and his supervisor had no expertise with children. All of the work Fuggle did in the three years he spent in Croydon was done out of necessity on home visits because he had no access to a consulting room in a clinic. Like Frosh, he was eager to gain experience and he drove from one home to the next, seeing as many families as he could. He recalled the work as 'not a million miles away from a [contemporary] social work kind of caseload, probably with slightly milder cases … all sorts of behavioural and developmental difficulties.' There were few restrictions around practice and plenty of room for innovation; for example, he recalled that having read an article about using video in clinical sessions, he bought a camera which he and an assistant psychologist used to film mothers and babies playing together. Using video was a 'breakthrough' in helping parents to see how they were interacting with their children, but 'on the other hand,' he reflected, 'it was a bit cavalier, I wasn't getting specialist supervision or anything and I kind of made it up as I went along.' He enjoyed the freedom to 'just go out and do things.'[91]

The fragmentation of children's mental health services may have offered opportunities to some, but others found it deeply frustrating. For decades, psychiatrists had argued that as a mental health service, child guidance should operate under the NHS and there was 'endless confusion and

[90] Interview with Frosh.

[91] Interview with Fuggle.

wrangling about certain clinics and attempts by psychiatrists such as Bowlby to reclaim what they saw as lost territory.'[92] The child guidance model was attacked as inefficient; hospital-based child psychiatrists asked why there were three types of practitioners—psychiatrist, educational psychologist and social worker—when one skilled person could deliver the service.[93] They pushed for the relocation of mental health services for children to the NHS where they believed there could be closer co-operation with medical and nursing practitioners in, for example, general practice, paediatrics, neurology, medicine and general psychiatry. Psychiatrist Dora Black argued that those with more severe or persistent problems 'stemming from psychiatric illness or complex familial problems' would be under the watchful eye of 'doctors as highly trained and experienced in child and adolescent psychiatry as are other consultants in the health service.' In this imagined future service structure, local authority social workers and educational psychologists would be trained in family and behaviour therapy and could deal with 'milder behaviour and learning problems.'[94] In the early 1970s, the Court Committee proposed an integrated Child and Adolescent Psychiatry Service instead of local authority-run child guidance clinics and the separate hospital-based psychiatric services,[95] but it would be more than a decade before significant structural change occurred.

Another challenge was that the current delivery model was not meeting children's needs. Rutter and his colleagues had estimated that one fifth of adolescents had a psychiatric disorder and that one in six children had some sort of physical, educational or psychiatric disorder.[96] Only a tiny proportion (an estimated one per cent of children) were seen by either

[92] Stewart, "'The Dangerous Age of Childhood": Child Guidance in Britain C.1918–1955.'

[93] Jack Tizard, 'Maladjusted Children and the Child Guidance Service,' *London Educational Review* 2, no 2 (1973). These sorts of debates about 'role blurring,' generic working and professional identities continued into the 2000s in relation to multidisciplinary mental health teams. Brian Brown, Paul Crawford, and Jurai Darongkamas, 'Blurred Roles and Permeable Boundaries: The Experience of Multidisciplinary Working in Community Mental Health,' *Health & Social Care in the Community* 8, no 6 (2000).

[94] Dora Black, 'Are Child Guidance Clinics an Anachronism?,' *Archives of Disease in Childhood* 58, no 8 (1983): 644–655.

[95] John Stewart, 'The Dangerous Age of Childhood: Child Guidance and the "Normal" Child in Great Britain, 1920–1950' *Paedagogica Historica* 47, no 6 (Dec 2011): 785–803.

[96] Michael Rutter et al, 'Adolescent Turmoil: Fact or Fiction?,' *Journal of Child Psychology and Psychiatry* 17, no 1 (1976): 35–36.

child guidance or a child psychiatric service in the early 1970s.[97] There was a chronic shortage of inpatient beds available for children with serious psychiatric problems.[98] Rutter's Isle of Wight studies showed geographical variations in the rates of mental disorders implying that levels of poverty and deprivation had an impact on children's mental health. Naomi Richman's Waltham Forest study had demonstrated that behaviour problems in the pre-school years were often indicators of later disorders,[99] but services were failing to reach very young children. This sorts of research was presented as an evidence base to convince the government that there should be a specific strategy to improve children's mental health outcomes and that 'systematic, standardised methods and measurement' were needed in order to measure improvements.[100]

When the NHS Health Advisory Service's *Bridges Over Troubled Waters* report about 'services for disturbed adolescents' was published in 1986, it listed more than one hundred recommendations for improvements. Psychoanalysis was completely out of favour, obliterated by the 'scientific approach.' John Steiner, Chairman of the Association for Psychoanalytic Psychotherapy in the NHS, protested against the committee's bias, epitomised by its failure to mention psychotherapy even once. According to Steiner, the report was not only partisan, but its recommendations that every psychiatric unit should provide a 'total psychiatric service' and adopt an 'eclectic' approach were unworkable.[101] A single unified Child and Adolescent Mental Health Services (CAMHS) service was introduced in 1987 but there was to be no national strategy until 1995.[102]

[97] S. T. Morton and Israel Kolvin, 'Services for the Adolescent in the United Kingdom,' in *Health Care of Mothers and Children in National Health Services: Implications for the United States*, ed. Helen Wallace (Cambridge, Mass: Ballinger Publishing Company, 1975).

[98] Barrett notes this as a problem in the 1980s. It was not resolved by any ensuing CAMHS strategies. Susan Barrett, 'From Adult Lunatic Asylums to CAMHS Community Care: The Evolution of Specialist Mental Health Care for Children and Adolescents 1948–2018,' *Revue Française de Civilisation Britannique [Online]*, XXIV-3 (2019); House of Commons Health Committee, 'Children's and Adolescents' Mental Health and CAMHS: Third Report of Session 2014–15.'

[99] Jacqueline McGuire and Naomi Richman, 'Outcome of Behaviour Problems in the Preschool Setting,' *Child: Care, Health and Development* 13, no 6 (1987): 403–414.

[100] Barrett, 'From Adult Lunatic Asylums to CAMHS Community Care.'

[101] John Steiner, 'Bridges over Troubled Waters,' *Bulletin of the Royal College of Psychiatrists* 10, no 9 (Sept 1986): 246.

[102] 'Together We Stand: The Commissioning, Role and Management of Child and Adolescent Mental Health Services,' ed. Richard Williams and NHS Health Advisory Service (London: HMSO, 1995).

The government introduced a four-tier system within CAMHS that was designed to increase early intervention, improve the integration between hospitals and community provision and deliver a more effective service. Tier 1 would be a universally available service delivered by GPs, school nurses, health visitors, teachers, social workers and youth offending teams. Their early intervention might prevent problems escalating and requiring specialist (and more expensive) input. At Tier 2, counsellors or psychologists were to deliver early intervention services to those at risk of developing mental health problems; at Tier 3, multidisciplinary mental health teams would deliver assessment and treatment to those with more complex or severe disorders. Many of the services at Tier 2 were delivered in community settings such as schools or GP practices; Tier 3 services were usually based in a hospital or a community health clinic. Tier 4 included children with the most severe problems (sexual abuse was included here) and included day- and in-patient settings.

These structural changes left CAMHS practitioners in a similar position to that experienced by GPs, health visitors and social workers in the 1970s and 1980s. They had been fractious and preoccupied with structural changes, engaged in frequent arguments about their own and each other's roles and responsibilities in ways which affected their ability to be vigilant about child sexual abuse in the family. A decade later, structural changes monopolised their energy and attention. Alongside the lack of specific training and a weak management structure, this is another reason why detecting and responding to child sexual abuse was not taken up as a key issue across the profession.

## Part 4: 'Specialists'

The clinical psychology profession had not, it seems, been stirred by the BPS Working Party's attempts to persuade them that child sexual abuse was a psychological matter and hence part of their core business. However, some practitioners did develop groundbreaking responses to child sexual abuse in the family, taking full advantage of the autonomous spaces they found in the shifting landscape of children's mental health services. Smith, Frosh and Warner participated in these sorts of innovative services. Smith joined Haringey Council in 1984, in the same year, Frosh became part of a new NHS specialist sexual abuse team at Lewisham. In Liverpool, Warner was hired straight after she qualified to set up a new sexual abuse service that would work right across the city.

In the mid-1980s, Haringey Social Services had become increasingly frustrated by the difficulties they were experiencing in getting children seen by the local child guidance clinic. They decided to take matters into their own hands. They established their own multidisciplinary community assessment service and, in a highly unusual move, directly employed a psychiatrist and a clinical psychologist alongside a local authority educational psychologist and social workers. The clinical psychologist was Smith. The team's purpose was to support families where there was a risk that their child would be excluded from school, taken into care or get involved in crime. She and another psychologist, Maria Mars, ran a child sexual abuse consultation service, which provided a safe space for staff from a wide range of agencies to discuss cases and they delivered a comprehensive training programme, working on the basis that preventing sexual abuse was everyone's concern.

Smith recalled that they had great success in raising awareness about sexual abuse. For example, the health visitors they had trained put posters about sexual abuse above the weighing scales in baby clinics so 'every mother of a baby would see this information.' Anti-racist practice was high on their agenda. They made leaflets about sexual abuse available in a wide range of community languages. Smith remembered that she and Mars were cognisant of the level of denial of sexual abuse in Black communities. Mars delivered an Afro-Caribbean consultation service, Smith assisted. When the numbers of children on the child protection register for sexual abuse rose, the team felt it was due to the good work they had done in increasing 'the sensitivity of our network to notice the signs and symptoms of possible sexual abuse.' They were disappointed to be told, 'you need to get those figures down,' rather than asking 'why aren't other people picking it up in the same way that Haringey is?'[103]

Frosh was also working in a new type of service. In 1984, psychiatrist Danya Glaser decided to set up a specialist sexual abuse team in Forest Hill and invited colleagues to join her, and Frosh volunteered for one day per week. There was no advance planning or needs assessment, Glaser 'just said I'm going to set up this team and see what comes' and many referrals arrived from health visitors, community paediatricians and social workers. The team delivered assessment and therapeutic work to families and

[103] Interview with Smith. Smith thought that the disapproval of the 'high' figures came from the Social Services Inspectorate and in discussion with London Area Child Protection Committees. Personal correspondence with Smith by author, 30 Jan 2024.

offered consultations to other organisations. There was plenty of professional development; they got together to discuss cases; and they learned a lot about how to communicate with and interview children,[104] including using the 'so-called anatomically correct dolls.' The work 'went right across the board' from 'suspicion of sexual abuse to children in foster care with sexualised behaviour.' They 'even saw some abusers.'[105]

As soon as she finished her clinical training, Warner was asked by the Liverpool Psychology Service to develop multiagency sexual abuse provision across the city. She had prior earlier experience at Taboo, but this was a job with greater scope and responsibility. Although she 'had an abundance of confidence,' she decided to exercise some caution and spent six months scoping out what was needed and whether she could deliver. After that, she was formally appointed to a specialist multiagency post working to develop multiagency responses to children where sexual abuse was suspected or there had been a disclosure. She reported to the Head of the Psychology Department, but most of her contact was with other services across the area, particularly social work. She delivered consultation, training under the auspices of the Area Child Protection Committee, joint and direct work with children and non-abusing parents, usually mothers. Much of her time was spent containing the anxieties of non-abusing carers and social workers; and working directly with children to help them find a 'breathing space' and work out what support would be most helpful for them.[106]

While certain people and teams were increasingly seen as 'specialists' in child sexual abuse, Warner remembered other psychologists and psychiatrists saying, 'oh I never work around sexual abuse.' She thought 'well that is only because you're making it really clear, you don't want to hear about that.' She thought that people were uncomfortable having conversations about sexual abuse and that there was a tendency to refer children on to other services very quickly. Sexual abuse was

[104] Glaser was an adviser to the 'Bexley Joint Investigation project' which sought to improve police and social services joint investigations of child sexual abuse within the family. The project developed procedures and training in child interviewing techniques. Metropolitan Police and Bexley Social Services, 'Child Sexual Abuse: Joint Investigative Project: Final Report,' (London: HMSO, 1987).

[105] Oral history interview with Danya Glaser by author, 20 Jul 2020.

[106] Interview with Warner.

> spoken about as if it was something special, as if it was something different from any other form of abuse so people, even within mental health, would avoid it, they would push it on.[107]

The lead psychiatrist in the Child Mental Health Service in Liverpool referred anything to do with sexual abuse to Warner's multiagency team rather than holding it in the NHS. She 'didn't feel confident … so anything sexual abuse, she would refer to me.' What that meant was that the psychiatrist-led hospital service did not take a curious stance in relation to sexual abuse in other (undisclosed or undetected) cases; they did not ask 'what's happened to you?' They were wedded to the question 'what's wrong with you? Can we diagnose it?'[108]

Unfortunately, another consequence of this tendency to refer sexual abuse work on to services like Warner's was that when funding was withdrawn or redirected, there was no one to do the work. Those who were nervous about sexual abuse and had pushed referrals away would not suddenly now pick it up. The clinical child psychologists to whom they had referred cases on in 'specialist' posts or teams began to disappear. There had been a number of posts and services established to work specifically with sexual abuse in statutory and voluntary sector agencies (e.g. Barnardos, the NSPCC) in different parts of the country in the late 1980s and early 1990s, including, for example, Liverpool, Manchester, Preston, Cornwall, Leeds, Wrexham, Newcastle and a number of London boroughs. Now these were wound up or redefined for different client groups. When Warner left her Liverpool post in 1996, it was not re-advertised although the funding was still in place. And, she recalled, 'over time, all those posts went away.'[109] In Lewisham, Glaser ran her clinic together with another psychiatrist until the mid-1990s, but after she left its remit widened to include other forms of child abuse.[110] Probably due in large part to the government's 1998 Quality Protects programme,[111] which set out to achieve better outcomes for children in the care of the local authority,

[107] Interview with Warner.

[108] Interview with Warner.

[109] Interview with Warner.

[110] Interview with Glaser.

[111] Alan Rushton and Cherilyn Dance, 'Quality Protects: A Commentary on the Government's Agenda and the Evidence Base,' *Child and Adolescent Mental Health* 7, no 2.

the money was redirected into looked after children's posts.[112] The consequence, Warner believed, was that 'you were only able to deliver within the context of prolonged and entrenched difficulties.' The opportunity to work with children who did not have a specific mental health diagnosis, or with families that were not entrenched in an array of child protection issues, to do that 'early doors' work, was lost.[113]

The length of time practitioners could work with children and families was also shortened. Increasingly from the 2000s, interest in time-limited interventions such as CBT grew within child and adolescent services.[114] Critics saw the 'over-emphasis on short-term interventions' as a way of coping with high volumes of referrals[115] or, as Warner put it, 'getting people through and out the door as quickly as possible.' Warner felt that assessing and managing risk, as well as supporting emotional regulation had become the core business of CAMHS. Whether through medication or 'some form of CBT,' Warner described it as 'pushing down extreme feelings so whether you're too high or too low, it's about managing people's emotional arousal.' In terms of sexual abuse, she pointed out, this approach did not 'invite disclosure' because it was 'absolutely not about exploring the things that underlie those extremes of emotions' and it did not allow practitioners the flexibility to work with traumatised children over long periods of time.[116] Critics within mental health services were concerned too about the way resources were targeted on children with less severe difficulties 'and a particular view of Evidence Based Practice' which resulted in services neglecting the 'types of severe and enduring difficulties in children and young people that are an increasing concern to society and most costly in their use of resources.'[117] Critics of Evidence Based Practice

[112] The term 'looked after' was introduced through the Children Act 1989 and refers to children aged under eighteen who are in the care of the local authority.

[113] Interview with Warner.

[114] Courtney L. Benjamin et al, 'History of Cognitive-Behavioral Therapy in Youth,' *Child and Adolescent Clinics of North America* 20, no 2 (2011): 179–189.

[115] Written evidence submitted to the Inquiry into CAMHS by the NHS Northern School of Child and Adolescent Psychotherapy (CMH0143), 18 Mar 2014. https://committees.parliament.uk/writtenevidence/49616/pdf/. Accessed 24 Sep 2024.

[116] Interview with Warner. For a helpful critique of the NHS Talking Therapies IAPT (Improving Access to Psychological Therapies) model and its 'McDonaldization,' see James Binnie, 'Do You Want Therapy with That? A Critical Account of Working within IAPT,' *Mental Health Review Journal* 20, no 2 (2015): 79–83.

[117] Written evidence submitted to the Inquiry into CAMHS by the NHS Northern School of Child and Adolescent Psychotherapy.

have argued that publication bias tends to minimise negative results; and even leaders in CBT have viewed the dominance of randomised control trials as a problem, stating that it seemed 'unlikely that it will ever be appropriate to exclusively consider the management of psychosocial problems in this way.'[118]

Even though the specialist services they led or worked in were closed down, the early vanguard of clinical child psychologists made important contributions to individual children and families' lives through their skills in creating the conditions for disclosure, identifying child sexual abuse, providing assessments and therapeutic interventions to children. They made a broader contribution, too, in the ways they supported, trained and nurtured other practitioners. They were generous in passing on the theoretical knowledge and clinical skills they built up via their writings and the training courses they put on for others.[119]

## Part 5: The 2000s Onward: Generic Services

By the early 2000s, there were few health or local authority services delivering psychological support aimed specifically at children who had experienced sexual abuse; the provision that was available was more typically located in the voluntary or for profit sectors. There were long waiting lists. In order to respond to supposedly 'new' types of risk to children such as child sexual exploitation or criminal exploitation, policy makers and

[118] Marks, 'Psychologists as Therapists: The Development of Behavioural Traditions in Clinical Psychology,' 203–204.

[119] Gerrilyn Smith, *The Protectors' Handbook: Reducing the Risk of CSA and Helping Children Recover* Handbook Series (London: The Women's Press, 1995); *Systemic Approaches to Training in Child Protection* (London: Routledge, 2018); Sam Warner, *Understanding Child Sexual Abuse: Making the Tactics Visible* (Gloucs: Handsell, 2000); 'Disrupting Identity through Visible Therapy: A Feminist Post-Structuralist Approach to Working with Women Who Have Experienced Child Sexual Abuse,' *Feminist Review* 68, no 1 (2001); Paula Reavey and Sam Warner, *New Feminist Stories of Child Sexual Abuse Sexual Scripts and Dangerous Dialogues* (London; New York: Taylor & Francis, 2003); Sam Warner, *Understanding the Effects of Child Sexual Abuse: Feminist Revolutions in Theory, Research, and Practice* (London; New York: Routledge, 2009); Stephen Frosh, 'Issues for Men Working with Sexually Abused Children,' *British Journal of Psychotherapy* 3, no 4 (1987); Danya Glaser and Stephen Frosh, *Child Sexual Abuse*, Second edition ed. (Basingstoke: Macmillan Education, 1993); Dickon Bevington and Peter Fuggle, 'Supporting and Enhancing Mentalization in Community Outreach Teams Working with "Hard-to Reach" Youth: The AMBIT Approach,' in *Minding the Child: Mentalization-Based Interventions with Children, Young People and Their Families*, ed. Nick Midgley and Ioanna Vrouva (New York: Routledge, 2013).

commissioners diverted funds away from child sexual abuse in the family. Funding priorities shifted to such an extent that practitioners increasingly found that one of the only ways to get access to support services for a child who had been sexually abused in the family context was to mention 'sexual exploitation,' it was 'one of the few ways of getting them some support.'[120] Danger on the streets had returned to centre stage; assailants with ready access to their own children in the home were once again sub-rosa.

One of the only locations in the NHS where CAMHS practitioners might provide support services specifically to sexually abused or sexually exploited children was in a Sexual Assault Referral Centres (SARC). These came out of the criminal justice system rather than having medical or psychosocial origins. The early SARCs did not support children, but children's SARCs were established, particularly in urban areas, e.g. The Rainbow Centre at Alder Hey and St Mary's in Manchester. The Child House model piloted at the Lighthouse in London from 2018 included swift access to therapeutic support in a child-friendly location as one of its aims and had clinical psychologists on staff. Their focus was on post-disclosure or identification and they required a police or social work referral. Their relevance here is because one of the effects of funding SARCs was that sexual abuse services largely disappeared from the NHS and local authorities.[121] That meant that most CAMHS practitioners no longer had any experience of working in a service designated for sexually abused children. NHS-employed clinical child psychologists and counsellors were deployed in a broad array of settings, including multidisciplinary services at tiers 2, 3 and 4 of CAMHS and in multiagency teams located in other agencies. These included services in early years, those for children who were in residential or foster settings or at high risk of admission to local

[120] Di McNeish, Liz Kelly, and Sara Scott, 'Effectiveness of Services for Sexually Abused Children and Young People. Report 1: A Knowledge Review,' (Centre of Expertise on Child Sexual Abuse, 2019), 5, 16.

[121] Jo Lovett, Linda Regan, and Liz Kelly, 'Sexual Assault Referral Centres: Developing Good Practice and Maximising Potentials. Home Office Research Study 285,' (Child and Woman Abuse Studies Unit, London Metropolitan University, 2004); Andrea Goddard, Emma Harewood, and Lauren Brennan, 'Review of Pathway Following Sexual Assault for Children and Young People in London,' (London: The Havens, Kings College Hospital London, on behalf of NHS England, 2015); Children's Commissioner, 'Barnahus: Improving the Response to Child Sexual Abuse in England,' (2016); 'Strategic Direction for Sexual Assault and Abuse Services: Lifelong Care for Victims and Survivors: 2018–2023,' (NHS England, 2018); Claire Bethel, 'Child House in a Box Toolkit,' (London: RedQuadrant for MOPAC, Undated, c2021).

authority care, or youth offending. CAMHS staff delivered targeted and specialist mental health assessment and interventions, often using cognitive behavioural therapy as well as behavioural and family therapy approaches. Their ongoing training in, and experiences of, responding to child sexual abuse in practice varied, depending on the function of the service in which they were located, the composition and culture of the team and their own level of awareness and interest.

In 2009, Rahman joined Haringey Council's multidisciplinary team for children looked after by the local authority. The borough's social work service was by this time in chaos, having been condemned by the media and politicians following the death of seventeen-month-old Peter Connolly in 2007. The adults who should have cared for him were responsible for this death, but much of the public ire was directed at practitioners, especially social workers. Rahman recalled that in the aftermath, Haringey found it almost 'impossible' to recruit staff, they had to look overseas and, because of this, she worked with 'lots of bewildered Americans.'[122] She spent half of her week in a CAMHS clinic and, on the other days, was integrated into the leaving care team.[123] There she found that many of the young people had been subjected to abuse and she 'had to think much more directly' about it than in her previous roles.

In the mid-1990s, clinical child psychologists could work in specialist sexual abuse teams, but in the late 2000s (as Warner had described) they were situated in teams supporting children who often had long histories of multiple forms of abuse and neglect. One consequence of this was that it removed the early intervention aspect of the work; CAMHS practitioners were no longer in the types of roles where they could spread awareness about sexual abuse and deliver training to community services (as Smith and Warner had done in Haringey and Liverpool, and Glaser had done in Lewisham). Another consequence was that the skills of psychologically minded practitioners were largely confined to cases of known abuse; their ability to communicate sensitively with children and help them to disclose was not utilised more widely, nor were their skills in encouraging less confident practitioners to act on any suspicions about abuse.

There were still some opportunities to raise other practitioners' consciousness, however. For example, when Rahman subsequently worked in

[122] Interview with Rahman by author, 18 May 2021.

[123] In an example of how institutional memory is lost, Rahman was unaware that Haringey had been at the vanguard in integrating psychologists alongside social workers in the 1980s.

a service supporting children to stay in school, she was able to bring the expertise she had gained in Haringey with her. Based in a local authority school inclusion team, she felt that part of her role was to encourage staff to think about what a child might be feeling, what they might be experiencing at home and might be trying to communicate through their behaviour. 'What might be going on' for the child included sexual abuse and she promoted discussion about that in supervision and clinical team meetings. She was usually called in to consult on a case when it was at a crisis point and that, she thought, made it difficult for staff to think beyond the child's 'immediate behaviours.' She would ask them, 'is there something that you're particularly worried about?' But she reflected that there was 'a process to getting to that point where people can even consider naming or even wondering about might this be going on,' which she thought was related to the professionals feeling safe and held. She felt that she and other clinicians could have a role in helping to create that sense of safety in the network.

> So, you know I'm using the words tentative, gently, sensitive, because those are the—those are what enable people to be able to face some pretty—really complex, distressing—Things that really—people don't necessarily go into these various professions thinking about. So, a teacher wouldn't necessarily be going into teaching thinking how am I going to manage supporting a child who might be at risk of or experiencing sexual abuse.[124]

Equally, her position as a clinician from a different discipline in a team made up mainly of social workers could enable her to 'maybe ask some challenging questions which might be heard differently.' Rahman thought that when co-located in multidisciplinary teams, CAMHS practitioners had enough knowledge of the team's processes, culture and the language they used to be a part of difficult conversations, but at the time they could be 'slightly independent ... slightly external to the organisation but yet is very much accessible and known.' In a pressurised space, where the network could easily fracture and push teams and individuals apart, the clinician could play a role in 'slow[ing] the network down.' The clinician could say, 'hang on a minute, I know there's a crisis going on, but actually making decisions in ways where we're not really reflecting on ...what's behind

[124] Interview with Rahman.

all of this will lead to possibly some unhelpful decision making or not good enough decision making.'

In Rahman's experience, practitioners, whether social workers, teachers or others, often dismissed their own emotional responses in thinking about what might be behind a child's distress. They thought 'Oh, that's not—why is my emotional response to this—how's that relevant or how is that related?' Part of the clinical role was to support practitioners to recognise that their feelings were part of the information to be pieced together in order to make sense of the child's situation.

> You know, these children might be bringing something to us and putting some of that emotion into us in order that …we can be responsive to that and where we're missing those cues, … those social and emotional communications from children because actually we're not paying attention to how that leaves us feeling. Then that is part of the block of why we might not be getting to that point of recognising, 'oh, this is an indicator, this is a potential risk of child sexual abuse that this child is kind of communicating to me.'[125]

However, there was a need to have collegiate support, safe spaces and systems to raise concerns and take what 'just starts with a feeling' to the point where you can work out what exactly is causing those feeling and 'put words to it.'[126]

In Underhill's first job post-qualification, the impact of child sexual abuse was unmistakable. She worked in a secure adolescent intensive care unit as part of a large NHS team. It was a small unit of six or seven beds; the patients were self-harming and at high risk of suicide. Although the unit had good facilities and was nicely decorated, light and airy, closer examination revealed signs of coercion and control too: an isolation room where children could be locked in, which the young people used to call 'the padded cell;' things bolted to the floors in the rooms. There was spasmodic violence. She was not at work on the day a fourteen-year-old girl was brought in from police custody and 'kicked a nurse repeatedly so hard that she lost a kidney,' but she remembered the fear, distress and low morale that followed.

Out of the six young women who were resident on the ward when she left, five had reported sexual abuse within their family. For some, the abuse

[125] Interview with Rahman.

[126] Interview with Rahman.

was already part of the case history but 'it was something that [the girls] kept talking about.' Sometimes there were obvious reasons why they constantly repeated their stories; for example, one girl's mother refused to believe her daughter's disclosure and instead accepted what the male relative responsible for the abuse had told her. Her daughter was deeply distressed by her mother's ongoing denial and saw it as the cause of her mental distress. Underhill thought that the girls' feelings about being detained and obliged to take medication were similar to their emotional response to the sexual abuse; they were not in control of their own bodies while they lived on the unit; they felt as if their bodies were 'being taken over.' They were also, she believed, working out feelings of confusion and shame whilst hovering at the brink of childhood/adulthood, thinking 'did I ask for that [abuse]? Did I become a grown up too quickly? Is being a grown up really dangerous?'

In every one of her subsequent jobs, Underhill encountered sexual abuse disclosures. She worked on an NHS helpline service for people having their first mental health crisis. When the client made contact, she supported them for an hour or two. She recalled that she might be trying to calm a family member or their teenage son or daughter while they were 'tearing their room apart.' She remembered many calls from young people aged sixteen to twenty-one saying they would commit suicide, talking about negative experiences and abuse; the 'majority of that was young people phoning in at ten or eleven at night wanting to talk about their history of largely sexual abuse.'

In 2018, Underhill left specialist services to work as a counselling psychologist across a number of schools. She described it as

> sort of an experiment that actually maybe children who are referred for therapy, that should be in school rather than out in a clinical environment, and perhaps mental health teams should be working with teachers and parents more closely than they do with other clinicians.[127]

This approach came from proposals put forward by the government to establish Mental Health Support Teams in schools,[128] with the aims of delivering 'evidence-based' interventions for mild-to-moderate mental

[127] Interview with Underhill.

[128] Transforming Children and Young People's Mental Health Provision: A Green Paper (CM 9626), (London: Department of Health and Social Care, and Department for Education, 2017).

health issues; developing school-wide strategies to improve children's emotional wellbeing and mental health; and providing timely advice to school staff as well as liaison with specialist services where needed so that children could 'get the right support and stay in education.'[129] In the service Underhill joined, there was a disciplinary hierarchy: counsellors dealt with the mildest cases; psychotherapists with an intermediate level; and clinical psychologists worked with the most complex. Underhill's caseload included children who were refusing to come into school and those who were 'really truculent in school, having experienced a trauma.' She was asked to deal with many children who were waiting for a diagnostic assessment or in the process of diagnosis, often for Autism Spectrum Disorder (ASD). In her experience, 'schools loved pinning an ASD on children.' While the child was on the long CAMHS waiting lists for diagnosis, the clinicians would start to provide therapy to 'see what flushes out' and Underhill thought that 'fifty per cent of the time the ASD diagnosis goes away.' For example, a young woman in her early teens, whom Underhill had been seeing for therapy for about three months, said to her, 'after coming to therapy, there's something I think I want to tell mum and I just want to check it with you.' The girl told her,

> 'I think my dad needs to go to prison' and I said 'okay, well, that sounds really serious and I'm really shocked to hear that and I believe you. Do you think you can tell me a bit more about it?' And she said, 'I'm not sure if I can, I'm not sure if I can tell anyone but I think I need your help to tell mum.'[130]

After the girl's disclosure that her father had sexually abused her while she was staying with him, the behaviours which the school had presumed were symptoms of ASD disappeared. The girl had previously refused to go to class, now she explained why, stating 'I've been carrying around this secret and I thought people could see it.' Why then, wondered Underhill, did the school system jump to thinking that a child had autism or Attention Deficit Hyperactivity Disorder (ADHD) rather than wondering whether there was a traumatic incident in the child's life that was affecting their behaviour? She felt that in a large majority of those cases, 'some form of

[129] NHS England, 'Mental health support in schools and colleges,' https://www.england.nhs.uk/mental-health/cyp/trailblazers/ accessed on 8 Jan 2024.

[130] Interview with Underhill.

disclosure comes out and those behaviours fall away.' Underhill would work with primary school children for up to thirty sessions and saw most adolescents for twenty-five to thirty sessions. She believed that the model of being present in the school and in a position to offer sessions over an extended period allowed her to build trust with individual children.[131]

In the last twenty years, some psychologists like Rahman and Underhill have been attuned to the possibility that the children they worked with might have been subjected to some form of abuse, including sexual abuse. They had disclosures in services that worked with children considered at high risk of harming themselves or others and equally in universal settings that supported children that were categorised as having mild or moderate emotional and behavioural problems. They saw their roles as directly supporting children, young people and families as well as supporting practitioners from other disciplines. At the same time, many other clinical child psychologists identified cases of child sexual abuse rarely, if at all. They worked with some children for a limited number of sessions and with others for many months without hearing any disclosures.

## Conclusion

This chapter has looked at why, since the 1980s, most community-based CAMHS practitioners failed to hear what children and young people tried to tell them.[132] It explored why practitioners did not associate children's distress with what Johnstone referred to as 'all this trauma' in their young lives.[133] By engaging with the memories of six individuals, it has been possible to illustrate some of the shifting barriers to increasing early recognition. Clinical psychology, and particularly clinical *child* psychology, was a new discipline without a stable professional culture or leadership. Different

[131] Interview with Underhill.

[132] I have focused mainly on clinical child psychologists and assistants but there are also counsellors, family therapists, psychotherapists and more recently-introduced posts at lower grades, such as children's wellbeing practitioners and education mental health practitioners (EMHPs). The government is funding training EMHPs as part of the national Children and Young People's Improving Access to Psychological Therapies plan. Their training is funded by Health Education England. https://www.healthcareers.nhs.uk/explore-roles/psychological-therapies/roles-psychological-therapies/education-mental-health-practitioner accessed on 21 Jan 2024.

[133] Johnstone, *Users and Abusers of Psychiatry: A Critical Look at Psychiatric Practice*, 115–116.

disciplines and clinical approaches jostled for supremacy within child mental health. Individuals who could be tolerant and empathetic with patients often did not show the same qualities in battles about different clinical approaches including behavioural, psychoanalytical, cognitive behavioural and family therapy. Structures of service delivery shifted, and management lines were weak.

From the 1980s, some practitioners became deeply involved in child sexual abuse in terms of recognition, assessment and treatment; others had little interest in it and saw it as outside of their core remit. In her critique of the medical model of responding to psychological distress, Johnstone touched on clinical psychologists, noting that some were sceptical of not only the medical model but also of 'scientist-practitioner' approaches, but that it was 'comparatively rare for them to use their confidence and status to speak out.'[134] Was the reluctance to intervene early in the lives of children who had experienced sexual abuse within their families another symptom of this professional insecurity?

[134] *Users and Abusers of Psychiatry: A Critical Look at Psychiatric Practice*, 139.

CHAPTER 7

# Conclusion

Doctors, nurses and therapists are people we turn to for help. We meet them in a confidential space, often when we are at our most vulnerable. We have the opportunity to speak to them about our most private problems. We confide in them. We trust them to examine our bodies and understand the signs of injury or illness. We expect them to treat us with care. How puzzling then that sexually abused children or worried parents would not choose their doctor, health visitor or therapist as a safe person to talk to about abuse in the family. How peculiar that these practitioners did not see the physical signs of sexual abuse on children's bodies, or demonstrate greater curiosity about why children were distressed or behaving in unusual ways. This book examined how this situation came to be.

Survivors' testimonies are the cornerstone of this history, but they make up only a small portion of the book. That is because there are strict rules about access to personal records and sensitive information, which work against historical research that can centre the voices of children and adult survivors of abuse. The survivors' perspectives were by necessity gathered from disparate sources such as memoirs, letters to a public inquiry, and snippets from published accounts. In June 2022, however, I was contacted by a survivor called Suzy who had heard that I was researching health practitioners' responses to child sexual abuse. She had recently obtained her own medical records and wondered if I would be interested in 'the various descriptions' of her mental health issues over forty years. We recorded her oral history over two sessions in 2022 and 2023, and this



R. Beecher, *Community Health Practitioners and Child Sexual Abuse in the Family, 1970s–2010s*, Genders and Sexualities in History, https://doi.org/10.1007/978-3-031-80052-8_7

provided a rare opportunity to compare health practitioners' contemporaneous notes about Suzy with her own memories decades later.

Suzy was born in 1958. Her father was a policeman, a powerful figure at home and in the small town where she lived. He insisted that his family must be models of propriety, 'so you didn't want anything bad coming to the house or anything that would show up the family.' On her thirteenth birthday, she was raped by an eighteen-year-old in her neighbourhood. She had no memory of disclosing this to anyone, but when she met up with a school friend some years ago, the woman told her, 'I remember you when we were at first year at school, we were sitting next to each other in English and you told me what happened to you.' The woman said that she wished she had told her own mother back then. Suzy did not blame her friend. Suzy's own mother, she thought, had not been aware of the abuse either, but her brother 'knew something had happened to me, but nothing had ever really been discussed. So it was all shrouded in a kind of shame and uncertainty and talking in euphemisms.' As other survivors' testimonies in this book have highlighted, it was not uncommon for children to try to tell someone, or signal to them that something was wrong in the hope that they would ask questions. Suzy was no exception; she told her friend, and her brother also knew. In a statement he later made to the police, he said that Suzy had 'changed overnight' and that she 'even looked different.' And yet, none of the three children who knew about the abuse had an adult in their lives who asked questions about the signs, nor did they trust anyone enough to speak about what had happened to Suzy.

At eighteen, Suzy went to see a GP to get help. She wanted to start 'an intimate relationship' with her boyfriend, but 'it was agony.' She could not remember exactly what she told the young, male doctor, but she felt he had not asked her any questions. He wrote only three words in her notes. On a video call, she read those words out to me, 'what it actually says is "narrowed introitus"—which I believe is vagina—question mark, and then a word that looks like "webbing" and I have absolutely no idea what any of that means.' She recalled that she experienced the physical examination as 'incredibly uncomfortable both physically and mentally.' It took place without any nurse or chaperone in the room, and she remembered the intimate examination accompanied by a feeling that 'this isn't right.' She felt she was 'reliving the sexual abuse and a sort of lack of control all over again.' The examination was painful and 'it went on for a little bit longer than [she] felt it should have done.'

In fact, one of the reasons that Suzy had requested her medical records was because a memory of this examination had come back to her after hearing about a doctor who was struck off the medical register for inappropriate behaviour. Survivors have spoken to the Independent Inquiry into Child Sexual Abuse about similar assaults taking place 'under the cover of clinical examinations' by healthcare providers, usually male GPs. Children sought 'treatment, care and recovery,' often relating to abuse they suffered at home, and instead were subjected to further violations by healthcare professionals.[1] This GP's physical examination of Suzy was at best callous and at worst abusive. It demonstrates that we cannot separate child sexual abuse simplistically into different settings and types, as well as reminding us that predators seek out young people who are vulnerable and take advantage of them. But even if this GP had not assaulted Suzy, he did not help her in any way.

The doctor did not ask Suzy any questions about whether anything bad had happened to her, he failed to explain what might be causing her symptoms and what the treatment could be, and he denied her any comfort or reassurance about her physical and mental health. Did he consider in his own mind that Suzy might have been a victim of sexual abuse? Did he deliberately deny it as a possibility? Or perhaps he was merely irritated, like many of the GPs of the 1970s, by having to deal with 'unhappy women' with 'gynae problems.' Whichever it was, his behaviour was not uncommon. As I have shown in this book, prior to the 1980s, practitioners often turned away from the possibility of child abuse, even when there was irrefutable evidence that an underage child had been raped: a pregnancy or miscarriage. In later decades, these overt physical signs were less common, but survivors still spoke of sending out signals and getting no response from health practitioners.

Suzy experienced two years of sexual abuse, followed by forty years during which she made tenacious efforts to get the help she needed. Although her medical records from 1983 demonstrate that mental health services knew then that she had been repeatedly raped as a thirteen-year-old, many entries downplayed the abuse and adultified her by referring to a 'sexual relationship,' while at the same time acknowledging that she was a child going to 'play with a friend.' She was implicitly blamed for perpetuating the abuse because she returned to the same spot to play with that friend. She was referred to as 'needy,' 'dependent,' 'attention seeking,' and in many other pathologising terms. Her depression and sexual problems were associated by therapists with her early family relationships rather than with the sexual abuse. She did not meet a mental health practitioner who

[1] Julienne Zammit et al., 'Truth Project Thematic Report: Child Sexual Abuse in Healthcare Contexts,' (London: IICSA, 2020).

asked her about what had happened to her until nearly twenty years after the abuse. That clinical psychologist encouraged her to write a letter to the rapist. She still had the letter when we spoke in 2022 and remembered what happened when she showed it to her therapist:

> I wrote it down. And it was shocking. But I remember he took it and he looked at it and he was really visibly shaken. And he said, 'I know, I'm not supposed to say anything here, but I hope they've had a bloody awful life.' [Suzy laughs]. You know, so, I know that therapists aren't meant to get involved, but he really did look quite green. Because I put everything and it was quite visceral, I didn't leave anything out. And he was sickened by it. And at last, it was like, somebody is actually understanding for the first time in my life. So it took me to 1994 or 1995 to get there.[2]

Perhaps it was no coincidence that the first time a mental health practitioner took Suzy's past seriously was in the mid-1990s, at a time when personal testimonies increasingly appeared in the media and when the National Commission into the Prevention of Child Abuse drew public and political attention to survivors' accounts of the impact of childhood abuse.

Over the decades, Suzy was described as a 'very mixed up frightened young woman.' In another document, she was said to be 'a rather sad lady … rather a fragile person.' Reflecting back, Suzy wondered why practitioners described her in these ways given that 'they must have thought, "well, she's had a terrible time but look at what she's doing now, she can't be that fragile. You know, holding down a job and being responsible."' Why, she wondered, did they not ask more questions?[3]

This book has demonstrated that in the last forty years, there has been no effective early intervention by health practitioners for children who were sexually abused in their families or close networks. Despite a great surge of optimism in the 1980s about the potential of the confluence of family doctors, public health nurses and mental health practitioners in bringing child sexual abuse 'out of the shadows,' that promise was not realised. Although these professions accepted (somewhat reluctantly) that they had a responsibility to intervene in cases of child abuse, there was no evidence of widespread intent to identify child sexual abuse or of concerted efforts to intervene.

Health practitioners were asked to deliver effective early intervention in families. This is defined today much as it was in the 1980s: the idea that a

[2] Oral history with Suzy by author, 13 Oct 2022 and 5 May 2023.

[3] Interview with Suzy.

practitioner can prevent problems from occurring, or 'tackle them head-on' when they do occur, before the situation gets worse.[4] But this was not applied to sexual abuse. Only a minority of individuals within these community-based professions ever succeeded in being strong allies to children who were victimised in this way. Few paid attention to children's distress signals, asked children direct questions, created the conditions in which children could begin to talk about what had been done to them, or took action to protect them. But when they did, their interventions could be very powerful. It often meant the abuse was curtailed, and the children could get access to appropriate medical and psychological help. Without it, as testimony like Suzy's demonstrates, children's ordeals were often prolonged for many years into adulthood.

## Not Our Job?

In the 2020s, some of the practitioners I approached to ask about their experiences in identifying and responding to child sexual abuse in the family did not seem to realise that it was or had ever been an expectation of their roles. They were somewhat hesitant to state categorically that it was not part of the job. After all, their mandatory safeguarding training courses taught them to remain vigilant to all forms of abuse. However, there was no sense that they were on the lookout for potential physical or behavioural indicators or thinking about ways to ensure children or protective parents would feel comfortable making a verbal disclosure of sexual abuse to them. My analysis of archival sources (journals, trade papers, training materials, organisational reports and newsletters) from the 1970s to the 2000s demonstrated that, contrary to those beliefs, GPs, mental health practitioners and health visitors were the recipients of strong messages, first from paediatricians, psychiatrists and charity leaders, and later from government officials, that early intervention in child sexual abuse in the family was a core professional responsibility. Although that responsibility remains in place today, they receive few disclosures, rarely raise suspicions of sexual abuse or make referrals. These low rates of identification seem to have remained static over decades. And yet, this failure to notice the signs and act to protect the child goes unremarked and unexamined. The net result is that early intervention in child sexual abuse in the family is

[4] 'What is early intervention?' https://www.eif.org.uk/why-it-matters/what-is-early-intervention, Early Intervention Foundation, Accessed 24 March 2024.

nominally a core responsibility of every community health practitioner, but it is an obligation that most evade, leaving children largely unprotected.

This book traced the history of community health practitioners' involvement in protecting children, mostly in the period between the 1970s and the 2010s. That history was not linear or neat. Looking back, practitioners tended to remember various barriers that prevented them from identifying sexual abuse in the family and perceived those as fairly static. For example, a lack of resources meant there were too many patients and not enough time, or the political emphasis on performance management led services to prioritise activity (e.g. the number of visits made, or immunisations delivered) over time spent in building trusting relationships with family members. But this book has shown that these structural and cultural factors were not static. The ways doctors, nurses and mental health practitioners worked within their individual professions and across the disciplines changed. Often their physical locations were transformed (e.g. single to group practices for GPs), governance shifted from the NHS to local authority or vice versa for health visitors and child mental health, and new legislation or statutory guidance affected them. National policies shifted and the resources attached to their adoption had to be spent in particular ways.

Ironically, prior to the 1990s, many of the conditions that might have enabled doctors, nurses and mental health practitioners to respond to the signs of sexual abuse were in place. 'Continuity of care,' is something GPs aspire to deliver today, but in those years it was closer to the norm. GPs and health visitors had ongoing connections with families that lasted many years. All the professionals had far greater autonomy to manage their own schedules and decide who they would prioritise and what interventions they would deliver than they do in the 2020s. Complaints about 'rationing' of services and 'postcode lotteries' were still to come.[5] Each of the professional groups were less pressured than they are today in terms of the numbers of families using their services. However, the capacity to do the work was almost irrelevant because practitioners lacked awareness and there was very little training available.

In any case, we cannot idealise those decades. Doctors, health visitors and child guidance practitioners were affected by changes in policy at the national and local levels, which had implications for the way they were

[5] Satpal Singh Shekhawat and Faisel Baig, 'Commissioning: Important for All GPs,' *British Journal of General Practice* 69, no 685 (2019); Lucina Rolewicz and William Palmer, 'What Health and Care Need from the Next Government: NHS Staffing. Briefing Paper 1,' (London: Nuffield Trust, 2024).

deployed and the content of their jobs. There were arguments about disciplinary boundaries, professional autonomy and status. Doctors and health visitors; health visitors and social workers; hospital and community-based psychiatrists; medical officers for health and paediatricians; paediatricians and police surgeons—many roles associated with children and families were contested in these years. Debates about how services should best be delivered and who should assume leadership were constant. Doctors were reluctant to absorb social problems into their remit. Health visitors were unsure as to whether their role was to deliver light-touch public health services to all the families in their 'patch,' or to concentrate more on the 'needy' families. They also feared losing their professional identity and being used as GPs' assistants under government proposals for group practices and GP attachment. At the same time, they were resentful of the better-paid social workers in the new social services departments. There were fierce debates about the best way to provide services for the many children with mental health needs that went unmet, while questions were asked about the efficacy and efficiency of the child guidance triumvirate of psychiatrist, psychiatric social worker and education psychologist.

This was the backdrop for another clash, this time between two strong pressure groups advocating for children who were sexually abused in their families: feminists / survivors and medics/ psychiatrists. They were heavily influenced by their counterparts in the United States. In both countries, there were deep ideological differences between the two factions. The most generous interpretation of the motives of the paediatricians and psychiatrists involved was that they wanted to demonstrate that child sexual abuse had a devastating and life-long negative impact that could not be addressed through a purely juridical response. The criminal justice system could only punish perpetrators, it left their sexual interest in children untreated and they were likely to abuse again on release. Meanwhile, the child and other family members lost a father figure and were usually not provided with any medical or social support. However, what is clearly demonstrated through the historical evidence is that, in an attempt to bring about policy change and investment in treatment services for the whole family, medics objectified and pathologised adult survivors as 'damaged goods.' Gendered stereotypes of the 'seductive child' and the 'collusive mother' proliferated in their concepts of sexual abuse and how it should be treated. Their dismissal of feminist theorising and survivors' perspectives was mirrored in the mainstream media and in practitioner training, where the emerging medical and psychiatric 'experts' were given a platform and survivors were silenced.

My examination of practitioners' professional education, on-the-job training, guidance and support demonstrated the lack of investment by each profession's leadership in equipping their staff to respond to child sexual abuse. Professional leaders allowed the internecine rivalries and rhetoric about disciplinary boundaries, status and authority referred to above to proliferate, rather than develop a clear child-centred vision in relation to child sexual abuse in the family. When it came to investment in training, most practitioners had no specific training in child abuse at all until the 1990s. Medical, nursing and clinical psychology education did not comprehensively address child abuse until the mid-2000s and even then child sexual abuse was not addressed thoroughly or thoughtfully.

In terms of professional education, doctors probably had the best foundation for the child abuse work because of the emphasis within their training on professional curiosity, physical examination, asking questions about the patient's history and symptoms and making differential diagnoses. By the 1990s, their roles in relation to child sexual abuse were also more clearly defined than those of health visitors or child and adolescent mental health staff. Ironically, the very public criticism of the Cleveland paediatricians and the subsequent public inquiry in 1987 was a catalyst for greater clarity in paediatrics and general practice about what was to be the remit of specialist paediatricians as opposed to that of general practitioners and other types of doctor.

Health visitors, on the other hand, had extensive training but it was not tailored towards child protection. As a profession, they were not well prepared to confront child sexual abuse within the family. Their training was wholly inadequate. There was no vision or clarity from their leadership as to what their role should be in relation to child sexual abuse in the family. Both the archival sources and the oral histories suggested that the profession was reluctant to confront the corporeality of child sexual abuse. The failure on the part of senior health visitors to articulate the strengths of the profession and demonstrate its value to other professional groups meant that the specific knowledge, experience and skills of the health visitor were not used to benefit sexually abused children.

In common with other community-based health practitioners, clinical child psychologists had little training in child sexual abuse. Unlike medicine and nursing, however, it was a relatively new profession which swiftly extended its influence across children's services over this forty-year period. The lack of interest from professional leadership at the British Psychological Society, the strong behavioural focus of the Institute of Psychiatry which had widespread influence on the training of clinical psychologists across

Britain, and the move towards short term interventions like CBT thwarted recognition of child sexual abuse in the family in terms of early intervention. And yet within clinical child psychology, there was a significant minority of feminist practitioners who realised the potential of the discipline and developed innovative approaches and services for sexually abused children.

## Cultures of Misogyny

This book has shown clearly that responding effectively to child abuse in the family setting has had a complicated history in Britain over the last forty years. It is a history that has been profoundly affected by cultures of misogyny in medicine and inflected by gendered assumptions and conflict at every turn. Suzy's medical records demonstrated that not only did psychiatric practitioners ignore the unequal power dynamics in the sexual abuse inflicted upon her, but they also repeatedly deployed tired misogynistic tropes about her mental health that echoed the experiences of countless other survivors, not only in relation to their own personal care, but also to their activism.

The inter- and intra-professional arguments about role and remit within medicine and nursing that started in the 1970s in relation to child abuse were also heavily gendered. The impact of feminism, along with increasing numbers of women entering medicine and psychiatry and moving gradually into positions of greater seniority generated fierce and often mean-spirited debate. Misogynistic attitudes to women's expertise in the professional environment were often mirrored by gendered stereotypes about women and girls' behaviour in the family home. Professional behaviours and processes were also subjected to a kind of gendered thinking that placed a mantle of authority on male doctors and psychiatrists, which extended to accepting the theories they espoused as 'scientific' and 'reliable' even when they rested on the flimsiest of evidence. The theories and opinions of certain women (survivors of sexual abuse and feminists) came under far greater scrutiny and were liable to be discounted as emotional and irrational.

Within the professions, the almost entirely female health visiting profession was subjected to a pervasive sexism and their views were disparaged in very similar ways to survivors. This severely undermined their ability to be allies to children in relation to sexual abuse in the family. Health visitors were silenced when they tried to introduce talk of emotion into discussions about possible child sexual abuse. And yet as clinical psychologist Natasha Rahman* pointed out, every practitioner needed to be able to connect with their own feelings and ask what those were telling them. Many health visitors were like Jane Bramwell who described that she had 'grave concerns,' and that it was 'more a feeling,' that 'there was something not quite right' in a family.[6] Rather than dismissing such emotional responses as sentiment or unreasoned opinion, practitioners needed to

> recognise that that's very much part of the information that helps us to make sense of what we're experiencing with these children and these children's responses. You know, these children might be bringing something to us and putting some of that emotion into us in order that we can be responsive to that. And where we're missing those social and emotional communications from children because actually we're not paying attention to how that leaves us feeling. Then that is part of the block of why we might not be getting to that point of recognising, 'oh, this is an indicator, this is a potential risk of child sexual abuse that this child is communicating to me.'[7]

Rahman conceptualised practitioners' emotional reactions as important sources of intelligence that they should draw upon in relation to the child's circumstances and presentation. But, as she went on to point out, teams were needed to help make the connection between the feeling and the 'really deep concerns.' Facilitation from a supervisor, a manager or a colleague enabled practitioners to 'make some connection or to be able to put words to it,' to help them work out what was it they noticed about the child's behaviour that left them with that 'funny feeling.' Paediatrician Michelle Cutland and others also spoke of creating time and space for reflection in underresourced, overburdened and highly pressurised contexts. Psychologist Kim Underwood said she

> made relationships with people who were with me being confronted [by child sexual abuse disclosures]. And perhaps we've processed that as our own trauma… the stuff you hear is pretty shocking and you have to work through that together.[8]

Some practitioners, including psychiatrists Judith Trowell, Arnon Bentovim and Danya Glaser, recognised that they occupied positions of privilege. They had supportive teams around them and access to personal therapy which helped them to persevere with this work over many years.

[6] Interview with Bramwell.

[7] Interview with Rahman.

[8] Interview with Underwood.

Practitioners also spoke of a connection that alerted them to child sexual abuse either through a personal experience of sexual violence (Sam Warner, Gerrilyn Smith, Michelle Cutland) or through contact with someone who raised their awareness, often at the beginning of their careers. Underwood remembered an early encounter with a young man in a paediatric intensive care unit who described to her how his brother sexually abused him for years. She recalled 'the language he used that—that I couldn't—I had—it was—even now it just makes—it makes my—it makes my skin crawl a little bit.' She felt it was 'so confronting,' but it altered her frame of reference and perhaps that was why throughout her career she 'always had children disclosing' to her. She described it 'almost like the stopper was removed early on, so you were willing to have these difficult conversations.'

Perhaps it was the same in terms of noticing the signs. GP Stephen Amiel recalled a young woman who came to see him for a cervical smear. He was 'pretty sure' he offered her a chaperone, but she declined. When he asked her to go into lithotomy position (lie on her back with knees at 90 degrees) for the examination, she recoiled and he 'thought well, this is—I need to stop.' He remembered

> there was a look absolutely of a kind of rabbit in the headlights type of terror actually. It was palpable and quite shocking, and it made me feel absolutely dreadful that I was able to elicit that in her although there was no inkling that it was anything other than something that she'd asked for and come for. Anyway, I didn't proceed with the smear and obviously said, 'I'm sorry, that was really distressing for you, is there anything you want to talk about as to, you know, how we can make it easier or why it's so difficult?'[9]

Amiel's response was perhaps what Suzy might have hoped for. But it was not straightforward. The woman disclosed to him that her father had abused her over many years. Amiel tried to find her a therapist, but she was not happy with any of the practitioners he recommended. Eventually, one of the therapists he approached recognised that he had become quite enmeshed as a 'rescuer' in this situation, helped him to step away and began counselling the survivor. Amiel felt grateful for that, reflecting that 'therapists need their supervisors to unpick all of this which is something that isn't there for doctors, there is nowhere for us to go…'[10] But he described encounters with adult survivors that sensitised him and made him more vigilant.

[9] Interview with Amiel.
[10] Interview with Amiel.

There is no neat end point in relation to the recent histories of health practitioner responses to child sexual abuse in the family. These histories are as messy, complicated and contested as the phenomena itself. There is no straightforward narrative of progress and improvement for children. What this book has shown is that, in every decade, the majority of practitioners in community health settings were unable to reach out to children and non-abusing parents and act as their allies and that there was no great pressure on them to do so from their own leadership or wider societal expectations. The book also provided numerous examples of the ways that certain health practitioners made themselves accessible to children, despite a lack of vision and leadership in their professions, and sometimes a lack of structural and institutional support. Can these individual examples of allyship be transformed to a stronger collective everyday practice? Perhaps it is time to revisit the strong feminist message of Gerrilyn Smith's *Protectors' Handbook* published nearly thirty years ago in which she argued that all adults must take a stronger protecting stance towards children, with 'all the skills and information necessary to recognise the signs of sexual abuse, and to know what to do if it occurs.'[11] To be a passive non-abuser is not enough. All adults must be active protectors.

[11] Gerrilyn Smith, *The Protectors' Handbook: Reducing the Risk of CSA and Helping Children Recover* Handbook Series (London: The Women's Press, 1995), 8.

# Bibliography


Abnett, Helen, James Bowles, and John Mohan. 'The Role of Charitable Funding in the Provision of Public Services: The Case of the English and Welsh National Health Service.' *Policy & Politics* 51, no. 2 (2023): 362–384.

Abram, Jan. 'Donald Woods Winnicott (1896–1971): A Brief Introduction.' *The International Journal of Psychoanalysis* 89, no. 6 (2008): 1189–1217.

Abrams, Lynn. *Oral History Theory*. Abingdon: Routledge, 2010.

Adisa, Olumide, Megan Hermolle, and Fiona Ellis. 'Denial, Disbelief and Delays: Examining the Costs on the NHS of Delayed Child Sexual Abuse Disclosures in England and Wales.' Suffolk: Survivors in Transition and University of Suffolk, 2023.

Agathonos, Helen. 'Report of Meeting: First European Congress on Child Abuse and Neglect, Rhodes, Greece, April 6–10, 1987.' *Child Abuse & Neglect* 12 (1988): 123–128.

Ahmad, Bandana, and Race Equality Unit - Personal Social Services. *Black Perspectives in Social Work*. Birmingham: Venture Press, 1990.

Ahmed, Sara. *Complaint!*. North Carolina: Duke University Press, 2021.

Alaggia, Ramona, Delphine Collin-Vézina, and Rusan Lateef. 'Facilitators and Barriers to Child Sexual Abuse (CSA) Disclosures: A Research Update (2000–2016).' *Trauma, Violence & Abuse* 20, no. 2 (2019): 260–283.

Allnock, Debra, and Pam Miller. 'No One Noticed, No One Heard: A Study of Disclosures of Childhood Abuse.' London: NSPCC, 2013.

Anderson, Deborah. 'Touching: When Is It Caring and Nurturing or When Is It Exploitative and Damaging?'. *Child Abuse & Neglect* 3, no. 3 (1979): 793–794.




R. Beecher, *Community Health Practitioners and Child Sexual Abuse in the Family, 1970s–2010s*, Genders and Sexualities in History, https://doi.org/10.1007/978-3-031-80052-8

Anderson, Lorna M., and Gretchen Shafer. 'The Character-Disordered Family: A Community Treatment Model for Family Sexual Abuse.' *American Journal of Orthopsychiatry* 49, no. 3 (1978): 436–445.

Angelides, Steven. *The Fear of Child Sexuality: Young People, Sex, and Agency.* Chicago: The University of Chicago Press, 2019.

Angelou, Maya. *I Know Why the Caged Bird Sings.* London: Virago, 1984.

'Appendix 4: Selected Workforce Data.' In *Clinical Psychology in Britain: Historical Perspectives*, edited by John Hall, David Pilgrim and Graham Turpin, 390. Leicester: The British Psychological Society, 2015.

Armstrong, Louise. *Rocking the Cradle of Sexual Politics: What Happened When Women Said Incest.* London: Women's Press, 1996.

August, Andrew. 'A Culture of Consolation? Rethinking Politics in Working-Class London, 1870–1914.' *Historical Research* 74, no. 184 (2001): 193–219.

Azzopardi, Corry, Ramona Alaggia, and Barbara Fallon. 'From Freud to Feminism: Gendered Constructions of Blame across Theories of Child Sexual Abuse.' *Journal of Child Sexual Abuse* 27, no. 3 (2018): 254–275.

Bamford, Frank, and Raine Roberts. 'Child Sexual Abuse - II.' In *ABC of Child Abuse*, edited by Roy Meadow, 31–36. London: BMA Publications, 1989.

Barnes, Josephine. 'Forensic Medicine and Toxicology: Rape and Other Sexual Offences.' *British Medical Journal* 2, no. 5547 (1967): 293–295.

Barrett, Susan. 'From Adult Lunatic Asylums to CAMHS Community Care: The Evolution of Specialist Mental Health Care for Children and Adolescents 1948–2018.' *Revue Française de Civilisation Britannique [Online]*, XXIV-3 (2019).

Bass, Ellen, and Laura Davis. *The Courage to Heal: A Guide for Women Survivors of Child Sexual Abuse.* New York: Perennial Library, 1988.

Beecher, Ruth. 'Children, Sexual Abuse and the Emotions of the Community Health Practitioner in England and Wales, 1970–2000.' *Journal of the History of Medicine and Allied Sciences* 78, no. 4 (2023): 365–380.

Behlmer, George K. *Child Abuse and Moral Reform in England, 1870–1908.* Stanford, Ca: Stanford University Press, 1982.

Bender, Lauretta, and Abram Blau. 'The Reaction of Children to Sexual Relations with Adults.' *American Journal of Orthopsychiatry* 7, no. 4 (1937): 500–518.

Benjamin, Courtney L., Connnor M. Puleo, Cara A. Settipani, Douglas M. Brodman, Julie M. Edmunds, Colleen M. Cummings, and Philip C. Kendall. 'History of Cognitive-Behavioral Therapy in Youth.' *Child and Adolescent Clinics of North America* 20, no. 2 (Apr 2011): 179–189.

Bentovim, Arnon. 'Commentary on Kempe C.H. 1978 Sexual Abuse, Another Hidden Pediatric Problem: 1977 C. Anderson Aldrich Lecture.' In *C. Henry Kempe: A 50 Year Legacy to the Field of Child Abuse and Neglect*, edited by Richard D. Krugman and Jill E. Korbin, 205–214. Netherlands: Springer, 2013.

Bentovim, Arnon, Anne Elton, Judy Hildebrand, Marianne Tranter, and Eileen Vizard, eds. *Child Sexual Abuse within the Family: Assessment and Treatment*. London: Wright, 1988.

Berger, Michael. 'Towards a History of Clinical Child Psychology.' In *Clinical Psychology in Britain: Historical Perspectives*, edited by John Hall, David Pilgrim and Graham Turpin, 221–236. Leicester: The British Psychological Society, 2015.

Bernstein, D. M., and E. F. Loftus. 'How to Tell If a Particular Memory Is True or False.' *Perspectives on Psychological Science* 4 , no. 4 (2009): 370–374.

Bethel, Claire. 'Child House in a Box Toolkit.' London: RedQuadrant for MOPAC, Undated, c2021.

Bevington, Dickon, and Peter Fuggle. 'Supporting and Enhancing Mentalization in Community Outreach Teams Working with "Hard-to Reach" Youth: The AMBIT Approach.' In *Minding the Child: Mentalization-Based Interventions with Children, Young People and Their Families*, edited by Nick Midgley and Ioanna Vrouva. New York: Routledge, 2012.

Bingham, Adrian. "It Would Be Better for the Newspapers to Call a Spade a Spade': The British Press and Child Sexual Abuse, C. 1918–90.' *History Workshop Journal* 88 (2019): 89–110.

Binnie, James. 'Do You Want Therapy with That? A Critical Account of Working within IAPT.' *Mental Health Review Journal* 20, no. 2 (2015): 79–83.

Black, Dora. 'Are Child Guidance Clinics an Anachronism?'. *Archives of Disease in Childhood* 58, no. 8 (1983): 644–655.

Bluestone, Joanne B., and James Robertson. 'Hospitals, Children and Their Families: The Report of a Pilot Study by Margaret Stacey, Rosemary Dearden, Roisin Pill, and David Robinson.' *Journal of Health and Social Behavior* 12 (1971): 180–182.

Bolen, Rebecca M., and Maria Scannapieco. 'Prevalence of Child Sexual Abuse: A Corrective Metanalysis.' *Social Service Review* 73, no. 3 (1999): 281–313.

Bond, Emma, Fiona Ellis, and Jenny McCusker. 'I'll Be a Survivor for the Rest of My Days. Adult Survivors of Child Sexual Abuse and Their Experience of Support Services.' Suffolk: Survivors in Transition and University Campus Suffolk, 2018.

Boughton, John. *Municipal Dreams: The Rise and Fall of Council Housing*. London: Verso, 2018.

Bourke, Joanna. *Disgrace: Global Reflections on Sexual Violence*. London: Reaktion Books, 2022.

———. *Rape: A History from 1860 to the Present Day*. London: Virago, 2012.

Bowlby, John. *Attachment and Loss: Vol. I Attachment*. London: Penguin, 1971.

Boyle, Mary, and Lucy Johnstone. *A Straight Talking Introduction to the Power Threat Meaning Framework: An Alternative to Psychiatric Diagnosis*. Straight Talking Introductions. Monmouth, UK: PCCS Books, 2020.

Brattfjell, Maria Larsen, and Anna Margrete Flåm. '"They Were the Ones That Saw Me and Listened." from Child Sexual Abuse to Disclosure: Adults' Recall of the Process Towards Final Disclosure.' *Child Abuse & Neglect* 89 (2019): 225–236.

Brennan, Patricia A. W. 'The Medical and Ethical Aspects of Photography in the Sexual Assault Examination: Why Does It Offend?'. *Journal of Clinical Forensic Medicine* 13, no. 4: 194–202.

Brown, Brian, Paul Crawford, and Jurai Darongkamas. 'Blurred Roles and Permeable Boundaries: The Experience of Multidisciplinary Working in Community Mental Health.' *Health & Social Care in the Community* 8, no. 6 (2000): 425–435.

Brownmiller, Susan. *Against Our Will: Men, Women, and Rape.* New York: Bantam, 1975.

Brumberg, Joan Jacobs. '"Ruined" Girls: Changing Community Responses to Illegitimacy in Upstate New York, 1890–1920.' *Journal of Social History* 18, no. 2 (1984): 247–272.

Buckley, Peter J. 'Historical Research Approaches to the Analysis of Internationalisation.' *Management International Review* 56, no. 6 (2016): 879–900.

Burton, Lindy. *Vulnerable Children: Three Studies of Children in Conflict.* London: Routledge and Kegan Paul, 1968.

Butler-Sloss, Elizabeth. 'Report of the Inquiry into Child Abuse in Cleveland 1987 : Presented to the Secretary of State for Social Services by the Right Honourable Lord Justice Butler-Sloss.' London: HMSO, 1988.

Cameron, J. M., H. R. Johnson, and F. E. Camps. 'The Battered Child Syndrome.' *Medicine, Science and Law*, no. 6 (1966): 2–21.

Campbell, Beatrix. *Secrets and Silence: Uncovering the Legacy of the Cleveland Child Sexual Abuse Case.* Bristol: Bristol University Press and Policy Press, 2023.

Carter, Jan, ed. *The Maltreated Child.* London: Priory Press, 1974.

Carver, Vida, ed. *Child Abuse: A Study Text.* Milton Keynes and New York: The Open University Press, 1978.

Child Protection*: Guidance for Senior Nurses, Health Visitors and Midwives.* London: HMSO, 1988.

'Childhood Matters: Report of the National Commission of Inquiry into the Prevention of Child Abuse. Volume I.' London: The Stationery Office, 1996.

Children's Commissioner. 'Protecting Children from Harm: A Critical Assessment of Child Sexual Abuse in the Family Network in England and Priorities for Action.' 2015.

Children's Commissioner. 'Barnahus: Improving the Response to Child Sexual Abuse in England.' 2016.

CIBA Foundation. *Child Sexual Abuse within the Family.* Cambridge: Tavistock Publications, 1984.

Clark, Gillian. 'The Role of Mother and Baby Homes in the Adoption of Children Born Outside Marriage in Twentieth-Century England and Wales.' *Family & Community History* 11, no. 1 (2008): 45–59.

Clayden, G. S. 'Anal Appearances and Child Sexual Abuse.' *The Lancet* 8533 (1987): 620–621.

Clyde, James J. *The Report of the Inquiry into the Removal of Children from Orkney in February 1991.* Edinburgh: HMSO, 1992.

Cohen, Sol. 'The Mental Hygiene Movement, the Commonwealth Fund, and Education, 1921–1933: Every School a Clinic.' In *Counterpoints: Challenging Orthodoxies: Toward a New Cultural History of Education*, 185–202. New York: Peter Lang, 1999.

Collin-Vézina, Delphine, Mireille De La Sablonnière-Griffin, Andrea M. Palmer, and Lise Milne. 'A Preliminary Mapping of Individual, Relational, and Social Factors That Impede Disclosure of Childhood Sexual Abuse.' *Child Abuse & Neglect* 43 (2015): 123–134.

'Colposcopy.' *British Medical Journal (Clinical Research Edition)* 282, no. 6260 (1981): 250–251.

Cook, Hera. *The Long Sexual Revolution: English Women, Sex, and Contraception, 1800–1975.* Oxford: Oxford University Press, 2004.

Corwin, David L., and Erna Olafson. 'Videotaped Discovery of a Reportedly Unrecallable Memory of Child Sexual Abuse: Comparison with a Childhood Interview Videotaped 11 Years Before.' *Child Maltreatment* 2, no. 2 (1997): 91–112.

Coulter, Rebecca Priegert. 'Gender Equity and Schooling: Linking Research and Policy.' *Canadian Journal of Education / Revue canadienne de l'éducation* 21, no. 4 (1996): 433–452.

Court, S. D. M. 'Fit for the Future : Report of the Committee on Child Health Services.' London: HMSO, 1976.

Crane, Jennifer. *Child Protection in England, 1960–2000: Expertise, Experience, and Emotion.* Cham, Switzerland: Palgrave Macmillan, 2018.

Crozier, Ivan Dalley. 'The Medical Construction of Homosexuality and Its Relation to the Law in Nineteenth-Century England.' *Medical History* 45, no. 1 (2001): 61–82.

Davidson, Roger. "This Pernicious Delusion:' Law, Medicine, and Child Sexual Abuse in Early Twentieth-Century Scotland.' *Journal of the History of Sexuality* 10, no. 1 (2001): 62–77.

Davies, Carolyn, and Harriet Ward. *Safeguarding Children across Services : Messages from Research.* Safeguarding Children across Services Series. London: Jessica Kingsley London, 2012.

Davis, Joseph E. *Accounts of Innocence: Sexual Abuse, Trauma, and the Self.* Chicago, London: University of Chicago Press, 2004.

Dean, Janet G., I. A. G. MacQueen, Ross G. Mitchell, and C. Henry Kempe. 'Health Visitor's Role in Prediction of Early Childhood Injuries and Failure to Thrive.' *Child Abuse & Neglect* 2, no. 1 (1978): 1–17.

Delap, Lucy. "Disgusting Details Which Are Best Forgotten:' Disclosures of Child Sexual Abuse in Twentieth-Century Britain.' *Journal of British Studies* 57, no. 1 (2018): 79–107.

Denov, Myriam S. 'The Myth of Innocence: Sexual Scripts and the Recognition of Child Sexual Abuse by Female Perpetrators.' *The Journal of Sex Research* 40, no. 3 (2003): 303–314.

Department of Health. *Child Abuse: A Study of Inquiry Reports 1980–1989*. London: HMSO, 1991.

———, Home Office, and Department for Education and Employment. 'Working Together to Safeguard Children.' London: The Stationery Office, 1999.

Department of Health and Social Security. *Child Abuse: A Study of Inquiry Reports 1973–1981*. London: HMSO, 1982.

———. 'Diagnosis of Child Sexual Abuse: Guidance for Doctors.' London: HMSO, 1988.

———. 'Report of the Committee of Inquiry into the Care and Supervision Provided in Relation to Maria Colwell.' London: HMSO, 1974.

'The Development of Child and Adolescent Psychiatry from 1960 until 1990.' Witness Seminar Centre for the History of Medicine, University of Glasgow, 2009.

Dingwall, Robert. "In the Beginning Was the Work:' Reflections on the Genesis of Occupations.' *The Sociological Review* 31, no. 4 (1983): 605–624.

Dominelli, Lena. *Anti-Racist Social Work : A Challenge for White Practitioners and Educators*. Basingstoke: Macmillan Education, 1988.

Dorling, Daniel. *Poverty, Wealth and Place in Britain, 1968 to 2005*. Bristol: Policy Press, 2007.

Driver, Emily. 'Through the Looking Glass: Children and the Professionals Who Treat Them.' In *Child Sexual Abuse: Feminist Perspectives*, edited by Emily Driver and Audrey Drioisen. Basingstoke: Macmillan, 1989.

Driver, Emily, and Audrey Droisen, eds. *Child Sexual Abuse: Feminist Perspectives*. Basingstoke: Macmillan, 1989.

Dutt, Ratna, Melanie Phillips, and Race Equality Unit. 'Race, Culture and the Prevention of Child Abuse.' In *Childhood Matters: Report of the National Commission of Inquiry into the Prevention of Child Abuse*. Vol 2: Background Papers. London: The Stationery Office, 1996.

Eagles, John M., and Sam Wilson. 'The Feminisation of Psychiatry: Changing Gender Balance in the Psychiatric Workforce.' *Psychiatric Bulletin* 30, no. 9 (2006): 321–323.

*The Ealing Battered Baby Conference: Proceedings of a One Day Conference Organised by the Health Department of the London Borough of Ealing*. London: Edsall and Co. Ltd., 1975.

Easton, Scott D. 'Disclosure of Child Sexual Abuse among Adult Male Survivors.' *Clinical Social Work Journal* 41, no. 4 (2013): 344–355.

El Saadawi, Nawal. *Woman at Point Zero*. London: Zed Books, 1983.

El-Mallakh, Rif, and K. L. Walker. 'Hallucinations, Pseudohallucinations, and Parahallucinations.' *Psychiatry* 73, no. 1 (2010): 34–42.

Elliott, Michele. *Dealing with Child Abuse : The Kidscape Training Guide*. London: Kidscape, 1989.

Evans, Bonnie, Shahina Rahman, and Edgar Jones. 'Managing the "Unmanageable:" Interwar Child Psychiatry at the Maudsley Hospital, London.' *History of Psychiatry* 19, no. 76 (2008): 454–475.

'Explanation of Special Colour Plate.' *British Medical Journal* 1, no. 2349 (1906): 16–18.

Eysenck, Hans J. 'The Effects of Psychotherapy: An Evaluation. 1952' *Journal of Consulting Clinical Psychology* 60, no. 5 (1992): 659-663.

———. 'Learning Theory and Behaviour Therapy.' *Journal of Mental Science* 105, no. 438 (1959): 61–75.

Fairburn, A. C., and A. C. Hunt. 'Caffey's "Third Syndrome:" a Critical Evaluation ("the Battered Baby").' *Medicine, Science and Law*, 4 (1964): 123–126.

Faller, Kathleen Coulborn. 'The Child Sexual Abuse Disclosure Controversy: New Perspectives on an Abiding Problem.' *Child Abuse & Neglect* 99 (2020): 104285.

Ferguson, Harry. 'Protecting Children in Time: A Historical Sociological Study of the Abused Child and Child Protection in Cleveland from 1880 to the 'Cleveland Affair' of 1987.' University of Cambridge, 1992.

———. *Protecting Children in Time: Child Abuse, Child Protection and the Consequences of Modernity*. Hampshire: Palgrave Macmillan, 2004.

Finkelhor, David. 'Risk Factors in the Sexual Victimization of Children.' *Child Abuse & Neglect* 4, no. 4 (1980): 265–273.

———. *Sexually Victimized Children*. New York: Free Press, 1979.

Finkelhor, David, and Lisa Jones. 'Have Sexual Abuse and Physical Abuse Declined since the 1990s?' New Hampshire: Crimes against Children Research Centre, 2012.

Finkelhor, David, Anne Shattuck, Heather A. Turner, and Sherry L. Hamby. 'The Lifetime Prevalence of Child Sexual Abuse and Sexual Assault Assessed in Late Adolescence.' *Journal of Adolescent Health* 55, no. 3 (Sep 2014): 329–333.

Franklin, Alfred White. 'British Association for the Study and Prevention of Child Abuse and Neglect.' *Child Abuse & Neglect* 5, no. 1 (1981): 69–70.

Frosh, Stephen. 'Issues for Men Working with Sexually Abused Children.' *British Journal of Psychotherapy* 3, no. 4 (1987): 332–339.

Frude, Neil, Anne Peake, Jean Sambrooks, and Peter Stratton. 'British Psychological Society Report: Psychologists and Child Sexual Abuse.' *The Psychologist*, 1990, 344–348.

Furniss, Tilman, Liza Bingley-Miller, and Arnon Bentovim. 'Therapeutic Approach to Sexual Abuse.' *Archives of Disease in Childhood* 59, no. 9 (Sep 1984): 865–870.

Garbarino, J., and D. Sherman. 'High-Risk Neighborhoods and High-Risk Families: The Human Ecology of Child Maltreatment.' *Child Development* 51, no. 1 (1980): 188–198.

Garry, M., C. G. Manning, E. F. Loftus, and S. J. Sherman. 'Imagination Inflation: Imagining a Childhood Event Inflates Confidence That It Occurred.' *Psychonomic Bulletin and Review* 3 (1996): 208–214.

Gekoski, A, J C Davidson, and M A H Horvath. 'The Prevalence, Nature, and Impact of Intrafamilial Child Sexual Abuse: Findings from a Rapid Evidence Assessment.' *Journal of Criminological Research, Policy and Practice* 2, no. 4 (2016): 231 – 243.

Giarretto, Henry. 'A Comprehensive Child Sexual Abuse Treatment Program.' *Child Abuse & Neglect* 6, no. 3 (1982): 263–278.

———. 'A Comprehensive Child Sexual Abuse Treatment Programme.' In *Sexually Abused Children and Their Families*, edited by Patricia Beezley Mrazek and C. Henry Kempe, 179–198. Oxford: Pergamon, 1981.

Gladstone, David, ed. *British Social Welfare: Past, Present and Future*. London: UCL Press, 1995.

Glaser, Danya, and Stephen Frosh. *Child Sexual Abuse*. Basingstoke: Macmillan Education, 1988.

———. *Child Sexual Abuse*. Second edition. Basingstoke: Macmillan Education, 1993.

Goddard, Andrea, Emma Harewood, and Lauren Brennan. 'Review of Pathway Following Sexual Assault for Children and Young People in London.' London: The Havens, Kings College Hospital London, on behalf of NHS England, 2015.

Goodwin, Jean. *Sexual Abuse: Incest Victims and Their Families*. Boston: J Wright, 1982.

Gordon, Linda. *Heroes of Their Own Lives: The Politics and History of Family Violence Boston, 1880–1960*. London: Virago, 1989.

———. 'The Politics of Child Sexual Abuse: Notes from American History.' *Feminist Review*, 28, no. 1 (1988): 56–64.

Gorey, Kevin M, and Donald R Leslie. 'The Prevalence of Child Sexual Abuse: Integrative Review Adjustment for Potential Response and Measurement Biases.' *Child Abuse & Neglect* 21, no. 4 (1997): 391–398.

Gorey, Kevin M., and Donald R. Leslie. 'Debate with Authors. Working toward a Valid Prevalence Estimate of Child Sexual Abuse: A Reply to Bolen and Scannapieco.' *Social Service Review* 75, no. 1 (2001): 151–158.

Gould, Lynette, and Stephen Richards. *Heart of Darkness: How I Triumphed over a Childhood of Abuse*. London: John Blake Publishing Ltd, 2007.

Griffiths, Melanie, and Colin Yeo. 'The UK's Hostile Environment: Deputising Immigration Control.' *Critical Social Policy* 41, no. 4: 521–544.

Haaken, Janice. *Pillar of Salt: Gender, Memory, and the Perils of Looking Back*. London: Free Association, 1998.

Hacking, Ian. 'The Making and Moulding of Child Sexual Abuse.' *Critical Inquiry* 17, no. 2 (1991): 253–288.

Hallett, Christine, and Olive Stevenson. *Child Abuse: Aspects of Interprofessional Co-operation*. London Boston: Allen & Unwin, 1980.

Hamblin, Angela and Romi Bowen. 'The Sexual Abuse of Children.' In *Women against Violence against Women*, edited by Dusty Rhodes and Sandra McNeill. London: Onlywomen Press, 1985.

Hanley, Anne. '"I Caught It and Yours Truly Was Very Sorry for Himself:" Mapping the Emotional Worlds of British VD Patients.' In *Patient Voices in Britain, 1840–1948*, edited by A. Hanley and J. Meyer. Social Histories of Medicine, 299–337. Manchester, England: Manchester University Press, 2021.

'Health of Children: Prevention of Break-up of Families.' Ministry of Health, 1954.

Hechler, David. *The Battle and the Backlash: The Child Sexual Abuse War*. Lexington, Mass.: Lexington Books, 1988.

Heger, Astrid, S. Jean Emans, and Carole Jenny. *Evaluation of the Sexually Abused Child : A Medical Textbook and Photographic Atlas*. New York: Oxford University Press, 1992.

Helfer, Ray E. 'The Responsibility and Role of the Physician.' In *The Battered Child*, edited by Ray E. Helfer and C. Henry Kempe. Chicago, London: University of Chicago Press, 1968.

Hendrick, Harry D. *Child Welfare: England: 1872–1989*. London: Routledge, 1994.

Henriques, Basil, and Nesta H. Wells. 'Sexual Assaults on Children.' *British Medical Journal* 2, no. 5267 (1961): 1628–1633.

Herman, Judith Lewis, and Lisa Hirschman. *Father-Daughter Incest*. Cambridge, Mass: Harvard University Press, 1981.

Hildebrand, Judy, and Constanze Forbes. 'Group Work with Mothers Whose Children Have Been Sexually Abused.' *British Journal of Social Work* 17, no. 3 (1987): 285–304.

Hobbs, C. J., and J. M. Wynne. 'Sexual Abuse of English Boys and Girls: The Importance of Anal Examination.' *Child Abuse & Neglect* 13, no. 2 (1989): 195–210.

Hobbs, Christopher J., Helga Hanks, and Jane M. Wynne. *Child Abuse and Neglect: A Clinician's Handbook*. Edinburgh, New York: Churchill Livingstone, 1993a.

Hobbs, Christopher J., and Jane Wynne. 'Buggery in Childhood: A Common Syndrome of Child Abuse.' *The Lancet* 328, no. 8510 (1986): 792–796.

Hobbs, Christopher J., Jane M. Wynne, and J. E. S. Fortin. *Child Abuse (Bailliere's Clinical Paediatrics)*. London; Philadelphia: Bailliere Tindall, 1993b.

Hobson, W. 'What Is Social Medicine.' *British Medical Journal* 4619, no. 2 (1949): 125–130.

Hooper, Carol-Ann. 'Child Sexual Abuse and the Regulation of Women: Variations on a Theme.' In *Gender Violence: Interdisciplinary Perspectives*, edited by Laura L. O'Toole, Jessica R. Schiffman and Marge L. Kiter Edwards, 342–359. New York: New York University Press, 2007.

Hotaling, Gerald T., David Finkelhor, John T. Kirkpatrick, and Murray A. Straus, eds. *Coping with Family Violence: Research and Policy Perspectives*. Newbury Park, Beverly Hills, London, New Delhi: Sage Publications, 1988.

House of Commons Health Committee. 'Children's and Adolescents' Mental Health and CAMHS: Third Report of Session 2014–15.'

Hunter, Mark. 'Physical Signs of Sexual Abuse in Children.' *Archives of Disease in Childhood* 78, no. 3 (Mar 1998): 288.

Hunter, Sally V. 'Disclosure of Child Sexual Abuse as a Life-Long Process: Implications for Health Professionals.' *Australian and New Zealand Journal of Family Therapy* 32, no. 2 (2013): 159–172.

'Incest and Family Disorder.' *British Medical Journal* 2, no. 5810 (1972): 364–365.

Irish, Leah, Ihori Kobayashi, and Douglas L Delahanty. 'Long-term physical health consequences of childhood sexual abuse: a meta-analytic review.' Journal of Pediatric Psychology 35, no. 5 (2010): 450–61.

Jackson, Graham. 'Child Abuse Syndrome: The Cases We Miss.' *British Medical Journal* 2, no. 5816 (1972): 756–757.

Jackson, Louise A. *Child Sexual Abuse in Victorian England*. London: Routledge, 2000.

Jay, Alexis. 'Independent Inquiry into Child Sexual Exploitation in Rotherham 1997–2013.' Rotherham Metropolitan Borough Counci, 2014.

Jeffreys, Sheila. *The Spinster and Her Enemies: Feminism and Sexuality, 1880–1930*. London: Pandora Press, 1985.

Jenkins, Philip. *Intimate Enemies: Moral Panics in Contemporary Great Britain*. New York: Aldine de Gruyter, 1992.

———. *Moral Panic: Changing Concepts of the Child Molester in Modern America*. New Haven and London: Yale University Press, 1998.

Johnstone, Lucy. *Users and Abusers of Psychiatry: A Critical Look at Psychiatric Practice*. 2nd. London: Routledge London, 2000.

Jones, Helen, and Kate Cook. *Rape Crisis: Responding to Sexual Violence*. Dorset, UK: Russell House Publishing Ltd, 2008.

Kelly, Liz. 'Continuum of Sexual Violence.' In *Women, Violence and Social Control*, edited by J. Hanmer and M. Maynard, 46–60. London: Macmillan Press Ltd, 1987.

Kelly, Liz, and Kairika Karsna. 'Measuring the Scale and Changing Nature of Child Sexual Abuse and Child Sexual Exploitation - Scoping Report.' London: Centre of Expertise on Child Sexual Abuse, London Metropolitan University, 2021.

Kempe, C. H. 'Sexual Abuse, Another Hidden Pediatric Problem: The 1977 C. Anderson Aldrich Lecture.' *Pediatrics* 62, no. 3 (1978a): 382–389.

Kempe, C. Henry. 'Recent Developments in the Field of Child Abuse.' *Child Abuse & Neglect* 2, no. 4 (1978b): 261–267.

Kempe, C. Henry, F. N. Silverman, B. F. Steele, W. Droegemueller, and H. K. Silver. 'The Battered-Child Syndrome.' *JAMA* 181, no. 1 (1962): 17–24.

Kempe, Ruth S., and C. Henry Kempe. *Child Abuse*. The Developing Child. Edited by Jerome Bruner, Michael Cole and Barbara Lloyd. London: Fontana/ Open Books, 1978.

———. *The Common Secret: Sexual Abuse of Children and Adolescents* New York: W. H. Freeman, 1984.

Kendler, Kenneth S., Cynthia M. Bulik, Judy Silberg, John M. Hettema, John Myers, and Carol A. Prescott. 'Childhood Sexual Abuse and Adult Psychiatric and Substance Use Disorders in Women: An Epidemiological and Cotwin Control Analysis.' *Archives of General Psychiatry* 57, no. 10 (2000): 953–959.

Kincaid, James R. *Erotic Innocence: The Culture of Child Molesting*. Durham: Duke University Press, 1998.

Kinsey, Alfred C., Wardell B. Pomeroy, Clyde E. Martin, and Paul H. Gebhard. *Sexual Behavior in the Human Female*. Philadelphia: Saunders, 1953.

Kitzinger, Jenny. 'Defending Innocence: Ideologies of Childhood.' *Feminist Review*, 28, no. 1 (1988): 77–87.

———. 'Media Templates: Controversial Allegations and Analogies.' In *Framing Abuse: Media Influence and Public Understanding of Sexual Violence against Children*, 54–78. London: Pluto Press, 2004.

Kluemper, Nicole S. 'Published Case Reports: One Woman's Account of Having Her Confidentiality Violated.' *Journal of Interpersonal Violence* 29, no. 18 (2014): 3232–3244.

Kolvin, I, H Steiner, F Bamford, M Taylor, J Wynne, D Jones, and H Zeitlin. 'Child Sexual Abuse: Principles of Good Practice.' *British Journal of Hospital Medicine* (1988): 54–61.

Krugman, Richard D. 'Chapter 20 Introduction and Commentary: Child Sexual Abuse.' In *C. Henry Kempe: A 50 Year Legacy to the Field of Child Abuse and Neglect*, edited by Richard D. Krugman and Jill E. Korbin, 177–178. Netherlands: Springer, 2013.

———. 'Editorial: The More We Learn, the Less We Know "with Reasonable Medical Certainty"?' *Child Abuse & Neglect* 13, no. 2 (1989): 165–166.

Krystalli, Roxani, and Philipp Schulz. 'Taking Love and Care Seriously: An Emergent Research Agenda for Remaking Worlds in the Wake of Violence.' *International Studies Review* 24, no. 1 (2022).

Kunzel, Regina G. *Fallen Women, Problem Girls: Unmarried Mothers and the Professionalization of Social Work, 1890–1945.* Yale Historical Publications. New Haven: Yale University Press, 1993.

Lambert, Michael. '"Problem Families" and the Post-War Welfare State in the North West of England, 1943–74; Volume One.' Lancaster University, 2017.

Landig-Hevezi, Suzanne. 'Biological Mothers and Intrafamilial Sexual Abuse,' University of Arizona, 1982.

Lavender, Tony, and Graham Turpin. 'The Development and Training of the Clinical Psychology Workforce.' In *Clinical Psychology in Britain: Historical Perspectives*, edited by John Hall, David Pilgrim and Graham Turpin, 93–110. Leicester: The British Psychological Society, 2015.

Leathard, Audrey. *Health Care Provision: Past, Present and into the 21st Century.* Second edition. Stanley Thornes, 2000.

Ledray, Linda E. 'Review of the Common Secret: Sexual Abuse of Children and Adolescents, Ruth S. Kempe, Henry Kempe.' *The American Journal of Nursing* 85, no. 8 (1985): 930.

'Letter to the Editor.' *Child Abuse & Neglect* 22, no. 5 (1998): 337.

Lindsay, Geoff. 'Educational Psychology in England and Wales.' *Journal of School Psychology* 23, no. 4 (1985): 305–317.

Loftus, E. F., and M. J. Guyer. 'Who Abused Jane Doe? The Hazards of the Single Case History: Part 1.' *Skeptical Inquirer* 26, no. 3 (2002): 24–32.

Loftus, E. F., and J. E. Pickrell. 'The Formation of False Memories.' *Psychiatric Annals* 25, no. 12 (1995): 720 - 725.

Loftus, Elizabeth F., and Katherine Ketcham. *The Myth of Repressed Memory: False Memories and Allegations of Sexual Abuse.* New York: St. Martin's Press, 1994.

London, K., M. Bruck, S. Ceci, and D. Shuman. 'Disclosures of Sexual Abuse: What Does the Research Tell Us About the Ways That Children Tell?'. *Psychology, Public Policy, and Law* 11, no. 1 (2005): 194–226.

London Rape Crisis Centre. *Sexual Violence: The Reality for Women.* London: Women's Press, 1984.

Loughran, Tracey, Kate Mahoney, and Daisy Payling. 'Reflections on Remote Interviewing in a Pandemic: Negotiating Participant and Researcher Emotions.' *Oral History* 50, no. 1 (2022).

Lovett, Jo, Linda Regan, and Liz Kelly. 'Sexual Assault Referral Centres: Developing Good Practice and Maximising Potentials. Home Office Research Study 285.' Child and Woman Abuse Studies Unit, London Metropolitan University, 2004.

Lukianowicz, Narcyz. 'Incest.' *British Journal of Psychiatry* 120, no. 556 (1972): 301–313.

MacLeod, Mary, and Esther Saraga. 'Challenging the Orthodoxy: Towards a Feminist Theory and Practice.' *Feminist Review*, 28, no. 1 (1988): 16–55.

Marks, Sarah. 'Psychologists as Therapists: The Development of Behavioural Traditions in Clinical Psychology.' In *Clinical Psychology in Britain: Historical Perspectives*, edited by John Hall, David Pilgrim and Graham Turpin, 194–207. Leicester: The British Psychological Society, 2015.

Masson, Jeffrey M. *The Assault on Truth: Freud's Suppression of the Seduction Theory.* London: Faber, 1984a.

———. 'Freud and the Seduction Theory: A Challenge to the Foundations of Psychoanalysis.' *The Atlantic*, February 1984b.

Mathews, Ben. 'The Context of Child Sexual Abuse, and Points of Departure.' In *New International Frontiers in Child Sexual Abuse: Theory, Problems and Progress.* Switzerland, Cham: Springer Nature, 2019.

McCann, John, Joan Voris, Mary Simon, and Robert Wells. 'Perianal Findings in Prepubertal Children Selected for Nonabuse: A Descriptive Study.' *Child Abuse & Neglect* 13, no. 2 (1989): 179–193.

McCormick, Leanne, Sean O'Connell, John Privilege, and Olivia Dee. *Mother and Baby Homes and Magdalene Laundries in Northern Ireland, 1922–1990.* London: Department of Health, 2021.

McElvaney, Rosaleen. 'Disclosure of Child Sexual Abuse: Delays, Non-Disclosure and Partial Disclosure. What the Research Tells Us and Implications for Practice.' *Child Abuse Review* 24, no. 3 (2013): 159–169.

McGuire, Jacqueline, and Naomi Richman. 'Outcome of Behaviour Problems in the Preschool Setting.' *Child: Care, Health and Development* 13, no. 6 (1987): 403–414.

McManus, I. C., Diana N. J. Lockwood, and J. K. Cruickshank. 'The Preregistration Year: Chaos by Consensus.' *The Lancet* 309, no. 8008 (19 Feb 1977): 413–416.

McMillan, Lesley, and Deborah White. 'The Missing and Imagined Perpetrator in Rape Prevention Efforts.' *Women's History Review* 32, no. 7 (2023): 1040–1058.

McNeish, Di, Liz Kelly, and Sara Scott. 'Effectiveness of Services for Sexually Abused Children and Young People. Report 1: A Knowledge Review.' Centre of Expertise on Child Sexual Abuse, 2019.

Meadow, Roy, ed. *ABC of Child Abuse.* London: BMA Publications, 1989.

———. 'Video Recording and Child Abuse.' *British Medical Journal (Clinical Research Edition)* 294, no. 6588 (1987): 1629–1630.

Meadow, S. R., Jacqueline Y. Q. Mok, and Donna Rosenberg. *ABC of Child Protection.* 4th ed. Chicester: John Wiley & Sons, 2009.

Mellon, Michael W., Stephen P. Whiteside, and William N. Friedrich. 'The Relevance of Fecal Soiling as an Indicator of Child Sexual Abuse: A Preliminary Analysis.' *Journal of Developmental and Behavioral Pediatrics* 27, no. 1 (2006): 25–32.

Metropolitan Police, and Bexley Social Services. 'Child Sexual Abuse: Joint Investigative Project: Final Report.' London: HMSO, 1987.

Miller, David, and Jon Brown. '"We Have the Right to Be Safe:" Protecting Disabled Children from Abuse.' London: NSPCC, 2014.

Mills, June D. 'Child Guidance Clinics (A Review of their Development, Present Structure and Future Trends).' *The Journal of the Royal Institute of Public Health and Hygiene* 31, no. 2 (1968): 38–52.

Ministry of Health: Central Health Services Council Standing Medical Advisory Committee. 'Child Welfare Centres: Report of the Subcommittee.' London: HMSO, 1967.

Mintz, Steven. 'Placing Childhood Sexual Abuse in Historical Perspective.' https://tif.ssrc.org/2012/07/13/placing-childhood-sexual-abuse-in-historical-perspective/.

Morrow, Jan, Catherine A. Yeager, and Dorothy Otnow Lewis. 'Encopresis and Sexual Abuse in a Sample of Boys in Residential Treatment.' *Child Abuse & Neglect* 21, no. 1 (1997): 11–18.

Morton, S. T., and Israel Kolvin. 'Services for the Adolescent in the United Kingdom.' In *Health Care of Mothers and Children in National Health Services: Implications for the United States*, edited by Helen Wallace, 135–153. Cambridge, Mass: Ballinger Publishing Company, 1975.

Mrazek, Patricia Beezley. 'Sexual Abuse of Children.' *Journal of Child Psychology and Psychiatry* 21, no. 1 (1980): 91–95.

Mrazek, Patricia Beezley, and C. Henry Kempe, eds. *Sexually Abused Children and Their Families.* Oxford: Pergamon, 1981.

Mrazek, Patricia J., Margaret A. Lynch, and Arnon Bentovim. 'Sexual Abuse of Children in the United Kingdom.' *Child Abuse & Neglect* 7, no. 2 (1983): 147–153.

Mumm, Susan. '"Not Worse Than Other Girls:" the Convent-Based Rehabilitation of Fallen Women in Victorian Britain.' *Journal of Social History* 29, no. 3 (1996): 527–546.

Murdoch, Lydia. Review of Child Sexual Abuse in Victorian England by Louise A. Jackson. *Victorian Studies* 44, no. 3 (2002): 541–543.

Nava, Mica. 'Cleveland and the Press: Outrage and Anxiety in the Reporting of Child Sexual Abuse.' *Feminist Review*, no. 28 (1988): 103–121.

Neale, Victor. *The British Paediatric Association. Vol 2: 1952–1968.* London: Pitman Medical, 1970.

Nelson, Sarah. *Incest: Fact and Myth.* 2nd edition. Edinburgh: Stramullion, 1987.

———. 'Preparing for the Special Challenge of Sexual Abuse.' In *Safeguarding Children in Primary Care*, edited by Julie Taylor and Markus Huber, 23–38. London: Jessica Kingsley Publishers, 2009.

———. 'Surviving Well.' Scotland: Wellbeing Scotland, 2020.

———. *Tackling Child Sexual Abuse: Radical Approaches to Prevention, Protection and Support.* Bristol, UK: Bristol University Press, 2016.

Norwich Consultants on Sexual Violence. 'Claiming Our Status as Experts: Community Organizing.' *Feminist Review*, 28, no. 1 (1988): 144–149.

Ofshe, R., and E. Watters. *Making Monsters: False Memories, Psychotherapy, and Sexual Hysteria*. New York: Charles Scribner, 1994.

Olafson, Erna, David L. Corwin, and Roland C. Summit. 'Modern History of Child Sexual Abuse Awareness: Cycles of Discovery and Suppression.' *Child Abuse & Neglect* 17, no. 1 (1993): 7–24.

Oliver, J. E., and A. H. Buchanan. 'Generations of Maltreated Children and Multi-Agency Care in One Kindred.' *British Journal of Psychiatry* 135, no. 4 (1979): 289–303.

Oosterhuis, Harry. 'Sexual Modernity in the Works of Richard Von Krafft-Ebing and Albert Moll.' *Medical History* 56, no. 2 (2012): 133–155.

Paice, Elisabeth, Fiona Moss, Shelley Heard, Belinda Winder, and I. C. McManus. 'The Relationship between Pre-Registration House Officers and Their Consultants.' *Medical Education* 36, no. 1 (2002): 26–34.

Parker, G E. 'The Battered Child Syndrome.' *Medicine, Science and Law*, 5, no. 3 (1965): 160–163.

Parker, Tony. *The People of Providence: A Housing Estate and Some of Its Inhabitants*. London: Hutchinson, 1983.

Parton, Nigel. 'Changing and Competing Conceptions of Risk and Their Implications for Public Health Approaches to Child Protection.' In *Re-Visioning Public Health Approaches for Protecting Children*, edited by B. Lonne et al. Child Maltreatment. Switzerland: Springer Nature, 2019.

———. 'Child Abuse, Social Anxiety and Welfare.' *British Journal of Social Work* 11, no. 1 (1981): 391–414.

———. *Governing the Family: Child Care, Child Protection and the State*. Hampshire: Palgrave, 1991.

———. 'The Natural History of Child Abuse: A Study in Social Problem Definition.' *British Journal of Social Work* 9, no. 4 (1979): 431–451.

———. *The Politics of Child Protection : Contemporary Developments and Future Directions*. Basingstoke: Palgrave Macmillan, 2014.

———. *Safeguarding Childhood : Early Intervention and Surveillance in a Late Modern Society*. Hampshire, New York: Palgrave Macmillan, 2006.

Parton, Nigel, and Corinne Wattam, eds. *Child Sexual Abuse: Responding to the Experiences of Children*, Wiley Series in Child Protection and Policy. Chichester: Wiley, 1999.

Patihis, L., L. Y. Ho, I. W. Tingen, S. O. Lilienfeld, and E. F. Loftus. 'Are the "Memory Wars" Over? A Scientist-Practitioner Gap in Beliefs About Repressed Memory.' *Psychological Science* 25, no. 2 (2014): 519–530.

Penketh, Laura. 'Three: CCETSW's Anti-Racist Initiative.' In *Tackling Institutional Racism*. Bristol, UK: Policy Press, 2000.

'Physical Signs of Sexual Abuse in Children: A Report of the Royal College of Physicians.' The Royal College of Physicians, 1991.

Pickett, John. 'The BASPCAN Founders.' *Child Abuse Review* 1, no. 1 (1992): 2–4.

Quinton, David, Michael Rutter, and Christine Liddle. 'Institutional Rearing, Parenting Difficulties and Marital Support.' *Psychological Medicine* 14, no. 1 (1984): 107–124.

Rachman, S. J. 'Learning Theory and Child Psychology: Therapeutic Possibilities.' *Journal of Child Psychology and Psychiatry* 3 (1962): 149–163.

Radford, Lorraine, and National Society for the Prevention of Cruelty to Children. 'Child Abuse and Neglect in the UK Today.' (2011).

Raz, Mical. 'Lessons from History: Parents Anonymous and Child Abuse Prevention Policy.' *Pediatrics* 140, no. 6 (2017).

Reavey, Paula, and Sam Warner. *New Feminist Stories of Child Sexual Abuse Sexual Scripts and Dangerous Dialogues*. London; New York: Taylor & Francis, 2003.

Reed, Judith. 'Working with Abusive Parents, a Parent's View. Interview with Jolly K.' *Children Today* 4, no. 3 (May–Jun 1975).

Renvoize, Jean. *Children in Danger: The Causes and Prevention of Baby Battering*. Third edition. Penguin Books, 1976.

'Report of the Committee on Nursing. Chairman: Professor Asa Briggs'. London: HMSO, 1972.

'The Report of the Inquiry into the Removal of Children from Orkney in February 1991.' London: HMSO, 1992.

Richardson, Sue, and Heather Bacon. *Child Sexual Abuse: Whose Problem? Reflections from Cleveland*. Birmingham: Venture Press, 1991.

Robertson, Stephen. *Crimes against Children: Sexual Violence and Legal Culture in New York City, 1880–1960*. Chapel Hill, NC: University of North Carolina Press, 2005.

Rodgers, Daniel T. 'In Search of Progressivism.' *Reviews in American History* 10, no. 4 (1982): 113–132.

Rogers, David, John Tripp, Arnon Bentovim, Anthony Robinson, David Berry, and Roy Goulding. 'Non-Accidental Poisoning: An Extended Syndrome of Child Abuse.' *British Medical Journal* (3 April 1976): 793–796.

Rolewicz, Lucina, and William Palmer. 'What Health and Care Need from the Next Government: NHS Staffing. Briefing Paper 1.' London: Nuffield Trust, 2024.

Rouf, Khadj. 'Who Looks and Sounds Like a Psychologist.' *The Psychologist*, 10 Sep 2020.

Rush, Florence. *The Best Kept Secret: Sexual Abuse of Children*. New York: McGraw-Hill, 1980.

———. 'The Freudian Cover-Up.' *Chrysalis* (1977): 31–45.

———. 'The Sexual Abuse of Children: A Feminist Point of View.' In *Rape: The First Sourcebook for Women*, edited by Noreen Connell and Cassandra Wilson, 64–75. New York: New American Library, 1974.

Rushton, Alan, and Cherilyn Dance. 'Quality Protects: A Commentary on the Government's Agenda and the Evidence Base.' *Child and Adolescent Mental Health* 7, no. 2: 60–65.

Russell, Diana E H. *The Politics of Rape: The Victim's Perspective*. New York: Stein and Day, 1974.

Russell, Diana E. H. 'The Long-Term Effects of Incestuous Abuse: A Comparison of Afro American and White American Victims.' In *Lasting Effects of Child Sexual Abuse*, edited by Gail Elizabeth Wyatt and Gloria Johnson Powell: Sage Publications Inc, 1988.

Rusterholz, Caroline. *Women's Medicine, Sex, Family Planning and British Female Doctors in Transnational Perspective (1920–70)*. Manchester: Manchester University Press, 2020.

Rutter, Michael, Philip Graham, O. F. D. Chadwick, and W. Yule. 'Adolescent Turmoil: Fact or Fiction?' *Journal of Child Psychology and Psychiatry* 17, no. 1 (1976): 35–56.

Sacco, Lynn. *Unspeakable : Father-Daughter Incest in American History*. Baltimore. Md: Johns Hopkins University Press, 2009.

Sanders, Deidre. *The Woman Book of Love and Sex*. London: Sphere Books Limited, 1985.

———. *The Woman Report on Men*. London: Sphere Books Limited, 1987.

Sayal-Bennett, Anuradha. 'Equal Opportunities - Empty Rhetoric?' *Feminism and psychology* 1, no. 1 (1991): 74–77.

Schachter, C. L., C. A. Stalker, E. Teram, G. C. Lasiuk, and A. Danilkewich. *Handbook on Sensitive Practice for Health Care Practitioners: Lessons from Adult Survivors of Childhood Sexual Abuse*. Ottawa: Public Health Agency of Canada, 2008.

Scott Brown, M. 'Father-Daughter Incest: A Model for Treatment.' In *Current Issues in Clinical Psychology: Volume 3*, edited by Eric Karas, 79–85. Boston, MA: Springer US, 1987.

Sgroi, Suzanne M., ed. *Handbook of Clinical Intervention in Child Sexual Abuse*. Lexington, MA: Lexington Books, 1982.

Sharma, A., and R. Sunderland. 'Increasing Medical Burden of Child Abuse.' *Archives of Disease in Childhood* 63, no. 2 (Feb 1988): 172–175.

Sharman, Ruth. *Child Abuse: A Discussion Paper*. London: Council for the Education and Training of Health Visitors, 1983.

Sheftel, Anna, and Stacey Zembrzycki. 'Only Human: A Reflection on the Ethical and Methodological Challenges of Working with "Difficult" Stories.' *The Oral History Review* 37, no. 2 (2010): 191–214.

Shekhawat, Satpal Singh, and Faisel Baig. 'Commissioning: Important for All GPs.' *British Journal of General Practice* 69, no. 685 (2019): 376–377.

Smart, Carol. 'A History of Ambivalence and Conflict in the Discursive Construction of the "Child Victim" of Sexual Abuse.' *Social & Legal Studies* 8, no. 3 (1999): 391–409.

Smith, Gerrilyn. 'Child Sexual Abuse.' In *The Secret Life of Vulnerable Children*, edited by Ved P. Varma, 130–156. London: Routledge London, 1992a.

———. '"Collusive Women: Power and Sexual Abuse in the Family." Paper Presented at the Institute of Family Therapy.' London: Unpublished, 1989a.

———. 'Essay Book Review.' *Journal of Family Therapy* 14 (1992b): 423–428.

———. *The Protectors' Handbook: Reducing the Risk of CSA and Helping Children Recover* Handbook Series. London: The Women's Press, 1995a.

———. '"Right Solution, Incorrectly Applied. Maladaptive Coping in Sexual Abuse." Paper Presented to the British Psychological Society Annual Conference.' In *British Psychological Society annual conference*: Unpublished, 1987.

———. *Systemic Approaches to Training in Child Protection*. London: Routledge, 2018.

———. 'The Traumatic Response Cycle: Working with Adult Survivors of Childhood Sexual Abuse.' *Clinical Psychology Forum* (22 Aug 1989b).

———. '"The Traumatic Response Cycle." Paper Presented to the North West Thames Division of Clinical Psychology.' Unpublished, 1988.

Smith, Jennifer. 'Illustrations from the Wellcome Institute Library: The Archive of the Health Visitors' Association in the Contemporary Medical Archives Centre.' *Medical History* 39, no. 3 (July 1995): 358–367.

Smith, Noel, Cristian Dogaru, and Fiona Ellis. *Hear Me. Believe Me. Respect Me. A Survey of Adult Survivors of Child Sexual Abuse and Their Experiences of Support Services.* Suffolk: Survivors in Transition and University Campus Suffolk, 2015.

Stafford, Jo Mary. *Light in the Dust*. Hants: Caric Press Ltd, 1990.

Starkey, Pat. 'The Medical Officer of Health, the Social Worker, and the Problem Family, 1943 to 1968: The Case of Family Service Units.' *Social History of Medicine* 11, no. 3 (1998): 421–441.

Steele, B. F. 'Violence within the Family.' In *Child Abuse and Neglect: The Family and the Community*, edited by Ray Eugene Helfer and C. Henry Kempe, 3-24. Cambridge, Mass.: Ballinger Publishing Co., 1976.

Steele, Brandt F., and Carl B. Pollock. 'A Psychiatric Study of Parents Who Abuse Infants and Small Children.' In *The Battered Child*, edited by Ray E. Helfer and C. Henry Kempe, 103–147. Chicago, London: University of Chicago Press, 1968.

Steiner, John. 'Bridges over Troubled Waters.' *Bulletin of the Royal College of Psychiatrists* 10, no. 9 (September 1986): 246.

Stevenson, Olive, ed. *Child Abuse: Public Policy and Professional Practice*. Herts: Harvester Wheatsheaf, 1989.

Stewart, John. 'The Dangerous Age of Childhood: Child Guidance and the "Normal" Child in Great Britain, 1920–1950. ' *Paedagogica Historica* 47, no. 6 (Dec 2011): 785–803.

Stewart, John. "The Dangerous Age of Childhood': Child Guidance in Britain C.1918–1955.' https://www.historyandpolicy.org/policy-papers/papers/the-dangerous-age-of-childhood-child-guidance-in-britain-c.1918-1955.

'Strategic Direction for Sexual Assault and Abuse Services: Lifelong Care for Victims and Survivors: 2018–2023.' NHS England, 2018.

Summit, Roland C. 'The Child Sexual Abuse Accommodation Syndrome.' *Child Abuse & Neglect* 7, no. 2 (1983): 177–193.

Sunderland, R. 'Physical Signs of Child Abuse.' *Archives of Disease in Childhood* 75, no. 4 (Oct 1996): 356.

The National Resource Center on Child Sexual Abuse. *Think Tank Report: Allegations of Sexual Abuse in Child Custody & Visitation Situations.* Huntsville, Alabama: National Children's Advocacy Center, 1989.

Thompson, Paul. 'The Voice of the Past: Oral History.' In *The Oral History Reader*, edited by Robert Perks and Alastair Thomson, 21–28. 3rd edition. London and New York: Routledge, 2003.

Thompson, Paul, and Joanna Bornat. *The Voice of the Past: Oral History.* Fourth edition. Oxford: Oxford University Press, 2017.

Thomson, Mathew. *Lost Freedom: The Landscape of the Child and the British Post-War Settlement.* Oxford: Oxford University Press, 2013.

Tierney, Kathleen J., and David L. Corwin. 'Exploring Intrafamilial Child Sexual Abuse.' In *The Dark Side of Families: Current Family Violence Research*, edited by David Finkelhor, Richard Gelles, Gerald T. Hotaling and Murray A. Straus, 102–115. Beverly Hills: Sage, 1983.

Tizard, Jack. 'Maladjusted Children and the Child Guidance Service.' *London Educational Review* 2, no. 2 (1973): 22–37.

'Together We Stand: The Commissioning, Role and Management of Child and Adolescent Mental Health Services.' edited by Richard Williams and NHS Health Advisory Service. London: HMSO, 1995.

Transforming Children and Young People's Mental Health Provision: *A Green Paper* (Cm 9626). London: Department of Health and Social Care, and Department for Education, 2017.

van Damme, I., R. L. Kaplan, L. J. Levine, and E. F. Loftus. 'Emotion and False Memory: How Goal-Irrelevance Can Be Relevant for What People Remember.' *Memory* 25, no. 2 (2017): 201–213.

van der Horst, Frank C. P., and René van der Veer. 'Changing Attitudes Towards the Care of Children in Hospital: A New Assessment of the Influence of the Work of Bowlby and Robertson in the UK, 1940–1970.' *Attachment & Human Development* 11, no. 2 (2009): 119–142.

'The Victoria Climbié Inquiry: Summary Report of an Inquiry by Lord Laming.' London: HMSO, 2003.

Vizard, Eileen. *Self Esteem and Personal Safety: A Guide for Professionals Working with Sexually Abused Children*. London: Tavistock Publications, 1986.

———. 'Self Esteem and Personal Safety: Comments on Secondary Prevention Work with Young Sexually Abused Children.' *Newsletter of the Association for Child Psychology and Psychiatry* 9, no. 2 (1987): 16–22.

Vizard, Eileen, Arnon Bentovim, and Marianne Tranter. 'Interviewing Sexually Abused Children.' *Adoption & Fostering* 11, no. 1 (1987): 20–25.

Vizard, Eileen, and Marianne Tranter. 'Chapter 4 Recognition and Assessment of Child Sexual Abuse.' In *Child Sexual Abuse within the Family: Assessment and Treatment*, edited by Arnon Bentovim, Anne Elton, Judy Hildebrand, Marianne Tranter and Eileen Vizard. London: Wright, 1988.

Walker, Alice. *The Color Purple*. London: The Women's Press, 1986.

Walker, Janet. 'The Traumatic Paradox: Documentary Films, Historical Fictions, and Catacylismic Past Events.' *Signs* 22, no. 4 (1997): 803–825.

Wardle, Christopher J. 'Twentieth-Century Influences on the Development in Britain of Services for Child and Adolescent Psychiatry.' *British Journal of Psychiatry* 159, no. 1 (1991): 53–68.

Warner, Sam. 'Disrupting Identity through Visible Therapy: A Feminist Post-Structuralist Approach to Working with Women Who Have Experienced Child Sexual Abuse.' *Feminist Review* 68, no. 1 (2001): 115–139.

———. *Understanding Child Sexual Abuse: Making the Tactics Visible*. Gloucs: Handsell, 2000.

———. *Understanding the Effects of Child Sexual Abuse: Feminist Revolutions in Theory, Research, and Practice*. London; New York: Routledge, 2009.

Warrington, Camille, Helen Beckett, Elizabeth Ackerley, Megan Walker, and Debbie Allnock. 'Making Noise: Children's Voices for Positive Change after Sexual Abuse.' Beds: University of Bedfordshire in partnership with the NSPCC, 2017.

Watkins, Bill, and Arnon Bentovim. 'The Sexual Abuse of Male Children and Adolescents: A Review of Current Research.' *Journal of Child Psychology and Psychiatry* 33, no. 1 (1992): 197–248.

Wattam, Corinne. *Making a Case in Child Protection*. Longman Group UK, 1992.

Wattam, Corinne, and Clare Woodward. 'And Do I Abuse My Children? No!' In *Childhood Matters: Report of the National Commission of Inquiry into the Prevention of Child Abuse. Vol 2: Background Papers*. London: The Stationery Office, 1996.

Welshman, John. 'In Search of the 'Problem Family': Public Health and Social Work in England and Wales 1940–70.' *Social History of Medicine* 9, no. 3 (1996): 447–465.

Weston, Janet. 'Sexual Crimes, Medical Cures: The Development of a Therapeutic Approach toward Sexual Offenders in English Prisons, C. 1900–1950.' *Canadian Journal of History* 49, no. 3 (2014): 395–492.

Wild, N. J. 'Sexual Abuse of Children in Leeds.' *British Medical Journal (Clinical Research Edition)* 292, no. 6528 (1986): 1113–1116.

Williams, Jennie, and Gilli Watson. 'Mental Health Services That Empower Women: The Challenge to Clinical Psychology.' *Clinical Psychology Forum* 1, no. 1 (1997): 11–18.

Wilmots, Eva, Nick Midgley, Lisa Thackeray, Shirley Reynolds, and Maria Loades. 'The Therapeutic Relationship in Cognitive Behaviour Therapy with Depressed Adolescents: A Qualitative Study of Good-Outcome Cases.' *Psychology and Psychotherapy: Theory, Research and Practice* 93, no. 2 (2020): 276–291.

Wilson, Melba. *Crossing the Boundary: Black Women Survive Incest.* London: Virago, 1993.

Wolff, Sula. *Children under Stress.* Second edition. Suffolk: Pelican Books, 1969.

Wood, Nick, and Nimisha Patel. 'Special Issue: Racism During Training in Clinical Psychology.' *Clinical Psychology Forum* 323 (2019).

'Working Party on Management Structure in the Local Authority Nursing Services.' London: DHSS, 1969.

Wyatt, Gail Elizabeth, and Gloria Johnson Powell, eds. *Lasting Effects of Child Sexual Abuse*: Sage Publications Inc, 1988.

Zammit, Julienne, Sarah Brown, Jamie-Lee Mooney, and Sophia King. 'Truth Project Thematic Report: Child Sexual Abuse in Healthcare Contexts.' London: IICSA, 2020.

# Index[1]



[1] Note: Page numbers followed by 'n' refer to notes.



R. Beecher, *Community Health Practitioners and Child Sexual Abuse in the Family, 1970s–2010s*, Genders and Sexualities in History, https://doi.org/10.1007/978-3-031-80052-8